RESPIRATORY CARE EXAM REVIEW

Review for the Entry Level and Advanced Exams

RESPIRATORY CARE EXAM REVIEW

Review for the Entry Level and Advanced Exams

Third Edition

GARY PERSING, BS, RRT
Program Director
Respiratory Care Program
Tulsa Community College
Tulsa, Oklahoma

Respiratory Review Workshops
Director
CRT/RRT Exam Review Workshops
866-206-1541
rrworkshop@gmail.com
www.respiratoryreviewworkshops.com

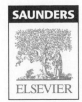

SAUNDERS
ELSEVIER

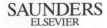

3251 Riverport Lane
Maryland Heights, Missouri 63043

RESPIRATORY CARE EXAM REVIEW: REVIEW FOR THE ENTRY LEVEL AND ADVANCED EXAMS, THIRD EDITION

ISBN: 978-1-4377-0674-1

NOTICE

Library of Congress Cataloging-in-Publication Data

Persing, Gary.
    Respiratory care exam review : review for the entry level and advanced exams / Gary Persing.—3rd ed.
        p. ; cm.
    Includes bibliographical references and index.
    ISBN 978-1-4377-0674-1 (pbk. : alk. paper)
    1. Respiratory therapy—Examinations, questions, etc.   I. Title.
    [DNLM: 1. Respiratory Therapy—methods—Examination Questions.   WF 18.2 P466r 2010]
    RC735.I5P453 2010
    615.8'36076—dc22

                                                                        2009038553

Publisher: Jeanne Olson
Managing Editor: Billie Sharp
Developmental Editor: Kathleen Sartori
Publishing Services Manager: Hemamalini Rajendrababu
Project Manager: Anand Kumar
Senior Designer: Kimberly E. Denando

Printed in United States of America

Last digit is the print number: 9 8 7 6 5 4 3 2

Thank you to Debbie, Lindsey, my parents and the faculty and students in the Respiratory Care Program at Tulsa Community College. I am truly blessed!

And thank you to my Lord and Savior Jesus Christ who has made all these blessings possible.

Philippians 4:6-7

REVIEWERS

Angie Cameron, MHS, RRT-NPS, AE-C, CPFT
Instructor
Louisiana State University Health Sciences Center
School of Allied Health Professions
Shreveport, Louisiana

Alan Clark, BA, RRT
Respiratory Therapy Program Director
NorthWest Arkansas Community College
Bentonville, Arkansas

Tonya Edwards, RRT, BSRC
Program Director
Respiratory Care
Weatherford College
Weatherford, Texas

Laurie Ann Freshwater, MA, RCP, RRT, RPFT
Director of Health Sciences
Carteret Community College
Morehead City, North Carolina

Julie A. Hopwood, MS, RRT
Director of Clinical Education
Respiratory Therapy Program
Central Piedmont Community College
Charlotte, North Carolina

Abe Johnson, ThM, RRT, RCP
Director Respiratory Care
Collin College
McKinney, Texas

Stacy Lewis-Sells EdM, RRT-NPS, CPFT
Program Coordinator for Respiratory Care
Southeastern Community College
West Burlington, Iowa

Maggie McMillin, MEd, RRT
Respiratory Care Program Director
Southwestern Illinois College/St. Elizabeth's Hospital
Belleville, Illinois

Joshua Neumiller, PharmD, CDE, GCP, FASCP
Assistant Professor
College of Pharmacy
Washington State University
Spokane, Washington

Charlotte L. Pasco, BA, RRT
Program Director for Respiratory Care
Southeast Community College
Lincoln, Nebraska

Randolph Regal, BS, PharmD
Clinical Assistant Professor
Adult Internal Medicine
University of Michigan Hospital and College of Pharmacy
Ann Arbor, Michigan

Dennis R. Wissing, PhD, RRT, AE-C
Professor of Medicine & Cardiopulmonary Science
Assistant Dean for Academic Affairs
School of Allied Health Professions
Louisiana State University Health Sciences Center
Shreveport, Louisiana

PREFACE

One of the most satisfying accomplishments that may be achieved by respiratory care practitioners is the successful completion of the Entry Level Certification Exam and/or the Advanced Practitioner Written Registry/Clinical Simulation Exam offered by the National Board for Respiratory Care (NBRC). The credential of Certified Respiratory Therapist (CRT) is awarded to individuals who score 75% or higher on the 140-question CRT exam. (Actually the test is composed of 160 questions, 20 of which do not count toward the final score.) Individuals attempting to obtain the credential of Registered Respiratory Therapist (RRT) must first be a CRT and then score 70% or higher on the 100-question Written Registry exam (actually, 115, 15 of which do not count toward the final score), as well as successfully complete the Clinical Simulation exam, which consists of 10 simulations (actually, 11, with one that does not count toward the final score).

The purpose of this text is to prepare you to successfully complete both the CRT and RRT exams. The NBRC provides a test matrix that indicates the areas tested on these exams. This matrix was used as a guideline for the material in this text to better prepare you for these exams. Because the NBRC exams may exclude more current types of therapy or equipment, the clinical practices reflected in this book are not necessarily the most current in your region.

This textbook and accompanying Evolve site with Evolve Exam Review **(http://evolve.elsevier.com/Persing/ respiratorycare/)** contain more than 800 questions, both multiple-choice questions and open-ended questions. Each chapter begins with a pre-test comprising several multiple-choice questions formatted like those found on the NBRC exams. After having completed the pre-test, study the chapter and then answer the open-ended post-chapter study questions. If you have to return to the chapter to find the answers to some of the questions, do not be discouraged. By going back through the chapter and recording your answers on the post-chapter questions, you are reinforcing the information that will help you to retain the material. The answers to the pre-test and post-chapter questions are located at the back of the book.

Evolve is an interactive learning environment designed to work in coordination with this text. Instructors may use Evolve to provide an Internet-based course component that reinforces and expands the concepts presented in class. For this book in particular, Evolve is a way for students to easily take practice tests to further simulate the NBRC credentialing examination. Students have the opportunity to take time-structured tests just like the real thing, or to tests themselves in a more leisurely manner using "study mode."

In each chapter, I have designated material that is exclusive to either the Entry Level exam or the Written Registry exam. This material is provided in boxes labeled *Exam Note*. As you go through the book, you will notice that the majority

of material will be found on both exams. Unless I have specifically stated that the material is exclusive to one exam, you should assume that the material may appear on both the CRT and RRT exams. About 85% of the material tested over on these exams overlap, or are found on both exams.

The major difference between the exams is that more "analysis" questions are asked on the RRT exam and more "application" questions are asked on the CRT exam. There are also more "recall" questions on the CRT exam, which require less of an understanding of the material. (See Complexity Level Boxes.)

Seventy-nine percent of the Written Registry exam is composed of analysis questions, whereas only 22% of the questions in the CRT exam fall into this category. Over half of the questions on the CRT exam are application questions.

New to this edition is the CRT and RRT Exam Content Matrix designations listed after each major section in each chapter. This will show you what part of the matrix the material is from. I encourage you to go to the NBRC website (nbrc.org) and download both the CRT and RRT Exam Content Matrix. It's a great study tool that provides all the topics that you could be tested over and how many questions may be asked from each specific content area. I use these matrices to update each edition of this book to make sure I cover all the topics on each matrix. A correlation guide to our book is also provided on Evolve.

Following the chapters is a 160-question Entry Level Certification Practice Exam and a 115-question Advanced

---

☑ **Complexity Levels for Entry Level Certification Exam**

Passing score: 120 correct answers (based on 75% of 160 questions)

Questions on the NBRC exams fall into three complexity levels.

- Recall questions: These questions require "the ability to recall or recognize specific respiratory care information." The Entry Level Certification Exam contains 35 recall questions.
- Application questions: These questions require "the ability to comprehend, relate, or apply knowledge to new or changing situations." The Entry Level Certification Exam contains 73 application questions.
- Analysis questions: These questions require "the ability to analyze information, put information together to arrive at solutions, or evaluate the usefulness of the solutions." The Entry Level Certification Exam contains 32 analysis questions.

Complexity Levels for Advanced Practitioner Written Registry Exam

Passing score: 81 correct answers (based on 70% of 115 questions)

Questions on the NBRC exam fall onto three complexity levels:

- Recall questions: These questions require "the ability to recall or recognize specific respiratory care information." The Advance Practitioner Written Registry Exam contains 7 recall questions.
- Application questions: These questions require "the ability to comprehend, relate, or apply knowledge to new or changing situations." The Advanced Practitioner Written Registry Exam contains 18 application questions.
- Analysis questions: These questions require "the ability to analyze information, put information together to arrive at solutions, or evaluate the usefulness of the solutions." The Advanced Practitioner Written Registry Exam contains 75 analysis questions.

Practitioner Written Registry Practice Exam. I have tried to make these exams as close to the actual NBRC exams as possible so that you will better know what to expect. Located on the Evolve site, the *Answer Key and Rationales to Text Pretests* section reveals the correct answer for each question and provides a detailed explanation for why the choice is correct. Also included is the complexity level of each question, which is described in the preceding boxes.

In addition to the Entry Level and Advanced Practitioner practice exams in the book Evolve Exam Review with inter-active practice exams for both CRT and RRT accompany the text.

Evolve also includes 11 clinical simulations with 167 questions. The simulations are written and developed in form and content to reflect those presented on the NBRC exam. Even if you are only preparing for the CRT exam, the simulations are good practice and beneficial preparation.

In the back of the book is an abbreviation list of commonly used terms found within the text, as well as a list of commonly used equations.

When you take the practice exams, find a quiet place and give yourself the appropriate time allotted for each exam. Take the exam as if it were the actual exam. This will give you an idea of how to pace yourself when you take the "real thing." After taking the exam, pay close attention to your areas of strength and weakness. Return to the study text chapters for further study, focusing more on your weak areas.

Proper preparation is essential to passing the NBRC exams. The NBRC provides excellent material to help you study for the credentialing exams. I highly recommend their self-assessment exams and practice clinical simulations and am sure you will find them very helpful. Over the course of your education in the field of respiratory care, you have surely accumulated many excellent textbooks and notes that are invaluable to your exam preparation. In this text, I have attempted to summarize, in a comprehensive and understandable way, the most important material necessary for you to understand in order to pass the NBRC CRT and registry exams. It is my sincere hope that whether you are preparing for the CRT or are already certified and working toward your RRT, this textbook will be beneficial to your preparation for the NBRC exams and you will be awarded the credential of Certified Respiratory Therapist or Registered Respiratory Therapist—whichever you are striving to achieve.

Gary Persing, BS, RRT

ACKNOWLEDGMENTS

I want to thank the staff at Elsevier for their dedicated work in the preparation of this manuscript. I especially want to thank Billie Sharp, Kathleen Sartori, and Mary Pohlman for their hard work on this project. You have made my job a lot easier. I also want to thank each educator who reviewed the manuscript and offered so many great suggestions. I am truly appreciative.

CONTENTS

1 **Oxygen and Medical Gas Therapy,** *1*
Pre-Test Questions, *1*
Review, *1*
Post-Chapter Study Questions, *21*

2 **Humidity and Aerosol,** *23*
Pre-Test Questions, *23*
Review, *23*
Post-Chapter Study Questions, *31*

3 **Assessment of the Cardiopulmonary Patient,** *32*
Pre-Test Questions, *32*
Review, *33*
Post-Chapter Study Questions, *48*

4 **Management of the Airway,** *49*
Pre-Test Questions, *49*
Review, *49*
Post-Chapter Study Questions, *67*

5 **Special Respiratory Care Procedures,** *69*
Pre-Test Questions, *69*
Review, *69*
Post-Chapter Study Questions, *74*

6 **Cardiopulmonary Resuscitation Techniques,** *75*
Pre-Test Questions, *75*
Review, *75*
Post-Chapter Study Questions, *83*

7 **Hyperinflation Therapy,** *85*
Pre-Test Questions, *85*
Review, *86*
Post-Chapter Study Questions, *95*

8 **Bronchopulmonary Hygiene Techniques,** *96*
Pre-Test Questions, *96*
Review, *96*
Post-Chapter Study Questions, *102*

9 **Cardiac Monitoring,** *103*
Pre-Test Questions, *103*
Review, *103*
Post-Chapter Study Questions, *120*

10 **ABG Interpretation,** *121*
Pre-Test Questions, *121*
Review, *121*
Post-Chapter Study Questions, *128*

11 **Ventilator Management,** *129*
Pre-Test Questions, *129*
Review, *129*
Post-Chapter Study Questions, *150*

12 **Disorders of the Respiratory System,** *151*
Pre-Test Questions, *151*
Review, *151*
Post-Chapter Study Questions, *165*

13 **Neonatal and Pediatric Respiratory Care,** *167*
Pre-Test Questions, *167*
Review, *167*
Post-Chapter Study Questions, *177*

14 **Respiratory Medications,** *179*
Pre-Test Questions, *179*
Review, *179*
Post-Chapter Study Questions, *186*

15 **Respiratory Home Care,** *187*
Pre-Test Questions, *187*
Review, *187*
Post-Chapter Study Questions, *190*

16 **Pulmonary Function Testing,** *191*
Pre-Test Questions, *191*
Review, *191*
Post-Chapter Study Questions, *198*

17 **Equipment Decontamination and Infection Control,** *199*
Pre-Test Questions, *199*
Review, *199*
Post-Chapter Study Questions, *203*

Entry Level Certification Exam: Practice Test, *204*

Advanced Practitioner Written Registry Exam: Practice Test, *224*

Pre-Test Answers and Rationales, *241*

Answers to Post-Chapter Study Questions, *248*

Index, *254*

Abbreviations, *272*

Commonly Used Equations, *274*

OXYGEN AND MEDICAL GAS THERAPY

PRETEST QUESTIONS

Answer the pretest questions before studying the chapter. This will help you determine your strong and weak areas in the material covered.

1. A patient is receiving oxygen from an "E" cylinder at 4 L/min through a nasal cannula. The cylinder pressure is 1900 psig. How long will the cylinder run until it is empty?

   A. 47 min
   B. 1.7 h
   C. 2.2 h
   D. 3.6 h

2. After setting up a partial rebreathing mask on a patient at a flow of 8 L/min, the reservoir bag collapses before the patient finishes inspiring. The respiratory care practitioner should do which of the following?

   A. Change to a 6-L/min nasal cannula.
   B. Decrease the flow.
   C. Change to a non-rebreathing mask.
   D. Increase the flow.

3. A patient with carbon monoxide (CO) poisoning can best be treated with which of the following therapies?

   A. Nasal cannula at 6 L/min
   B. Hyperbaric O_2
   C. Continuous positive airway pressure (CPAP)
   D. Non-rebreathing mask

4. The following blood gas levels have been obtained from a patient using a 60% aerosol mask.

pH	7.47
$PaCO_2$	31 mm Hg
PaO_2	58 mm Hg

   What should the respiratory care practitioner recommend at this time?

   A. Place the patient on CPAP.
   B. Increase the oxygen to 70%.
   C. Intubate and place the patient on mechanical ventilation.
   D. Change to a non-rebreathing mask.

5. Given the following data, what is the patient's total arterial O_2 content?

pH	7.41
$PaCO_2$	37 mm Hg
PaO_2	88 mm Hg
HCO_3^-	26 mEq/L
SaO_2	95%
Hb	14 g/dL

   A. 12 vol%
   B. 14 vol%
   C. 16 vol%
   D. 18 vol%

6. A patient is using a 30% Venturi mask at an O_2 flow of 5 L/min. The total flow delivered by this device is which of the following?

   A. 36 L/min
   B. 45 L/min
   C. 54 L/min
   D. 60 L/min

See answers and rationales at the back of the text.

REVIEW

I. **STORAGE AND CONTROL OF MEDICAL GASES**
   CRT Exam Content Matrix: IIA9a
   RRT Exam Content Matrix: IIA4d, IIC6
   A. Storage of Medical Gases and Cylinder Characteristics
      1. Cylinders are constructed of chrome molybdenum steel.
      2. Gas cylinders are stored at high pressures; a full O_2 cylinder contains 2200 psig pressure.
      3. Cylinders are constructed in various sizes. The most common sizes for O_2 storage are the "H" cylinder and the "E" cylinder.
         a. The "H" cylinder holds 244 cu ft (6900 L) of O_2.
         b. The "E" cylinder, used for transport, holds 22 cu ft (622 L) of O_2.

There are 28.3 L in 1 cu ft.

4. Valves on the cylinder allow attachment of regulators that release the gas at various flow rates. Cylinder and regulator safety systems dictate that the valves be constructed to allow the connection of only one type of gas regulator. For example, an O_2 regulator cannot be attached to a helium cylinder.
   a. Large cylinders use the American Standard Safety System. Each type of gas cylinder valve has a different number of threads per inch and a different thread size, and the cylinder may require either a right- or left-hand turning motion for attachment to the regulator.
   b. Small cylinders use the Pin Index Safety System. Each cylinder valve has two holes drilled in unique positions that line up with corresponding pins on the appropriate regulator. There are six different hole placement positions.
5. Safety relief devices on cylinder valves allow escape of excess gas if the pressure in the cylinder increases. There are two types of safety relief devices:
   a. Frangible disk—breaks at 3000 psig
   b. Fusible plug—melts at 208° to 220° F (caused by high ambient temperature or high pressure, which increase the temperature)
6. The Compressed Gas Association (CGA) developed a color code system for cylinders to distinguish the various gases.

Gas	Color of Cylinder
Oxygen	Green; white (internationally)
Helium	Brown
Carbon dioxide	Gray
Nitrous oxide	Light blue
Cyclopropane	Orange
Ethylene	Red
Air	Yellow
CO_2/O_2	Gray and green
He/O_2	Brown and green

7. Cylinder markings

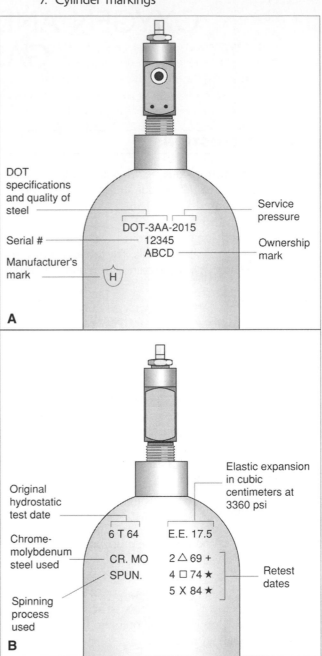

FIGURE 1-1   A, Cylinder markings. B, Cylinder markings.

8. Cylinder testing
   a. Cylinders are visually tested by dropping a lightbulb inside to look for corrosion.
   b. Cylinders are hydrostatically tested every 5 or 10 yr, depending on the cylinder marking. A "star" next to the latest test date means the next test must be done 10 yr from that date. Hydrostatic testing determines the amount or number of
      (1) Wall stress
      (2) Cylinder expansion
      (3) Leaks
9. Liquid gas systems
   a. 1 cu ft of liquid O_2 expands to 860 cu ft as it changes to a gas. Liquid O_2 is much more economical than gas.
   b. The liquid O_2 is stored in Thermos containers at a pressure not to exceed 250 psig and a temperature below $-297°$ F (the boiling point of O_2).
   c. Liquid O_2 is most commonly produced by the process of fractional distillation.
B. Control of Medical Gases
   1. Regulators are devices attached to the cylinder valve to regulate flow and reduce cylinder pressure to working pressure (i.e., 50 psig).
   2. Types of reducing valves
      a. Single-stage, which reduces the cylinder pressure directly to 50 psig and has one safety relief device
      b. Double-stage, which reduces the cylinder pressure to approximately 150 psig and then to 50 psig and has two safety relief devices
      c. Triple-stage, which reduces the cylinder pressure to approximately 300 psig, then to 150 psig, and finally to 50 psig and has three safety relief devices
   3. Regulators may be preset or adjustable.

a. Mechanics of a preset regulator:

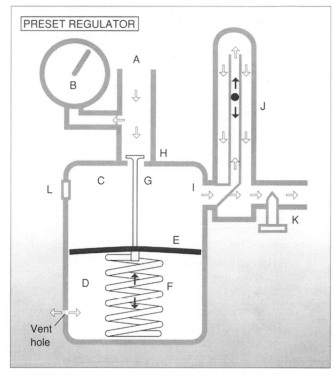

FIGURE 1-2   Gas under high pressure from the cylinder enters the inlet (*A*) of the reducing valve where cylinder pressure is read on the Bourdon gauge (*B*). Gas then passes through the inlet valve (*H*) into the pressure chamber (*C*) and pushes down on the diaphragm (*E*), spring (*F*), and valve stem (*G*) assembly, closing the valve and cutting off gas flow into the pressure chamber. At the moment the valve closes, the gas pressure is equal to the spring pressure in the ambient chamber (*D*). Then, as gas exits the pressure chamber through the outlet (*I*), pressure drops in the pressure chamber and the diaphragm assembly moves upward, which allows gas to enter the chamber again. In fact, the diaphragm assembly moves continually up and down, opening and closing the valve repeatedly, as gas passes through the chamber flowmeter (*J*) and needle valve (*K*). Excessive pressure in the pressure chamber is vented through a pressure relief valve (*L*). The spring tension on this regulator is preset at 50 psig.

b. Adjustable regulator:

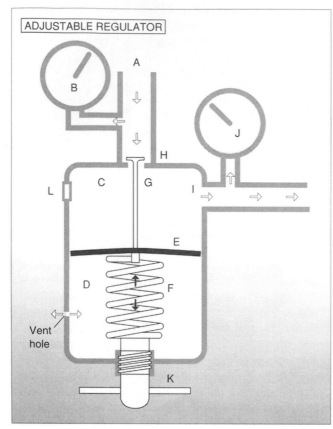

ADJUSTABLE REGULATOR

L

Vent hole

FIGURE 1-3 This is an example of a Bourdon gauge regulator. It works just as a preset regulator does, except the spring tension is adjustable by the user. The second gauge (*J*) indicates the pressure exerted by the spring. If a flowmeter or high-pressure hose leading to a ventilator is attached to the outlet of the regulator, the spring should be adjusted to 50 psig. The gauge may also be calibrated in L/min to read flow. This is called a *Bourdon gauge flowmeter*.

4. Technical problems associated with reducing valves and regulators
   a. Dust or debris entering the regulator from the cylinder valve may rupture the diaphragm. Always "crack" the cylinder before attaching a regulator. This is accomplished by turning the cylinder on and back off quickly to blow out the debris from the cylinder outlet.
   b. Constant pressure "trapped" in the pressure chamber after the cylinder is turned off may rupture the diaphragm. Always vent pressure in the regulator by turning the flowmeter back on after the cylinder is turned off.

c. A hole in the diaphragm will result in a continuous leak into the ambient chamber and out the vent hole (see diagram of regulator), causing failure of the regulator.
   d. A weak spring can result in diaphragm vibration and inadequate flows that are caused by premature closing of the inlet valve.
   e. When attaching a regulator to a small cylinder, make sure the plastic washer is in place or gas will audibly leak around the cylinder valve outlet and regulator inlet.
5. Calculating how long cylinder contents will last:

$$\frac{\text{Minutes remaining}}{\text{in cylinder}} = \frac{\text{cylinder pressure} \times \text{cylinder factor}}{\text{flow rate}}$$

Cylinder factors: "H" cylinder = 3.14 L/psig
"E" cylinder = 0.28 L/psig

EXAMPLE:

Calculate how long a full "H" cylinder will last running at 8 L/min.

$$\frac{2200\,\text{psig} \times 3.14\,\text{L/psig}}{8\,\text{L/min}} = \frac{6908}{8} = \frac{863.5\,\text{min}}{60} = 14.39\,\text{h}$$

EXAMPLE:

An "E" cylinder of O_2 contains 1800 psig. If the respiratory care practitioner runs the cylinder at 4 L/min through a nasal cannula, how long will it take for the cylinder to reach a level of 200 psig?

$$\frac{(1800\,\text{psig} - 200\,\text{psig}) \times 0.28\,\text{L/psig}}{4\,\text{L/min}} = \frac{448}{4}$$
$$= \frac{112\,\text{min}}{60} = 1.9\,\text{h}$$

---

6. Calculating the duration of flow for a liquid O_2 system

One liter of liquid oxygen weighs 2.5 lb (1.1 kg).

$$\text{Gas remaining} = \frac{\text{liquid wt (lb)} \times 860}{2.5\,\text{L/lb}}$$

$$\text{Duration of contents (min)} = \frac{\text{Gas remaining (L)}}{\text{Flow (L/min)}}$$

EXAMPLE:

A liquid oxygen tank contains 5 lb of liquid oxygen. The patient is receiving oxygen at 3 L/min through a nasal cannula. How long will the liquid oxygen last?

$$\text{Gas remaining} = \frac{5\,\text{lbs} \times 860}{2.5\,\text{L/lb}}$$

$$= \frac{4300}{2.5}$$

$$= 1720\,\text{L}$$

$$\text{Duration of contents} = \frac{1720\,\text{L}}{3\,\text{L/min}}$$

$$= 573\,\text{minutes};$$

$$\frac{573}{60} = 9.6\,\text{h or 9 h, 36 min}$$

Math shortcut: Because 860 and 2.5 are constants in the equation, cancel them out by dividing 860 by 2.5. The answer is 344. Now simply multiply **344** by the pounds of liquid oxygen. The answer will be the same as when you use the longer equation.

7. Flowmeters

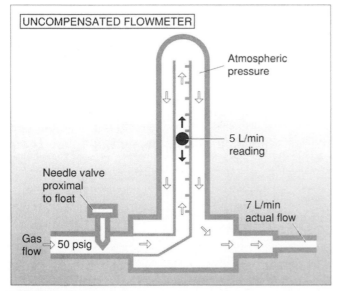

FIGURE 1-4

a. Uncompensated flowmeter:
(1) The needle valve is located proximal to (before) the float; therefore atmospheric pressure is in the Thorpe tube. Any back pressure in the tube affects the rise of the float.
(2) When a restriction, such as a humidifier or a nebulizer, is attached to the outlet, back pressure into the tube forces the float down and compresses the gas molecules closer together so that more molecules go around the float than what the float indicates. Therefore the flowmeter reading is lower than what the patient is actually receiving.
(3) Uncompensated flowmeters should not be used clinically.
b. Compensated flowmeter

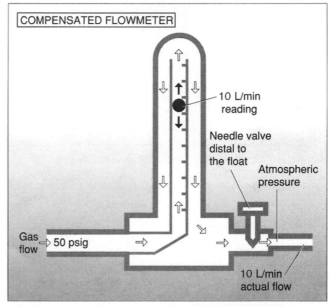

FIGURE 1-5

(1) The needle valve is located distal to (after) the float; therefore 50 psig is in the tube. Only back pressure that exceeds 50 psig will affect the rise of the float.
(2) The flowmeter reads accurately with an attachment, such as a humidifier or nebulizer on the outlet, or with any obstruction downstream. If the oxygen tubing is completely obstructed with no gas flowing to the patient, the flowmeter will reflect that with a flow reading of near zero.
(3) There are three ways to determine whether a flowmeter is compensated for pressure:
(a) It is labeled as such on the flowmeter.
(b) The needle valve is located after the float.
(c) The float jumps when the flowmeter, while it is turned off, is plugged into a wall outlet.
(4) Flowmeter outlets use the Diameter Index Safety System, as do all gas-administering equipment that operate at less than 200 psig, so that attachment to the wrong gas source is avoided.

(5) If the flowmeter is turned off completely but gas is still bubbling through the humidifier or is heard coming from the flowmeter, the valve seat is faulty and the flowmeter should be replaced.

c. Bourdon gauge flowmeter

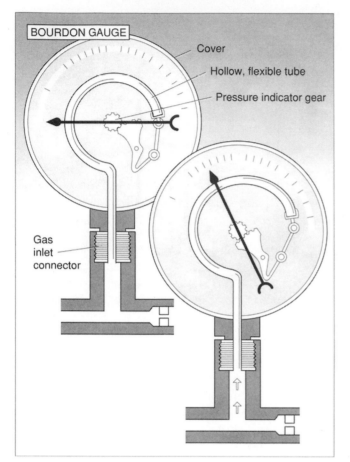

FIGURE 1-6

(1) The Bourdon gauge flowmeter is a pressure gauge that has been calibrated in liters per minute. It is uncompensated for back pressure.

(2) When a humidifier or nebulizer is attached to the outlet of the Bourdon gauge, back pressure is generated into the gauge (which measures pressure) and the gauge reading is higher than what the patient is actually receiving.

(3) Gas enters the hollow, flexible question mark–shaped tube, which tends to straighten as pressure fills it. A gear mechanism is attached to the tube, and as the tube straightens, it rotates a needle indicator that shows the pressure (flow).

(4) The advantage of the Bourdon gauge is that it, unlike Thorpe tube flowmeters, is not position dependent. It reads just as accurately in a horizontal position as it does in a vertical position.

(5) Because this gauge actually measures pressure, an obstruction to flow through the tubing attached to a Bourdon gauge flowmeter resulting in back pressure will cause the gauge reading to increase slightly. In other words, the gauge will indicate flow to the patient while the patient is receiving little or no oxygen.

8. Air compressors are used to provide medical air through either portable compressors or large medical air piping systems. Two types of air compressors are generally used:

a. Piston air compressor:

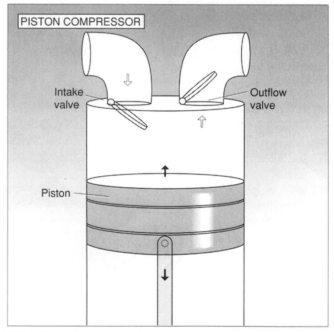

FIGURE 1-7

Air is drawn into the compressor, where it travels to a reservoir tank. From this tank, the air passes through a dryer to remove moisture and on to a pressure-reducing valve, which reduces the pressure to 50 psig to power a compressed-air wall outlet. As the piston drops, gas is drawn in through a one-way intake valve. On the upstroke, the intake valve closes and gas exits through a one-way outflow valve. Piston air compressors are seen most commonly on large medical air piping systems.

b. Diaphragm air compressor:

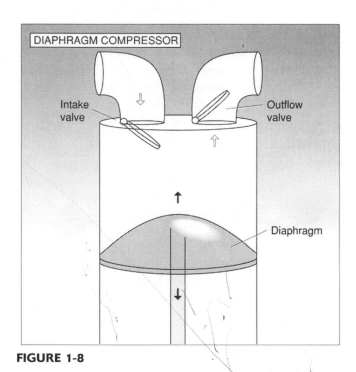

DIAPHRAGM COMPRESSOR

Intake valve

Outflow valve

Diaphragm

FIGURE 1-8

A diaphragm is used instead of a piston. On the downstroke, the flexible diaphragm bends downward, drawing air through a one-way intake valve. On the upstroke, air is forced out the one-way outflow valve. Diaphragm air compressors are commonly used on O_2 concentrators and portable air compressors.

II. **OXYGEN THERAPY**
   CRT Exam Content Matrix: IIA1a-c, IIA9a-b, IIA12a-b, IIID2d, IIID6, IIIE10, IIIF2d1-2, IIIG2c
   RRT Exam Content Matrix: IIA4b
   A. Indications for O_2 Therapy
      1. Hypoxemia
      2. Labored breathing or dyspnea
      3. Increased myocardial work
   B. Signs and Symptoms of Hypoxemia
      1. Tachycardia
      2. Dyspnea
      3. Cyanosis (unless anemia is present)
      4. Impairment of special senses
      5. Headache
      6. Mental disturbance
      7. Slight hyperventilation (tachypnea)
   C. Complications of O_2 Therapy
      1. Respiratory depression: The patient with chronic obstructive pulmonary disease (COPD) who is breathing with the "hypoxic drive" mechanism is most affected. Maintain PaO_2 between 50 and 65 mm Hg for these patients.

2. Atelectasis: High O_2 concentrations in the lung can wash out nitrogen in the lung and reduce the production of surfactant, which may lead to atelectasis. Maintain FiO_2 below 0.60.
3. Oxygen toxicity: High O_2 concentrations result in increased O_2 free radicals and therefore lung tissue toxicity. This may lead to acute respiratory distress syndrome (ARDS). Maintain FiO_2 below 0.60.
4. Reduced mucociliary activity: Maintain FiO_2 below 0.60. The beating of the cilia in the mucociliary blanket is not as active when high FiO_2 levels are used.
5. Neonatal retinopathy (retinopathy of prematurity): This is caused by high PaO_2 levels in infants and results in blindness. It is more common in premature infants. **Maintain PaO_2 below 80 mm Hg.** Normal level of PaO_2 in infants is **50 to 70 mm Hg**.

D. **Normal PaO_2 Values by Age**

Age (yr)	Normal PaO_2
≤60	80 mm Hg
70	70 mm Hg
80	60 mm Hg

E. Four Types of Hypoxia
   1. Hypoxemic hypoxia
      a. Caused by lack of O_2 in the blood as a result of
         (1) Inadequate O_2 in the inspired air: administering O_2 is beneficial.
         (2) Alveolar hypoventilation: administering O_2 alone may not be beneficial.
         (3) Diffusion defects (i.e., pulmonary edema, atelectasis, and pulmonary fibrosis): administering O_2 alone may not be beneficial.
         (4) A ventilation/perfusion mismatch: administering O_2 may be beneficial.
         (5) An anatomic right to left shunt: administering O_2 is not beneficial.
      b. If a normal PaO_2 level cannot be maintained with a 60% O_2 mask, a large shunt is probable and should not be treated with higher O_2 concentrations. CPAP should be administered provided that the $PaCO_2$ is at normal or below normal levels. If the $PaCO_2$ level is elevated in a patient with hypoxemia, mechanical ventilation should be initiated.

When given a patient using 60% oxygen or higher who is ventilating adequately (normal or low $PaCO_2$) but has hypoxemia, place the patient on CPAP. The exception to this rule is if the question states that the patient has hypotension, a low cardiac output, or an elevated intracranial pressure level. Positive pressure should not be administered because the increased intrathoracic pressure may worsen these conditions. Thus in these situations, increase the FiO_2.

2. Anemic hypoxia
   a. The blood's capacity to carry O_2 is reduced as a result of
      (1) A decreased hemoglobin (Hb) level.
         (a) Normal Hb level is 12 to 16 g/dL of blood.

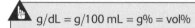 $g/dL = g/100\ mL = g\% = vol\%$

         (b) **The PaO_2 level may be normal, but because of the blood's reduced capacity to carry O_2, the tissues may be deprived of O_2. The Hb value must be determined to assess the patient's oxygenation status.**
         (c) The Hb content may be increased by administering packed red blood cells (RBCs).
      (2) CO poisoning
         (a) CO affinity for Hb is 200 to 250 times faster than O_2 and therefore occupies the iron-binding sites on Hb before O_2 can. This causes tissue hypoxia.
         (b) Because Hb releases the CO more readily when levels of PaO_2 are high, the patient should immediately be given 100% oxygen, usually via a non-rebreathing mask, which delivers high O_2 concentrations.

(c) Elevating the PaO_2 even higher to further increase the dissociation of Hb from CO may be achieved with hyperbaric O_2 therapy (discussed later in this chapter).
(d) Patients who have been involved in fires or who have been breathing car fumes must be treated immediately for CO poisoning.
(e) PaO_2 and Hb saturation (SaO_2) readings (discussed later in this chapter) may be within a normal range even though the patient has severe hypoxia.
(f) The level of CO bound to Hb (carboxyhemoglobin) may be determined with CO oximetry (discussed later in this chapter).
(g) The patient usually presents with a normal PaO_2 level and a low or normal $PaCO_2$ level. The pH level is usually low as a result of lactic acidosis (metabolic acidosis), caused by severe hypoxia. Lactic acid is produced as the body goes into anaerobic metabolism trying to provide more oxygen to the tissues.
(3) Excessive blood loss also may result in anemic hypoxia. Administering blood (RBCs) is the appropriate treatment.
(4) Methemoglobin may cause anemic hypoxia and is most commonly a result of nitrite poisoning. Treat by administering ascorbic acid or methylene blue, which removes the chemical (nitrite) from the system.
(5) Iron deficiency leads to anemia and is treated by increasing iron intake and administering blood.
   b. The blood carries O_2 in two ways
      (1) Bound to Hb: 1 g of Hb is capable of carrying 1.34 mL of O_2. To determine the milliliters of O_2 carried by Hb, use this formula: ($1.34 \times Hb \times SaO_2$).
      (2) Dissolved in plasma: 0.003 mL of O_2 dissolves in plasma for every 1 mm Hg of O_2 tension (PaO_2), or ($.003 \times PaO_2$).

If the question states the patient has been exposed to CO, always select the device that provides 100% oxygen, whether it's a non-rebreather, CPAP, or endotracheal (ET) tube flow-by.

The sum of these two mechanisms equals the total arterial O_2 content in mL/dL of blood, which is the **most effective method for determining the O_2-carrying capacity of a patient's blood.**

EXAMPLE:

Given the following information, calculate the patient's total arterial O_2 content.

Arterial Blood Gas Study Results
pH	7.42
PCO_2	41 mm Hg
PO_2	90 mm Hg
SaO_2	98%
Hb	15 g/dL

O_2 bound to Hb $= 1.34 \times 15 \times 0.98 = 19.7$ mL/dL

O_2 dissolved in plasma $= 0.003 \times 90 = 0.27$ mL/dL*

Total arterial O_2 content $= 19.7$ mL $+ 0.27$ mL $= 19.97$ mL/dL

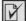 19.97 mL/dL may also be expressed as 19.97 vol%.

 *Exam Note

When calculating total O_2 content on the exam, it's not necessary to calculate O_2 dissolved in the plasma. The amount is always less than 1 mL. So take the answer you get after calculating the amount of O_2 bound to Hb and pick the answer that is closest to that number but just above it. The answers are far enough apart to still get the answer correct.

3. Stagnant (circulatory) hypoxia
   a. The O_2 content and carrying capacity is normal but capillary perfusion is diminished as a result of
      (1) Decreased heart rate
      (2) Decreased cardiac output
      (3) Shock
      (4) Embolism
   b. May be seen as a localized problem, such as peripheral cyanosis resulting from exposure to cold weather
4. Histotoxic hypoxia
   a. The oxidative enzyme mechanism of the cell is impaired as a result of
      (1) Cyanide poisoning
      (2) Alcohol poisoning
   b. Rarely accompanied by hypoxemia but is accompanied by increased venous PO_2 levels
F. **Oxygen Delivery Devices**
   1. Low-flow O_2 systems: an O_2 delivery device that does not meet the patient's inspiratory flow demands; therefore room air must make up the remainder of the patient's tidal volume (VT). The normal inspiratory flow rate is 25 to 30 L/min. The following devices are connected to humidifiers; however, in some institutions, humidifiers are not used if less than 5 L/min is being delivered.

 Exam Note

The FiO_2 delivered by these devices is dependent on the patient's ventilatory pattern. If the criteria listed below are not met, the delivered FiO_2 is inconsistent. (Deeper breaths, faster rate, and longer inspiratory time reduce FiO_2; shallower breaths, slower rate, and shorter inspiratory time increase FiO_2.)

   a. Transtracheal O_2 catheter

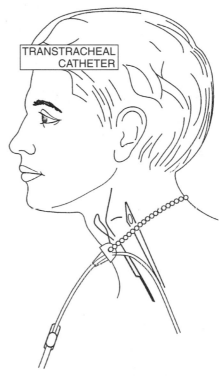

FIGURE 1-9   From Wilkins R, Stoller JK, Kacmarek R: *Egan's fundamentals of respiratory care,* ed 9, St Louis, 2009, Mosby.

   (1) The catheter is inserted directly into the midtrachea through an incision between the second and third tracheal rings to deliver low flow rates (1 to 3 L/min) of O_2.
   (2) Conserves O_2 for home patients by bypassing anatomic dead space, which results in a reduction in the work of breathing.
   (3) Possible complications include accidental removal of the catheter and irritation or infection at the insertion site and in the trachea.
   (4) The catheter should be cleaned routinely by instilling saline and inserting a cleaning wire into the catheter. The catheter should be replaced every 3 months before it becomes kinked, cracked, or obstructed by dry mucus.

b. Nasal cannula

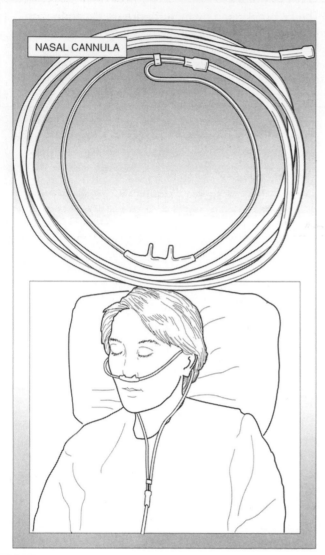

NASAL CANNULA

FIGURE 1-10

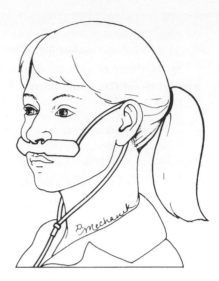

FIGURE 1-11   Nasal reservoir cannula. From Scanlan C, Wilkins R, Stoller J: *Egan's fundamentals of respiratory care,* ed 8, St Louis, 2003, Mosby.

(1) **Delivers 24% to 40% O₂ at flow rates of 1 to 5 L/min** (at about a 4% increase for every 1-L/min increase).

⚠️ Although a flow of 6 L/min is acceptable, according to the American Association for Respiratory Care Clinical Practice Guidelines, the maximum oxygen percentage obtainable with a nasal cannula is 40%.

(2) Much better tolerated by the patient

c. Nasal reservoir cannula

(1) The reservoir, which is positioned just below the nose, stores approximately

20 mL of O_2 that the patient inhales during the early part of inspiration.

(2) Because the patient receives more O_2 with each breath, the flow needed for a prescribed level of O_2 may be decreased, thus conserving O_2.

d. Pendant reservoir cannula

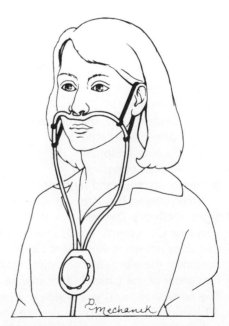

FIGURE 1-12   Pendant reservoir cannula. From Scanlan C, Wilkins R, Stoller J: *Egan's fundamentals of respiratory care,* ed 8, St Louis, 2003, Mosby.

(1) The pendant reservoir cannula uses a pendant-shaped inflatable reservoir that expands as the patient exhales, which forces the stored O_2 out of the pendant and up the cannula tubing to the patient.

(2) For this device to function properly, the patient must exhale through the nose so that the exhaled air passes through the cannula tubing to inflate the reservoir.

(3) Because the pendant may be hidden beneath clothing and the nasal reservoir is much larger than that of typical cannulas, the patient may prefer the pendant cannula.

e. Simple O_2 mask

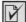 **Exam Note**

In place of O_2 flowmeters, **pulse-dose O_2 delivery systems** may be employed in conjunction with the nasal cannula, transtracheal catheter, and reservoir cannulas. Pulse-dose systems can supply oxygen to the cannula only during inspiration. The device, plugged into a 50-psig O_2 wall outlet, senses patient effort, and a solenoid valve opens, delivering a "pulse" of O_2 at the set flow rate. **These devices are typically used for home oxygen setups, such as with tanks or concentrators.**

   NOTE: Recently high-flow cannulas have become popular. See information on these in the "high-flow device" material later in this chapter.

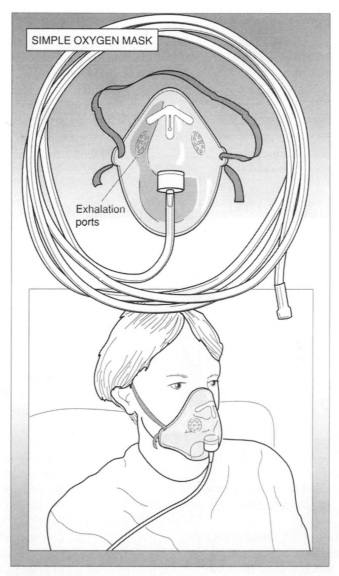

FIGURE 1-13

(1) **Delivers 35% to 50% O₂ at flow rates of 5 to 10 L/min.**
(2) Minimum flow rate of 5 L/min is required to prevent buildup of exhaled CO_2 in the mask.
  f. Partial rebreathing mask

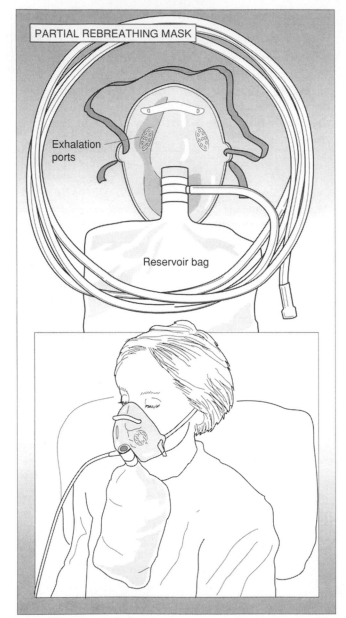

FIGURE 1-14

(1) Delivers 40% to 70% O_2 at flow rates of 8 to 15 L/min.
(2) The flow rate must be sufficient to keep the reservoir bag at least one-half full at all times.
(3) Ensure that the patient is not positioned so that the reservoir bag gets kinked or cuts off flow, which results in a lower FiO_2.

(4) Only the first part of the patient's exhaled gas enters the reservoir bag. This is gas that was left in the upper airway from the previous inspiration and is therefore high in O_2 and low in CO_2. It is gas that did not participate in gas exchange at the alveolar–capillary level.
  g. Non-rebreathing mask

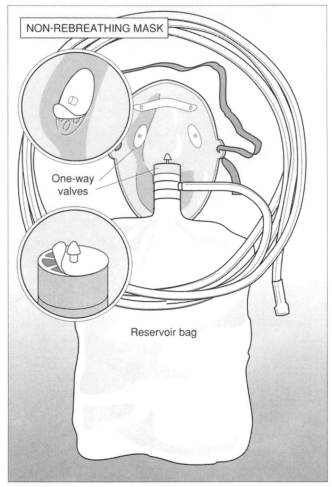

FIGURE 1-15

(1) **Delivers 60% to 80% O₂ at flow rates of 10 to 15 L/min.**
(2) Flow rate must be sufficient to keep the reservoir bag at least one-half full at all times.
(3) The non-rebreathing mask is equipped with a one-way valve between the mask and the reservoir bag, which prevents the patient's exhaled gas from entering the reservoir bag.
(4) One-way valves are located on either one or both exhalation ports of the mask to prevent room air entrainment. If only one exhalation port is covered with a

one-way valve, FiO$_2$ decreases because more room air can enter the mask. In this case, the mask is considered a low-flow mask; however, if both exhalation ports are covered by one-way valves, no air entrainment can occur, FiO$_2$ increases, and the mask is considered a high-flow device. Most commonly, only one exhalation port is covered by a one-way valve. Most manufacturers provide only one valve for the exhalation ports.

   (5) Ensure that the reservoir bag does not kink or cut off flow, especially if both exhalation ports have one-way valves, because no room air would be available to the patient. (For this reason, one valve is commonly left off.)

h. Low-flow O$_2$ devices are adequate O$_2$ delivery systems only when the patient meets the following criteria:

   (1) Regular and consistent ventilatory pattern
   (2) Respiratory rate of less than 25/min
   (3) Consistent VT of 300 to 700 mL (not fluctuating between 300 and 700 mL but consistent [e.g., a VT of 450 mL or 600 mL])
   (4) The percentage of O$_2$ delivered by a low-flow device is variable, depending on the patient's VT, respiratory rate, inspiratory time, and ventilatory pattern.

a. Air entrainment mask (Venturi mask)—provides 24% to 50% O$_2$.

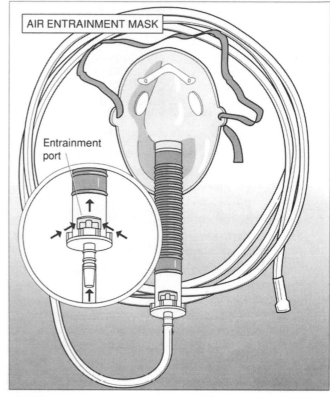

AIR ENTRAINMENT MASK

Entrainment port

FIGURE 1-16

---

(1) The jet size and entrainment port determine the FiO$_2$.
   (a) The larger the entrainment port, the more air entrained and the lower the FiO$_2$.
   (b) Likewise, the smaller the entrainment port, the less air entrained and the higher the FiO$_2$.
   (c) The larger the jet size, the less air entrained and the higher the FiO$_2$.
   (d) The smaller the jet size, the more air entrained and the lower the FiO$_2$.

2. High-flow O$_2$ delivery devices provide all of the inspiratory flow required by the patient at relatively accurate and consistent O$_2$ percentages. **Increasing the flow rate on high-flow devices will not increase FiO2**

⚠ The entrainment port must be prevented from becoming occluded (e.g., by the patient's hand or bedsheet) because this decreases the amount of air entrainment and thus increases the delivered O$_2$ percentage.

(2) Air/O$_2$ entrainment ratios

O$_2$ Percentage	Air/O$_2$ Entrainment Ratio
24%	25:1
28%	10:1
30%	8:1
35%	5:1
40%	3:1
45%	2:1
50%	1:7:1
60%	1:1

These ratios may be calculated by the following formula:

$$\frac{100 - x}{x - 20^*} = \frac{\text{parts of air entrained}}{1\,\text{part O}_2}$$

*Use 21 with percentages less than 40%.

EXAMPLE:

Calculate the air/O$_2$ ratio for 40% O$_2$.

$$(100 - 40)/(40 - 20) = (60/20) = (3/1) \text{ or } 3:1$$

This means that for every liter of O$_2$ (source gas) delivered from the flowmeter, 3 L of air is entrained into the device.

Another method to calculate air/O$_2$ ratios is the "magic box" method. It is not really magic, but most people like it better than the above equation.

20		60
	40	
100		20

1. Draw a tic-tac-toe box and place 20 or 21 (depending on the percentage you are calculating) in the upper left corner.
2. Place 100 in the lower left corner.
3. Place the percentage you are calculating in the middle box of the middle row (in this example, use 40).
4. Subtract 20 from 40 and place the answer in the lower right corner, and subtract 40 from 100 and place the answer in the upper right corner.
5. After subtracting, you should have 60 in the upper right corner (representing air) and 20 in the lower right corner (representing O$_2$). Now divide 60 by 20, which equals 3, or a 3:1 air/O$_2$ ratio.

---

(3) Calculating total flow

 Exam Note

If an air entrainment mask is set on 40% (3:1 ratio) with a flow rate of 12 L/min, the total flow delivered would be

$$\begin{array}{r} 12\,\text{L/min of O}_2 \\ + 36\,\text{L/min of air } (12 \times 3) \\ \hline 48\,\text{L/min of total flow} \end{array}$$

FASTER METHOD: Add the ratio parts together and multiply by the flow.

$$40\% \ (3:1\,\text{air/O}_2\,\text{ratio})$$

$$3 + 1 = 4 \text{ and } 4 \times 12 = 48\,\text{L/min}$$

EXAMPLE:

A Venturi mask is set on 24% O$_2$ with a flow of 4 L/min. Calculate the total flow.

$$\frac{100 - 24}{24 - 21} = \frac{76}{3} = \text{approx. } \frac{25}{1} = 25:1\,\text{air/O}_2\,\text{ratio}$$

$$\begin{array}{r} 4\,\text{L/min of O}_2 \\ + 100\,\text{L/min of air} \\ \hline 104\,\text{L/min of total flow} \end{array}$$

OR

Sum of the ratio of parts multiplied by flow:

$$[(25 + 1) = 26] \times 4 = 104\,\text{L/min}$$

EXAMPLE:

The physician has ordered a 40% aerosol mask to be placed on a patient who has a total inspiratory flow of 44 L/min. What is the minimum flow rate setting on the flowmeter that will meet this patient's inspiratory flow demands?

Because the air/O$_2$ ratio for 40% O$_2$ is 3:1, add the ratio parts together:

$$3 + 1 = 4$$

Set the flowmeter on the lowest L/min flow that multiplied by 4 delivers a total flow of at least 44 L/min, or $4 \times ? = 44$. Therefore, the flowmeter must be set at a minimum of 11 L/min.

☑ Exam Note

To determine a patient's inspiratory flow, use the following equation:

$$\text{Inspiratory flow} = \frac{VT\ (L)}{\text{inspiratory time (s)}}$$

The flow will be in L/s, so multiply by 60 to change to L/min.

b. Aerosol mask

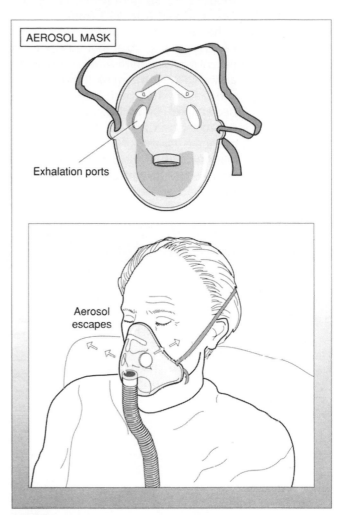

FIGURE 1-17

EXAMPLE:

The physician has ordered O_2 for a patient with a spontaneous VT of 550 mL and an inspiratory time of 1 s. The O_2 device must deliver what flow rate to meet the patient's inspiratory demands?

$$\text{Inspiratory flow} = \frac{0.55\,L}{1.0\,s} = 0.55\,L/s \times 60 = 33\,L/min$$

In other words, the O_2 delivery device used must be able to deliver a total flow of at least 33 L/min to meet the patient's inspiratory flow demands. Which of the following would produce the necessary flow?

A. 40% air entrainment mask at 8 L/min
B. 50% air entrainment mask at 12 L/min
C. 35% air entrainment mask at 6 L/min
D. 50% air entrainment mask at 10 L/min

Flow rates are A, 32 L/min; B, 32 L/min; C, 36 L/min; and D, 27 L/min. Choice "C" exceeds the patient's inspiratory flow demands and therefore is the correct choice.

(1) **This mask delivers 21% to 100% O₂ (depending on nebulizer setting) at flow rates of 8 to 15 L/min.**

(2) If the nebulizer is set on 100%, the device probably would not meet the patient's inspiratory flow demands. Room air would enter the mask through the exhalation ports during inspiration, decreasing FiO_2. In this case, two flowmeters must be used to provide adequate flow.

(3) **Mist should be visible at all times to ensure adequate flow rates.**

c. Face tent

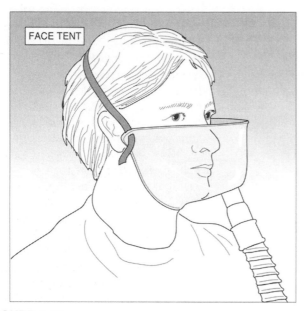

FIGURE 1-18

(1) **Delivers 21% to 40% O₂ (depending on nebulizer setting) at flow rates of 8 to 15 L/min**

(2) Used primarily for patients with facial trauma or burns or for those who cannot tolerate a mask

d. T-tube flow-by or Briggs adaptor

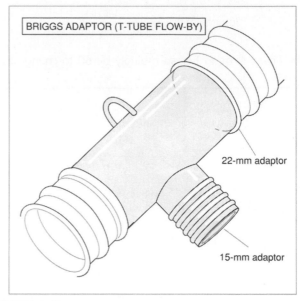

FIGURE 1-19

(1) **Delivers 21% to 100% O₂ (depending on nebulizer setting) at flow rates of 8 to 15 L/min.**

(2) Used on the intubated or tracheostomy patient.

(3) A 50-mL piece of reservoir tubing should be attached to the end of the T-piece (opposite from where the aerosol tubing from the nebulizer is attached). This prevents air from entering the T-piece during inspiration, and if the reservoir falls off, FiO_2 may decrease.

(4) **Adequate flows are ensured by visible mist flowing out of the 50-mL reservoir at all times.**

e. Tracheostomy mask (collar)

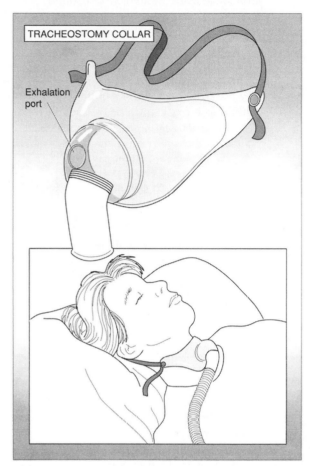

FIGURE 1-20

(1) **Delivers 35% to 60% O₂ (depending on nebulizer setting) at flow rates of 10 to 15 L/min.**
(2) **Adequate flows are ensured by visible mist flowing out of the exhalation port at all times.**
(3) Mask should fit directly over the tracheostomy tube.

f. Oxygen tent

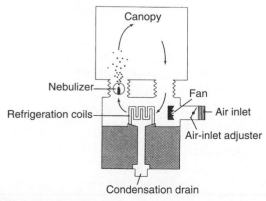

FIGURE 1-21   Oxygen tent.

(1) **Delivers 21% to 50% O₂ at flow rates of 10 to 15 L/min.**
(2) Used primarily on children with croup or pneumonia.
(3) Not an ideal O₂ delivery device because of the leakage and reduced O₂ delivery when the tent is opened for patient care.
(4) A fire hazard exists if electrical devices or friction toys, which may spark, are left in the tent.

g. High-flow cannula
(1) This cannula provides high-flow therapy (HFT) by the use of a thermally controlled humidification system. These devices provide close to 100% body humidity to infant, pediatric, and adult patients. **Flows of up to 8 L/min are used on infants and up to 40 L/min on adults and provide an oxygen percentage of up to 80%.** These flows are capable of meeting the patient's inspiratory flow demands and are therefore considered high-flow devices.
(2) Because the gas is delivered at body temperature and almost fully saturated, high flows are tolerable and even comfortable for the patient to breathe.
(3) Studies indicate that the high flow reduces anatomic dead space by washing out CO_2 from the nasopharynx. This increases alveolar PO_2 levels and results in increased PaO_2 and saturation levels.
(4) Another advantage is that oxygen through a cannula is better tolerated than oxygen through a mask. Communication is more difficult with a mask, and some patients experience claustrophobia, which results in poor patient compliance. Masks also limit the ability to eat and drink.

G. **Important Points Concerning High-Flow Devices**
1. High-flow O₂ devices set on 60% or higher may deliver a total flow rate of less than 25 to 30 L/min, thereby not meeting the patient's inspiratory flow demands and essentially acting as a low-flow device with the patient breathing in room air to make up the difference. When this happens, it means the O₂ percentage setting on the nebulizer is no longer accurate, and the patient is receiving less delivered O₂ than the setting suggests.
2. To ensure adequate flow rates on a device set on 60% or higher, use two flowmeters connected in line together.
3. To ensure adequate flow rates, set the flowmeter to a rate that delivers a total flow of at least 40 L/min.

4. **A restriction, such as kinked aerosol tubing or water in the tubing, causes back pressure into the nebulizer, decreasing the amount of air entrainment and therefore increasing the percentage of O_2.**

5. Increasing the flow on a high-flow device does not increase the delivered FiO_2. It only increases the total flow.

H. **Calculating FiO_2**

$$FiO_2 = \frac{O_2 \text{ flow} + (\text{air flow} \times 0.2)}{\text{total flow}}$$

EXAMPLE:

A nebulizer set on 40% dilution mode and connected to an O_2 flowmeter running at 10 L/min has an air bleed-in rate of 6 L/min downstream. Calculate the FiO_2.

O_2 flow $= 10$ L/min

Air flow $= 30$ L/min (entrained through nebulizer)

Air flow $= 6$ L/min (bleed-in)

Total flow $= 46$ L/min

$$FiO_2 = \frac{10 + (36 \times 0.2)}{46} = \frac{10 + 7.2}{46} = \frac{17.2}{46} = 0.37 \text{ or } 37\%$$

I. **Oxygen Blender**

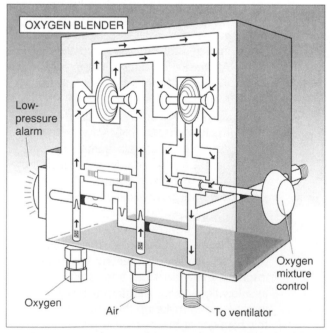

FIGURE 1-22

1. These devices use 50-psig gas sources to mix or blend O_2 and compressed air proportionately to deliver 21% to 100% O_2 at flow rates of 2 to 100 L/min.

2. A blender consists of pressure-regulating valves that regulate O_2 and air inlet pressure, a

mixture control (precision metering device), and an audible alarm system, which sounds if there is a drop in inlet pressure.

3. Blenders provide a stable FiO_2 as long as the outlet flow exceeds the patient's inspiratory flow demands.

4. **When using a blender/nebulizer to provide oxygen, make sure the nebulizer is set on 100%.** As the gas from the blender enters the nebulizer, room air will be entrained, which dilutes the blender mixture to a lower percentage if the nebulizer is set to anything but 100%.

III. **ALVEOLAR AIR EQUATION**
CRT Exam Content Matrix: IB9k, IB10k
RRT Exam Content Matrix: IB10l

A. Alveolar PO_2 is calculated by the following formula:

$$PAO_2 = [(PB - 47 \text{ mm Hg})(FiO_2)] - (PaCO_2 \times 1.25)$$

(47 mm Hg is the level of water vapor pressure at body temperature)

$$PAO_2 = [(760 - 47 \text{ mm Hg})(0.21)] - 40 \text{ mm Hg} \times 1.25$$

$$PAO_2 = (713 \times 0.21) - 50$$

$$PAO_2 = 150 - 50 = \textbf{100 mm Hg}$$

B. This value is often compared with PaO_2 to determine the $P(A–a)O_2$ gradient, which refers to the difference between alveolar O_2 tension and arterial O_2 tension. **The normal gradient on room air is 4 to 12 mm Hg.**

☑ **Exam Note**

Because the exam generally uses a barometric pressure of 747 torr, the corrected barometric pressure (PB) is 700 torr. When multiplying 700 times 0.21, the math can be made simpler by multiplying 7 times 21. Furthermore, instead of multiplying the $PaCO_2$ by 1.25, simply add 10 to the $PaCO_2$. This does not provide an exact answer, but the answer is close enough to choose the correct answer on the exam. To make the math simpler and faster on the exam, use the equation below:

A patient using a 40% air entrainment mask has the following arterial blood gas (ABG) levels:

pH	7.39
$PaCO_2$	42 mm Hg
PaO_2	82 mm Hg

What is this patient's A–a gradient?
(PB = 747 mm Hg)

$$PAO_2 = (7 \times O_2\%) - (PaCO_2 + 10)$$

$$280 - 52 = 228 \text{ mm Hg}$$

$$P(A–a)O_2 = PAO_2 - PaO_2$$
$$= 228 - 82$$
$$= \textbf{146 mm Hg}$$

IV. MIXED GAS THERAPY

CRT Exam Content Matrix: IIIF2e1-2
RRT Exam Content Matrix: IB9k, IB10k, IIA8,
IIIF2c1-2

A. Helium/O_2 Therapy

1. Helium is the second lightest gas and therefore, when combined with O_2, decreases the total density of the gas. This allows the gas to pass through obstructions more easily.
2. Helium/O_2 mixtures (heliox) are stored in brown-and-green cylinders.
3. Helium does not support life and therefore must be mixed with O_2. Two common mixtures are
   a. 80% helium and 20% O_2
   b. 70% helium and 30% O_2
4. Running these gas mixtures through an O_2 flowmeter gives inaccurate readings because the gas is lighter than pure O_2. A correction factor may be used to make the reading accurate.
   a. For an 80:20 mixture of helium and O_2, multiply the flowmeter reading by 1.8 to determine the correct flow rate. To deliver a specific flow, divide the flow rate by 1.8.

EXAMPLE:

An 80:20 mixture of helium and O_2 is running through an O_2 flowmeter at 10 L/min. What is the actual flow rate?

$$10 \times 1.8 = 18\,L/min$$

EXAMPLE:

You want to deliver 12 L/min of an 80:20 mixture of helium and O_2 to the patient. What must you set the O_2 flowmeter on to deliver this flow rate?

$$\frac{12}{1.8} = 6.6\,L/min$$

---

   b. For a 70:30 mixture of helium and O_2, multiply the flowmeter reading by 1.6. Divide by 1.6 to obtain a specific flow rate. (See example above and substitute 1.6 for 1.8.)
5. Helium and O_2 mixtures must be delivered in a tightly closed system, such as a non-rebreathing mask, ET tube, or tracheostomy tube, to prevent this lighter gas from leaking out.
6. The only side effect of helium/O_2 therapy is distortion of the voice.
7. Extreme caution must be used when mixing heliox from a helium cylinder and an O_2 cylinder. Inaccurate flow readings may result in the patient receiving less than 21% O_2. A premixed helium/O_2 cylinder is recommended.
8. Helium/O_2 mixtures are safe and may be of benefit in the treatment of
   a. Obstruction from secretions
   b. Asthma (during episodes of bronchospasm)
   c. Airway obstructions (tumors, foreign bodies, tracheomalacia)

B. Nitric Oxide

1. Inhaled nitric oxide (NO) is a selective pulmonary vasodilator that improves blood flow to ventilated alveoli, which results in decreased intrapulmonary shunting and improved arterial oxygenation.
2. It is indicated in term or near-term neonates of more than 34 weeks' gestation who have evidence of persistent pulmonary hypertension of the newborn (PPHN).
3. Although ARDS is characterized by pulmonary hypertension and hypoxemia, studies have demonstrated only short-term improvement with NO inhalation. Inhaled NO may be beneficial in improving refractory hypoxemia in ARDS patients after chest trauma.
4. The normal starting dose is 20 parts per million (ppm). The dose is then weaned to the lowest effective dose and continued until the neonate's condition has improved.
5. Toxicity levels of NO are low when administered at this low concentration.
6. Patients must be weaned from NO to prevent rebound effects during withdrawal. The recommend guidelines include
   a. Use the lowest effective NO dose (5 ppm or less).
   b. Do not withdraw inhaled NO until the patient's clinical condition has improved sufficiently.
   c. Before discontinuing NO, the patient should be receiving a dose of 1 ppm for 30 min to 1 h.
   d. Before discontinuing NO, increase the patient's FiO_2 and be prepared to provide hemodynamic support if necessary.

V. HYPERBARIC OXYGEN THERAPY

Note: This therapy is no longer on the CRT or RRT exam content matrix. The material has been left in the text in case a question is asked on the exams.

A. Hyperbaric Chambers
   1. Fixed multiplace chamber

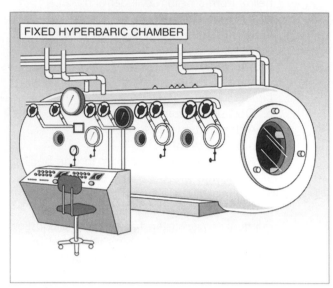

FIXED HYPERBARIC CHAMBER

FIGURE 1-23

   2. Portable monoplace chamber
B. Hyperbaric oxygen (HBO) therapy is the delivery of O_2 at greater than atmospheric pressure and is accomplished by placing the patient in a hyperbaric chamber.
C. The multiplace chamber is a walk-in unit that accommodates several people.
D. The monoplace unit accommodates only one person at a time.
E. The chambers are usually pressurized to 3 atm, or 3 times atmospheric pressure, as the patient breathes 100% O_2.
F. This increased pressure likewise increases the amount of O_2 in the blood and body tissues. While breathing room air at 1 atm, the patient has a PaO_2 of about 100 mm Hg with about 0.3 vol% O_2 dissolved in the plasma; however, while breathing 100% O_2 at 3 atm, the patient has a PaO_2 of about 1800 mm Hg with 6.2 vol% O_2 dissolved in the plasma.
G. Physiologic Effects of Hyperbaric O_2
   1. Elevated PaO_2 levels
   2. Vasoconstriction
   3. New capillary bed formation
   4. Metabolic alteration of aerobic and anaerobic organisms
   5. Reduction of nitrogen bubbles in the blood
H. Indications for Hyperbaric O_2 Therapy
   1. CO poisoning
   2. Cyanide poisoning

   3. Decompression sickness ("the bends")
   4. Gas gangrene
   5. Gas embolism
   6. Osteonecrosis
I. HBO treatments, or "dives" (as they are often called), usually require 90 min at 2 to 3 atm, two to four times a day.

VI. **OXYGEN ANALYZERS**
CRT Exam Content Matrix: IIA2,4, IIC2, IIIE10
RRT Exam Content Matrix: IIA10, IIC2
   A. **Galvanic Cell O_2 Analyzers**
      1. Electrolyte gel is used to chemically reduce O_2 to electron flow.
      2. A Clark electrode is used to measure O_2 concentration.
      3. The analyzer reading is affected by water, positive pressure, high altitude, a torn membrane, or lack of electrolyte gel.
   B. **Polarographic O_2 Analyzers**
      1. A battery polarizes the electrodes to allow O_2 reduction to occur, which gives off electron flow.
      2. The Clark electrode is used to measure O_2 concentration.
      3. The analyzer reading is affected by water, positive pressure, high altitude, a torn membrane, or lack of electrolyte gel.
      4. Electrodes last longer on the galvanic cell analyzer, but the polarographic analyzer has a quicker response time.

Other specialty gas analyzers may be used in the hospital setting. Helium and CO analyzers are seen in pulmonary function laboratories. Although much could be said about how these analyzers function, the most important aspect to remember for the examination is that these analyzers read zero when calibrated to room air.

VII. **OXYGEN SATURATION MONITORING (PULSE OXIMETRY)**
CRT Exam Content Matrix: IA7e, IB9c, o, IB10c, o, r, IC7, IIA20, IIIA1b5, IIIE3b, IIIE4d
RRT Exam Content Matrix: IA7e, IB9c, p, IB10c, q, IC8, IIIA1b5
   A. Use of the Pulse Oximeter
      1. Pulse oximeters are devices that measure SaO_2 by the principle of spectrophotometry. This is also referred to as "SpO_2."
      2. Light from the probe is directed through a capillary bed to be absorbed in different

amounts, depending on the amount of O_2 bound to Hb. The result is displayed on the monitor as a percentage of saturation.

3. The probe is noninvasive and may be attached to the finger, toe, or ear of adults and the ankle or foot of infants.
4. Pulse oximeters seem to be accurate, although some studies show they may be less accurate when used for "spot checks" rather than for continuous monitoring.
5. Pulse oximeters may be used during overnight sleep studies (polysomnogram) to detect oxygen saturation trends for several hours. Pulse oximeters can be useful in many sleep disorders, but they should not be used exclusively to diagnose sleep-related disorders. More comprehensive sleep studies should be done. (See Chapter 12 on disorders of the respiratory system.)

B. Causes of Inaccurate Readings
1. Low blood perfusion
2. CO poisoning. A pulse oximeter is not capable of determining what substance is being carried by hemoglobin. Therefore, a reading of 100% saturation doesn't reflect 100% oxygen saturation, but may actually be 60% oxygen and 40% CO. An oximeter should never be used on patients with suspected CO exposure since the reading may reflect an inaccurately high value.
3. Severe anemia
4. Hypotension
5. Hypothermia
6. Cardiac arrest
7. Nail polish, especially blue, green, brown, and black colors, may cause lower oximetry readings. Polish should be removed or the oximeter should be placed on the earlobe instead of the fingers.
8. Ambient light sources, such as direct sunlight, phototherapy, and fluorescent lights, affect the accuracy of the pulse reading. Wrapping the sensor site with a towel or gauze to block the light can eliminate this problem.
9. Dark skin pigmentation

VIII. **CO-OXIMETRY (HEMOXIMETRY)**
CRT Exam Content Matrix: IB10j, IIA24, IIC2, IIIE3c, IIIE4b
RRT Exam Content Matrix: IB9j, IB10j, IIA10, IIC2, IIIE3b
A. This procedure requires arterial blood to be obtained. The oximeter, part of the blood gas analyzer, is able to measure the amount of Hb, HbO_2, and HbCO in blood.

B. This procedure uses the principle of spectrophotometry to measure the blood level of CO bound to Hb (HbCO).
1. HbCO is usually expressed as a percentage of total Hb.
2. HbCO as high as 10% may be seen in heavy smokers, but higher levels are measured in patients who have inhaled large amounts of car fumes or smoke.
3. Patients with HbCO levels of less than 20% are usually asymptomatic.
4. HbCO levels of more than 20% result in nausea and vomiting. Fatal levels are 60% to 80%.

Transcutaneous oxygen monitoring is covered in Chapter 13 on neonatal and pediatric respiratory care.

POSTCHAPTER STUDY QUESTIONS

1. List the air/O_2 ratios for 60% O_2, 40% O_2, 35% O_2, 30% O_2, and 24% O_2.
2. Give four examples of high-flow O_2 delivery devices.
3. What is the primary benefit of using a reservoir cannula?
4. Calculate total O_2 content, given the following ABG test results:

pH	7.36
$PaCO_2$	40 mm Hg
PaO_2	82 mm Hg
SaO_2	96%
Hb	13 g/dL

5. What is the total flow delivered by an aerosol mask on 60% O_2, running at 12 L/min?
6. List the three ventilatory criteria that should be met by patients receiving O_2 from a low-flow device.
7. An 80:20 mixture of helium/O_2 running through an O_2 flowmeter at 6 L/min is delivering how much flow to the patient?
8. Calculate how long an "E" cylinder with 1900 psig will run at 5 L/min.
9. Give examples of three low-flow O_2 delivery devices.
10. List five conditions that affect the accuracy of pulse oximeters.
11. List five indications for the use of hyperbaric O_2 therapy.
12. How does water in the aerosol tubing of a mask affect the delivered FiO_2?
13. The physician orders O_2 therapy for a patient with a VT of 400 mL and an inspiratory time of 0.5 s. What flow must the mask deliver to meet this patient's inspiratory flow demands?

See answers at the back of the text.

BIBLIOGRAPHY

Cairo J, Pilbeam S: *Mosby's respiratory care equipment*, ed 8, St Louis, 2009, Mosby.

Fink J, Hunt G: *Clinical practice in respiratory care*, Philadelphia, 1999, JB Lippincott.

Hess D and others: *Respiratory care principles and practice*, ed 1, Philadelphia, 2002, Saunders.

Malley W: *Clinical blood gases: assessment and intervention*, ed 2, St Louis, 2005, Saunders.

Scanlan C, Wilkins R, Stoller J: *Egan's fundamentals of respiratory care*, ed 8, St Louis, 2003, Mosby.

Wilkins RL, Stoller JK, Kacmarek R: *Egan's fundamentals of respiratory care*, ed 9, St Louis, 2009, Mosby.

Wilkins RL, Stoller JK, Scanlan C: *Egan's fundamentals of respiratory care*, ed 8, St Louis, 2003, Mosby.

HUMIDITY AND AEROSOL

PRETEST QUESTIONS

Answer the pretest questions before studying the chapter. This will help you determine your strong and weak areas in the material covered.

1. Secretions tend to become thicker if the inspired air has which of the following characteristics?

   A. A relative humidity of 100% at body temperature
   B. 32 mg H_2O per liter of gas
   C. A water vapor pressure of 47 mm Hg
   D. 48 mg H_2O per liter of gas

2. A patient receiving 38 mg H_2O per liter of gas from a nebulizer has a humidity deficit of which of the following?

   A. 6 mg/L
   B. 9 mg/L
   C. 12 mg/L
   D. 18 mg/L

3. After connecting a nasal cannula to the humidifier outlet, you kink the tubing and hear a whistling noise coming from the humidifier. Which of the following most likely has caused this?

   A. The humidifier jar is cracked.
   B. The capillary tube in the humidifier is disconnected.
   C. The humidifier has no leaks.
   D. The top of the humidifier is not screwed on tightly.

4. You notice that the patient's secretions have become thicker and more difficult to suction since replacing the ventilator humidifier with a heat moisture exchanger. The respiratory therapist should recommend which of the following?

   A. Increase inspiratory flow.
   B. Increase the temperature to the heat moisture exchanger.
   C. Replace with a new heat moisture exchanger.
   D. Replace the heat moisture exchanger with a conventional heated humidifier.

5. Which of the following are indications for bland aerosol therapy?

   1. **A cough must be induced for sputum collection.**
   2. **Mobilization of secretions must be improved.**
   3. **Postextubation inflammation of the upper airway must be treated.**

   A. 1 only
   B. 1 and 2 only
   C. 2 and 3 only
   D. 1, 2, and 3

6. You notice that very little mist is being produced by a nebulizer attached to an aerosol mask. Which of the following could be responsible for this?

   1. **The liter flow is too high.**
   2. **The nebulizer jet is clogged with soap residue.**
   3. **The filter on the capillary tube is obstructed.**

   A. 1 only
   B. 2 only
   C. 1 and 3 only
   D. 2 and 3 only

See answers and rationales at the back of the text.

REVIEW

I. **HUMIDITY THERAPY**
   Note: Questions regarding humidity therapy appear on the CRT exam only.
   CRT Exam Content Matrix: IIA3, IIIB8, IIIF2, IIIF2g2
   A. **Humidity** is the quantity of moisture in air or gas that is caused by the addition of water in a gaseous state, or vapor. Also called *molecular water* or *invisible moisture*.

   The objective of humidity therapy is to make up for water loss that occurs when dry gas is delivered or when the upper airway is bypassed.

B. **Clinical Uses of Humidity**
   1. To humidify dry therapeutic gases
   2. To provide 100% body humidity of the inspired gas for patients with ET tubes or tracheostomy tubes
C. **Normal Airway Humidification**
   1. The nose warms, humidifies, and filters inspired air.
   2. The pharynx, trachea, and bronchial tree also warm, humidify, and filter inspired air.
   3. By the time inspired air reaches the oropharynx, it has been warmed to approximately 34° C and is 80% to 90% saturated with H_2O.
   4. By the time the inspired air reaches the carina, it has been warmed to body temperature (37° C) and is 100% saturated.
   5. When the inspired air is fully saturated (100%) at 37° C, it holds **44 mg H_2O per liter of gas and exerts a water vapor pressure of 47 mm Hg.**
D. **Absolute and Relative Humidity**
   1. **Absolute humidity** is the amount of water in a given volume of gas; its measurement is expressed in milligrams per liter.
   2. **Relative humidity** is a ratio between the amount of water in a given volume of gas and the maximum amount it is capable of holding at that temperature (capacity). Its measurement is **expressed as a percentage and is obtained with a hygrometer.**
   3.
   Relative humidity = absolute humidity capacity × 100

EXAMPLE:

The amount of moisture in a given volume of gas at 31° C is 24 mg H_2O per liter of gas. Calculate the relative humidity. (Note: At 31°C, air can hold 32.01 mg H_2O per liter.)

$$\text{Relative humidity} = \frac{24\,\text{mg/L}}{32.01\,\text{mg/L}} = 0.75 \times 100 = \textbf{75\%}$$

EXAMPLE:

A gas at 22°C has a relative humidity of 54%. Calculate the absolute humidity. (Note: At 22°C, air can hold 19.42 mg H_2O per liter.)

Absolute humidity = relative humidity × capacity

$$\text{Absolute humidity} = 0.54 \times 19.42\,\text{mg/L} = \textbf{10.5 mg/L}$$

E. **Body Humidity**
   1. Body humidity is the relative humidity at body temperature and is expressed as a percentage.
   2. $\text{Body humidity} = \dfrac{\text{absolute humidity}}{44\,\text{mg/L}} \times 100$

 The capacity of water at body temperature is 44 mg/L.

EXAMPLE:

If the gas that the patient is inspiring contains 21 mg of H_2O per liter of gas, what is the body humidity?

$$\text{Body humidity} = \frac{21\,\text{mg/L}}{44\,\text{mg/L}} = 0.48 \times 100 = \textbf{48\%}$$

---

   3. A 48% body humidity indicates that the inspired air is holding only 48% of the water it takes to fully saturate the gas in the airway at body temperature. The body's humidification system adds the other 52% by the time the air reaches the carina.
F. **Humidity Deficit**
   1. Inspired air that is not fully saturated at body temperature creates a humidity deficit. This deficit is corrected by the body's own humidification system.
   2. Humidity deficit may be expressed in milligrams per liter or as a percentage.
   3. **Humidity deficit = 44 mg/L − absolute humidity** or when expressed as a percent:

$$\frac{\textbf{Humidity deficit (mg/L)}}{\textbf{44 mg/L}} \times \textbf{100}$$

EXAMPLE:

A patient using T-tube flow-by is inspiring air from an Ohio nebulizer that contains 18 mg H_2O per liter of air. What is this patient's humidity deficit?

$$44\,\text{mg/L} - 18\,\text{mg/L} = \textbf{26 mg/L}$$

As a percentage:

$$\frac{26}{44\,\text{mg/L}} \times 100 = \textbf{59\%}$$

---

   4. This is why it is important to deliver humidified gas at body temperature to a patient with an artificial airway that bypasses the patient's upper airway.
   5. If adequate humidity is not provided, the patient's airway can dry out, which can lead to thickening of secretions and result in increased airway resistance.

6. Gas being delivered to a patient with an ET tube or tracheostomy tube that contains less than 44 mg H_2O per liter of gas or a water vapor pressure of **less than 47 mm Hg tends to dry secretions, making them thicker and more difficult to mobilize**.

G. **Efficiency of Humidifiers**

Depends on three important factors:

1. Duration of contact between the gas and water (longer duration results in increased humidity)
   a. The higher the flow rate used, the less time of contact between the gas and water and therefore the lower the humidity output.
   b. The lower the water level in the jar, the less time of contact between the gas and water and therefore the lower the humidity output.
2. Surface area of gas and water contact (greater surface area results in increased humidity)
3. Temperature of the gas and water (higher temperature results in increased humidity)

H. **Types of Humidifiers**

1. **Pass-over humidifier** (nonheated humidifier)

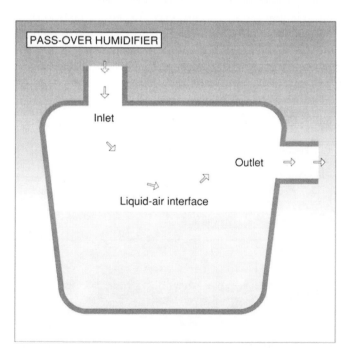

FIGURE 2-1

a. Gas simply passes over the surface of the water, picking up moisture and delivering it to the patient.
b. Produces low humidification because of the limited time of gas and water contact and the small surface area involved.
c. Provides a body humidity of approximately 25%.

2. **Bubble humidifier** (nonheated humidifier)

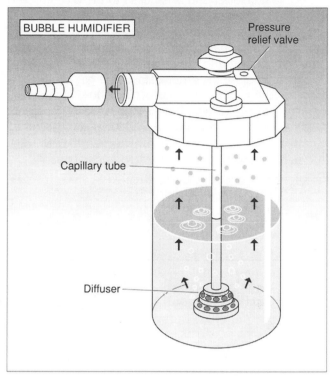

FIGURE 2-2

a. The most common type of humidifier used with oxygen delivery devices.
b. O_2 entering the humidifier travels through a tube under the surface of the water and exits through a diffuser at the lower end of the tube.
c. **Provides a body humidity of 35% to 40%.**

3. **Wick humidifier** (heated humidifier)

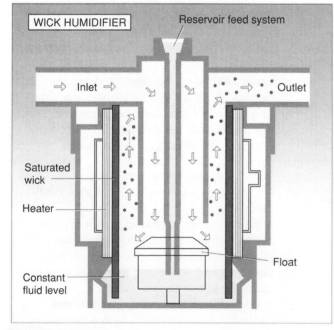

FIGURE 2-3

a. Gas from the flowmeter or ventilator enters the humidifier and is exposed to the wick (made of cloth, sponge, or paper), which is partially under the surface of the water.

b. As gas passes the wick, it absorbs water that is delivered to the patient.

c. Because the water bath or the gas is heated, a body humidity approaching 100% is delivered to the patient. This method is ideal for patients with artificial airways and those who receive mechanical ventilation.

4. **Cascade humidifier** (heated humidifier)

 Exam Note

The cascade humidifier is seldom used clinically, but questions regarding its use occasionally appear on the CRT exam.

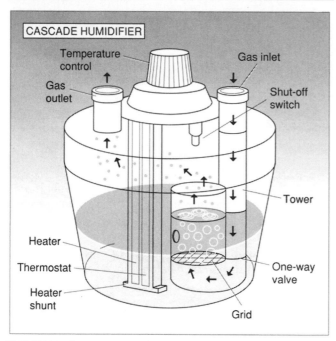

FIGURE 2-4

a. Gas travels down the tower and hits the bottom of the jar, which displaces the water upward over a grid, forming a liquid film. The gas travels back up through the grid (from underneath), picking up moisture and delivering it to the patient.

b. Because the humidifier is heated, this method is capable of delivering gas at **100% body humidity.**

c. If the humidifier is allowed to run dry, the thermostat automatically turns the heater off, which prevents the reservoir from being damaged and prevents hot dry gas from being delivered to the patient.

I. **Important Points Concerning Humidifiers**

1. Most nonheated humidifiers have a pressure pop-off valve set at **2 psi.** After the device is set

up, the tubing of the oxygen delivery device (e.g., cannula, mask) should be kinked to obstruct flow. If the pop-off sounds, there are no leaks. If no sound is heard, all connections, as well as the humidifier top, should be tightened.

2. Water levels of all humidifiers should be maintained at the levels marked on the humidifier jar to ensure maximum humidity output.

3. Condensation occurs in the tubing of heated humidifiers. This water should be discarded in a trash container or basin and should **never** be put back into the humidifier.

4. The temperature of inspired gas should be monitored continuously with an in-line thermometer when heated humidifiers are used. The thermometer should be as close to the patient's airway as possible.

5. Warm moist areas, such as heated humidifiers, are a breeding ground for microorganisms (especially *Pseudomonas* species). The humidifier should be replaced **every 24 hours.**

 Exam Note

Bacteria that grow in a heated humidifier probably will not be delivered to the patient (and cause a nosocomial infection) because the humidified particles are too small to carry the bacteria. Nebulizers are a more likely source of nosocomial infections because of the larger water particles produced, which are able to carry the bacteria to the patient.

J. **Heat Moisture Exchanger** (artificial nose)

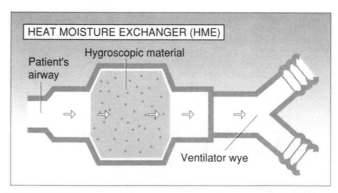

FIGURE 2-5

1. This device is placed in line between the patient's ET tube and the ventilator adapter of the ventilator circuit.

2. As the patient exhales, gas at body humidity and body temperature enters the heat moisture exchanger (HME), which heats the hygroscopic filter (made of felt, plastic foam, or cellulose sponge) and condenses water into it. During the next inspiration, gas passes through the HME and is warmed and humidified.

3. Under ideal conditions, the HME can produce 70% to 90% body humidity.

---

4. The HME may be used for temporary humidification during patient transport or for long-term humidification for ventilator-dependent patients. If ventilatory pressure begins to increase, check for water or secretions in the HME, and if there are obstructions, change to a new HME. If secretions are causing obstruction, a conventional heated humidifier should be used.

II. AEROSOL THERAPY

CRT Exam Content Matrix: IIA4, IIA12, IIA21, IIIC3, IIID5a, IIIF2c1-4

RRT Exam Content Matrix: IIIC3, IIID5a

A. **Aerosol** is defined as a suspension of water in particulate form (or a mist) in gas. Nebulizers produce aerosolized gas. Nebulizers are often referred to as aerosol generators.

B. **Clinical Uses for Aerosol Therapy**
   1. Laryngotracheobronchitis (LTB)
   2. To administer medications (via handheld nebulizer [HHN] or ultrasonic nebulizer [USN])
   3. Upper airway edema (cool aerosol)
   4. To hydrate the airway of a tracheostomy patient
   5. To induce a cough for sputum collection

C. **Hazards of Aerosol Therapy**
   1. Bronchospasm: administration of a bronchodilator may decrease the potential of this hazard.
   2. Overhydration
   3. Overheating of inspired gas
   4. Tubing condensation draining into the airway
   5. Delivery of contaminated aerosol to the patient

D. **Characteristics of Aerosol Particles**
   1. The ideal particle size for therapeutic use in respiratory care is 1.0 to 5.0 μm.
   2. Numerous factors affect the penetration and deposition of aerosol particles.
      a. **Gravitational sedimentation:** The larger a particle is, the more effect gravity has on it and the sooner it will deposit.
      b. **Brownian movement:** Affects particles of 0.1 μm or smaller in size, which will deposit too soon (possibly in the aerosol tubing).
      c. **Inertial impaction:** Larger particles have greater inertia, which keeps them moving in a straight line. Because they cannot make directional changes in the airway, they deposit sooner.

d. **Hygroscopic properties:** Aerosol particles are hygroscopic (retain moisture). As they travel down the airway, they may increase in size as they retain moisture, which may alter the time at which they deposit.

e. **Ventilatory pattern:** To obtain optimal particle penetration, the patient should be instructed to take **slow, moderately deep breaths** with a 2- to 3-second breath hold at end inspiration.

E. **Types of Nebulizers** (Pneumatic)
   1. **Jet nebulizer**

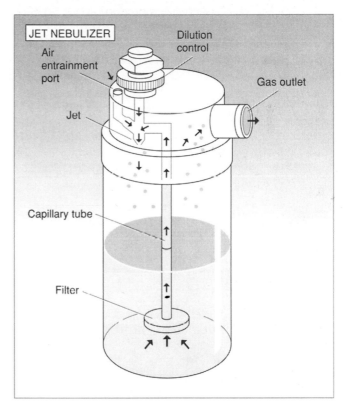

FIGURE 2-6

a. Uses viscous shear forces (see later note) to draw water up the capillary tube into the gas stream then to a baffle that breaks the water into fine aerosol particles.

b. Uses either a **Venturi** or **Pitot tube** for the entrainment of air to obtain various oxygen percentages.

   (1) **Venturi tube:** The objective is to allow air entrainment, increase flow, and restore postrestriction pressure toward prerestriction pressure.

   (2) **Pitot tube:** The objective is to maintain high forward velocity of the gas after air entrainment occurs, which results in a high forward pressure that is better able to counteract back pressure into the device and to maintain more stable oxygen

percentages of the gas. (Postrestriction lateral pressure is not restored to prerestriction levels.)

⚠️ Current theories in the literature suggest that the negative pressure created to entrain air is the result of viscous shear forces that occur as gas *passes through a restriction*. As the gas travels through a narrowed orifice, the flow becomes turbulent and the swirling of the gas causes a decrease in pressure, which allows air to be entrained in the area of lower pressure.

---

   c. Mechanical nebulizers produce about **50%** of their particles in the **0.5- to 3.0-μg** size range.

2. **Hydrosphere (Babington nebulizer)**

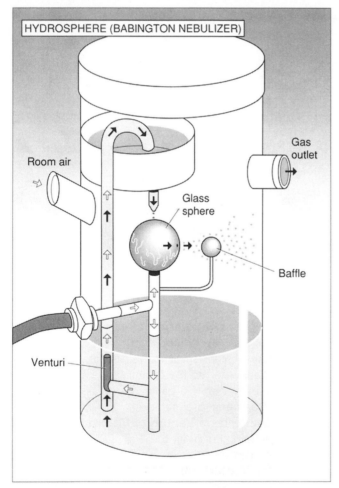

FIGURE 2-7

   a. Water is pumped up into a reservoir above a glass sphere and drops out of the reservoir onto the sphere. The sphere has a small hole with high-velocity gas coming through it that decreases the pressure pulling the water over the sphere. Water is hit by high-velocity gas,

producing an aerosol, and the particles hit a baffle, further reducing particle size.

   b. About 97% of the aerosol particles produced fall within the 1- to 10-μg size range, and 50% measure less than 5 μg.

   c. The hydrosphere is commonly used to deliver aerosol to an oxygen tent.

3. **Small-volume nebulizer**

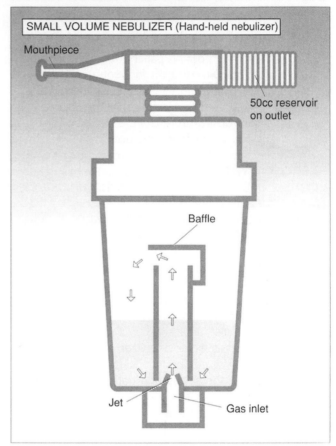

FIGURE 2-8

   a. Used as a handheld nebulizer or as a nebulizer on a ventilator or intermittent positive pressure breathing (IPPB) circuit to deliver medications.

   b. Usually holds 3 to 6 mL of liquid medications.

4. **Metered-dose inhaler**

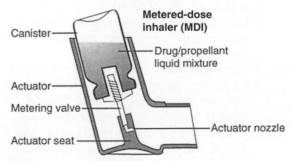

FIGURE 2-9 From Gardenhire DS: *Rau's respiratory care pharmacology*, ed 7, St Louis, 2008, Mosby.

a. This device delivers medication in aerosol form by squeezing the vial (in which the medication is stored) upward into the delivery port. This activates a small valve that allows the pressurized gas to nebulize the medication and deliver it to the patient.

b. Metered-dose inhalers (MDIs) have become a very popular method for delivering aerosolized drugs to the respiratory tract.

c. The particle size produced varies from 2 to 40 µg. Only about 10% of the dose actually reaches the lower respiratory tract.

d. The patient **must be instructed thoroughly and correctly** on the proper use of the MDI to ensure optimal aerosol particle penetration.

e. The following points should be emphasized in teaching the patient proper use of the MDI.

   (1) Do not place your lips around the delivery port, but keep your mouth opened wide so that the teeth and lips do not obstruct the flow of aerosol.

   (2) Hold the MDI about 1 inch from the mouth, with the delivery-port opening directed inside the mouth.

   (3) Inhale as slowly and as deeply as possible. **The MDI should be activated just after you start inhaling.**

   (4) Depending on the prescription, two or three aerosol doses (puffs) may be taken, waiting 30 s to 1 min between puffs.

   (5) Hold your breath at peak inspiration for **5 to 10 s** for optimal aerosol penetration.

f. MDIs are also used for ventilator-dependent patients by placement of the device directly into the inspiratory limb of the circuit and activation by the respiratory care practitioner. Ideally, the aerosol should be delivered during a sigh breath with an inspiratory hold.

g. Spacers and holding chambers, which are extensions placed on the outlet of the MDI, have proved to be effective in minimizing aerosol loss and increasing the evaporation of the propellant. This increases the stability of the aerosol and results in deeper penetration of the particles.

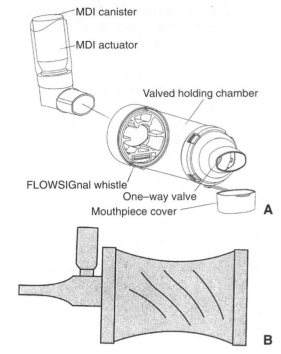

FIGURE 2-10   Types of spacers and holding chambers. **A,** From Monaghan Medical Corporation. **B,** From Gardenhire DS: *Rau's respiratory care pharmacology,* ed 7, St Louis, 2008, Mosby.

F. **Types of Nebulizers (Electric)**

   1. **Impeller nebulizer** (spinning disk or room humidifier)

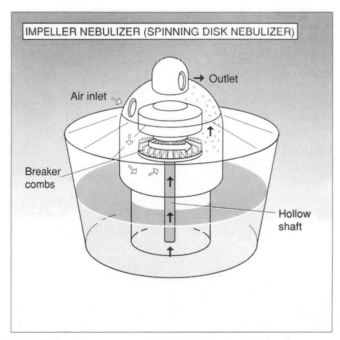

FIGURE 2-11

a. The disk rotates rapidly, drawing water up from the reservoir and throwing it through a slotted baffle, which reduces the size of the particles.

b. These devices are popular for home use, but clinically they do not produce adequate aerosol output.

c. These devices are difficult to keep clean.

2. **Ultrasonic nebulizer**
Note: The ultrasonic nebulizer is seldom used clinically, but questions regarding its use occasionally appear on the CRT exam.

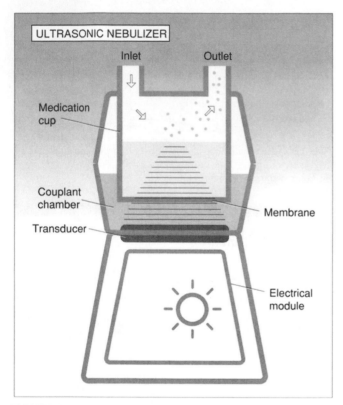

FIGURE 2-12

a. A piezoelectric transducer located in the bottom of the couplant chamber of the unit is electrically charged and produces high-frequency vibrations. These vibrations are focused on the bottom of the medication cup that sits in the couplant chamber. The vibrations break the medications in the cup into small particles, which are delivered to the patient.

b. **The frequency (which determines the particle size)** of the electric energy supplied to the transducer is approximately 1.35 Mc (1 Mc = 1 million Hz). Particle size cannot be adjusted by the user.

c. The couplant chamber contains **tap water** to help absorb mechanical heat and to act as a transfer medium for the sound waves to the medication cup.

d. The amplitude control determines the volume of the aerosol output. Volume may be as high as 6 mL/min, which is twice the output of pneumatic nebulizers, **making the ultrasonic nebulizer the best choice for patients with thick, retained sputum or when sputum induction is necessary for laboratory cultures.**

e. A built-in blower delivers 20 to 30 L/min of air to the medication cup to aid in aerosol delivery and help evacuate heat.

f. Ninety percent of the aerosol particles produced fall within the 0.5- to 3.0-μg range.

g. The temperature of the delivered aerosol is between 3° C and 10° C above room temperature during normal operation.

h. **Hazards of ultrasonic therapy**
   (1) Overhydration
   (2) Bronchospasm
   (3) Sudden mobilization of secretions
   (4) Electrical hazard
   (5) Water collection in the tubing
   (6) Swelling of secretions from the absorption of saline, which may obstruct the airway
   (7) Changes in drug dosage, caused by the drug reconcentrating because of the solvent in the medication cup, leading to an increasingly stronger dose as the treatment continues

G. **Important Points Concerning Nebulizers**

1. Of all respiratory equipment, heated nebulizers are the greatest source of delivery of contaminated moisture to the patient; *Pseudomonas* species are the most common contaminate. These nebulizers should be replaced every 12 to 24 h.

2. Make sure that jets and capillary tubes are clear of debris or buildup of minerals by cleaning after each use. If the nebulizer is not producing adequate mist, a clogged capillary tube or jet may be the cause.

3. Some older, nondisposable nebulizers have pressure pop-off valves that should be checked after the nebulizer is set up (valves are usually set at 2 psi). The pop-off valve is effective only when the nebulizer is set on 100% because an open entrainment port constitutes a leak in the nebulizer.

4. Keep water drained out of the aerosol tubing because this **increases** the percentage of oxygen delivered to the patient. Water in the tubing obstructs gas flow, resulting in back pressure into the nebulizer. As pressure increases in the nebulizer, less air is entrained in the entrainment port; therefore delivered FiO_2 increases, total flow

to the patient decreases, and less aerosol is delivered.

5. Keep the water level at the appropriate markings on the nebulizer to ensure optimal aerosol output.

6. Soap should not be used to clean the couplant chamber or medication cup of the ultrasonic nebulizer because residue interferes with the ultrasonic activity. If this occurs, a small amount of isopropyl alcohol in the couplant chamber or medication cup helps.

7. Make sure the filter at the end of the capillary tubes of pneumatic nebulizers are decontaminated properly. A dirty or clogged filter does not allow the fluid to be drawn up the tube adequately, which reduces aerosol output.

POSTCHAPTER STUDY QUESTIONS

1. List five hazards of aerosol therapy.
2. If the inspired air can hold 32 mg of H_2O per liter and is holding 8 mg/L, what is the relative humidity?
3. How much of a humidity deficit exists when a patient inspires air holding 30 mg of H_2O per liter?
4. Give an example of a humidifier that can deliver gas at 100% body humidity.
5. List four hazards of ultrasonic nebulizer therapy.
6. A clogged filter or capillary tube on a jet nebulizer has what effect on the operation of the device?
7. List five clinical indications for aerosol therapy.
8. How should a patient be instructed to breathe while a bronchodilating agent is being administered via a small-volume nebulizer?
9. An HME can produce a body humidity in what range?

See answers at the back of the text.

BIBLIOGRAPHY

Branson R, Hess D, Chatburn R: *Respiratory care equipment*, ed 2, Philadelphia, 1999, Lippincott.

Cairo J, Pilbeam S: *Mosby's respiratory care equipment*, ed 8, St Louis, 2010, Mosby.

Gardenhire DS: *Rau's respiratory care pharmacology*, ed 7, St Louis, 2008, Mosby.

Hess D and others: *Respiratory care principles and practice*, ed 1, Philadelphia, 2002, Saunders.

Wilkins RL, Stoller JK, Kacmarek, R: *Egan's fundamentals of respiratory care*, ed 9, St Louis, 2009, Mosby.

ASSESSMENT OF THE CARDIOPULMONARY PATIENT

PRETEST QUESTIONS

Answer the pretest questions before studying the chapter. This will help you determine your strong and weak areas in the material covered.

1. A patient coughs up yellow sputum after an IPPB treatment. Which one of the following statements is TRUE in regard to this sputum production?

   A. It is old and contains little water.
   B. It is termed *hemoptysis.*
   C. It contains white blood cells (WBCs).
   D. It is a normal color for sputum.

2. The term used to describe a condition in which a patient has difficulty breathing while in a supine position is which of the following?

   A. Orthopnea
   B. Hypoventilation
   C. Paroxysmal nocturnal dyspnea
   D. Kussmaul respirations

3. A patient enters the emergency department, and on initial examination the respiratory therapist observes paradoxical chest movement. Which of the following should the practitioner suspect?

   A. Pulmonary edema
   B. Pneumonia
   C. Flail chest
   D. Pleural effusion

4. Perfusion in the extremities may best be determined by which of the following methods?

   A. Obtaining ABG studies and determining the PaO_2 level.
   B. Assessing the SaO_2 level with a pulse oximeter.
   C. Assessing capillary refill.
   D. Palpating a brachial pulse.

5. While palpating the chest, the respiratory therapist determines that there are decreased vibrations over the right lower lobe. This may be the result of which of the following?

1. Pneumothorax
2. Pleural effusion
3. Pneumonia

   A. 1 only
   B. 2 only
   C. 1 and 2 only
   D. 2 and 3 only

6. A chest x-ray film obtained after ET intubation shows the tip of the ET tube is resting at the fourth rib. Which of the following actions should be taken?

   A. The tube should be advanced 2 cm.
   B. The tube should be advanced until equal breath sounds are heard.
   C. The tube should remain at this level.
   D. The tube should be withdrawn 3 cm.

7. A patient is suspected of having intrathoracic metastatic nodal disease. Which of the following imaging studies should the respiratory therapist recommend to determine, with the highest accuracy, whether disease is present?

   A. Positron emission tomography (PET)
   B. Magnetic resonance imaging (MRI)
   C. Computed tomography (CT)
   D. Pulmonary angiogram

8. Which of the following imaging studies may be useful in determining whether a pulmonary embolism is present?

1. MRI
2. PET
3. CT
4. Chest x-ray

   A. 1 and 3 only
   B. 1 and 2 only
   C. 1, 3, and 4 only
   D. 2, 3, and 4 only

See answers and rationales at the back of the text.

REVIEW

I. PATIENT HISTORY

CRT Exam Content Matrix: IA1, IB5a-f
RRT Exam Content Matrix: IA1

A. Patient Interview: Obtain the following information
1. Chief complaint
2. Symptoms that the patient has and when they started
3. Past medical problems
4. Occupation
5. Medications currently prescribed
6. Allergies
7. Exercise tolerance and daily activities
8. Living environment
9. Nutritional status
10. Social support systems available

B. Techniques for an effective patient interview
1. Introduce yourself and establish a rapport with the patient so that the patient feels comfortable and open to discussion.
2. Try to avoid leading questions, such as "Are you still short of breath?" These questions may elicit a different response than would "How is your breathing at this time?"
3. Always show respect for the patient's attitudes and beliefs.
4. Promote a relaxed atmosphere and avoid difficult medical terms that the patient may not understand.
5. To promote better understanding of the information discussed, the respiratory care practitioner (RCP) must be able to modify terminology to fit the age or educational level of the patient. Use simpler terms than the medical terms, which may be difficult for the patient.

EXAMPLE:

When describing the use of hyperinflation therapy, do not say, "This therapy will help you reach your inspiratory capacity and help prevent atelectasis." Do say, for example, "This therapy will help encourage you to breathe deeper to help prevent your lungs from collapsing."

II. ASSESSMENT OF SYMPTOMS

CRT Exam Content Matrix: IA2, IB1c, IB5a-f, IIIE5a
RRT Exam Content Matrix: IA2, IB1c, IB5a-e

A. **Common Symptoms in Patients with Pulmonary Disease**
1. **Cough**: aids in clearing the airway of secretions
    a. Nonproductive cough is caused by
       (1) Irritation of the airway
       (2) Acute inflammation of the respiratory mucosal membrane
       (3) Presence of a growth
       (4) Irritation of the pleura
       (5) Irritation of the tympanic membrane
    b. Productive cough: sputum color must be monitored:
       (1) White and translucent: contains normal mucus
       (2) Yellow: indicates infection and contains WBCs; called *purulent sputum*
       (3) Green: contains old, retained secretions
       (4) Green and foul smelling: indicates *Pseudomonas* species infection
       (5) Brown: contains old blood
       (6) Red: contains fresh blood

> ⚠ Foul-smelling sputum that often settles into several layers is characteristic of bronchiectasis. (See Chapter 12 on disorders of the respiratory system.)

    c. When a cough is productive, it is important to record the amount, consistency, odor, and color of sputum because changes in these qualities over 24 h are important in the diagnosis of pulmonary disease.
    d. Sputum collection and laboratory analysis are important parts of the pulmonary assessment. Steps in sputum collection
       (1) Explain to the patient the intent to collect a sample.
       (2) Good oral hygiene prevents the collection from being contaminated by oral secretions.
       (3) The sputum sample must be from a deep cough.

> ☑ **Exam Note**
>
> If a patient cannot cough adequately, nasotracheal suctioning for the sample may be necessary. To collect the sputum, a sputum trap or a Lukens tube catheter is necessary.

    e. Characteristics of a cough
       (1) Barklike cough usually indicates croup.
       (2) Harsh, dry cough with inspiratory stridor usually indicates upper airway problems.
       (3) Wheezing type of coughs usually indicate lower airway pathology.
       (4) Chronic productive coughs are indicative of chronic bronchitis.
       (5) Frequent hacking cough and throat clearing may be the result of smoking or sinus or viral infection.
2. **Dyspnea** is the patient's complaint of difficult or labored breathing.

a. It is a subjective symptom, meaning the patient expresses breathing difficulty, and can be influenced by the patient's reactions and emotional state.

✓ **Exam Note**

A patient who has dyspnea or tachypnea (elevated rate) is often said to be hyperventilating; however, the only way to determine whether someone is hyperventilating is to observe ABG results indicating a CO_2 level less than normal.

---

b. Causes of dyspnea
  (1) Increased airway resistance
  (2) Upper airway obstruction
  (3) Asthma and other chronic lung diseases
  (4) Decreased lung compliance
  (5) Pulmonary fibrosis
  (6) Pneumothorax
  (7) Pleural effusion
  (8) Abnormal chest wall
  (9) Anxiety state, when there is no physiologic explanation
c. Types of dyspnea
  (1) **Orthopnea** is dyspnea while lying down. The condition is usually seen in patients with heart failure and is caused by increased congestion of the lungs while lying down. It is often observed in patients with emphysema because of their inadequate diaphragmatic movement during ventilation.
  (2) **Paroxysmal nocturnal dyspnea** is sudden onset of shortness of breath after being in bed for several hours. It is seen in cardiac patients and results in acute pulmonary edema, which usually subsides quickly after the patient is positioned upright.
  (3) **Exertional dyspnea** is often seen in patients with cardiopulmonary disease. The severity is determined by the amount of exertion. It is important to determine at what point the patient experiences dyspnea: Does it begin after walking up a flight of stairs or after simply walking across the room?

3. **Hemoptysis** is coughing up blood from the respiratory tract.
  a. Blood-tinged or blood-streaked sputum is not hemoptysis.
  b. Hemoptysis is determined by the coughing up of a certain volume of blood; the amount indicates the severity of the symptom.
  c. Causes of hemoptysis
    (1) Pneumonia
    (2) Tuberculosis
    (3) Bronchiectasis
    (4) Lung abscess
    (5) Fungal lung infection: histoplasmosis
    (6) Neoplasms: bronchogenic carcinoma
    (7) Pulmonary embolism
    (8) Valvular heart diseases
    (9) Mitral valve stenosis
    (10) Trauma
  d. Patients may think they are "coughing up blood" from the lungs when the blood is from the gastrointestinal tract. The origin of the blood must be determined.

4. **Chest pain**
  a. The thoracic wall is the most common source of chest pain.
  b. The pain may be from nerves, muscles, or the skin or bones of the thoracic wall.
  c. The lung parenchyma is not sensitive to pain.
  d. The parietal pleura (layer lining the chest wall) is very sensitive to pain and is usually the source of pain associated with pneumonias, pleurisy, and other inflammatory processes.
  e. Chest pain may be associated with **pulmonary hypertension** caused by the increased tension on the walls of the vessels and increased workload on the right side of the heart.
  f. Chest pain may originate from the heart as a result of an inadequate blood supply. This pain is called **angina pectoris.**

g. Chest pain is also associated with a ruptured aorta, myocardial infarction, and esophageal problems.

III. OTHER PHYSICAL ASSESSMENTS

CRT Exam Content Matrix: IA2, IA6, IA8a-b, IB1a, IB2a-b, IB3, IB4a-c, IB7a-e, IB8, IC1, IIIA1b3, IIIE1, IIIE11

RRT Exam Content Matrix: IA2, IA6, IA8a-b, IB1a, IB2a-b, IB4a-c, IB7a-e, IB8, IC2, IIIA1b3, IIIE1

A. Breathing Patterns

1. **Eupnea:** the normal rate and depth of respirations, which is 10 to 20 breaths per minute.
2. **Bradypnea:** less than the normal respiratory rate. May be seen with respiratory center depression caused by head trauma or drug overdose.
3. **Apnea:** absence of breathing for a specific period of time (usually at least 10 s). Seen in patients with respiratory arrest caused by asphyxia, severe drug overdose, central and obstructive sleep apnea, and other central respiratory center disorders.
4. **Tachypnea:** faster than the normal respiratory rate but with the normal depth of breathing. May indicate decreased lung compliance and is associated with restrictive diseases, pneumonia, and pulmonary edema.
5. **Hypopnea:** shallow respirations (about half of normal depth) with slower than normal respiratory rate. Hypopnea is normal in well-conditioned athletes and is accompanied by a slow pulse rate. May be seen in patients with damage to the brainstem and is accompanied by a weak, rapid pulse.
6. **Hyperpnea:** deep, rapid, and labored breathing. Associated with conditions in which there is an inadequate oxygen supply, such as cardiac and respiratory diseases. Usually refers to hyperventilation.
7. **Kussmaul respiration:** increased rate and depth of breathing. Usually seen in patients with severe metabolic acidosis (diabetic ketoacidosis).

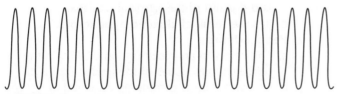

FIGURE 3-1   Kussmaul respirations.

8. **Biot respiration:** irregular breathing pattern characterized by short periods of deep, consistent volumes with periods of apnea. The apneic period may last 10 to 30 s. Associated with elevated ICP or meningitis.

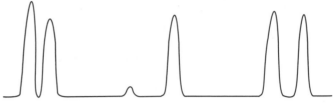

FIGURE 3-2   Biot respirations.

9. **Cheyne-Stokes respiration:** deep, rapid breathing followed by apnea. The breaths begin slow and shallow and gradually increase to above normal volume and rate, then gradually diminish in volume and rate, followed by apnea. Apnea may last 10 to 20 s before the cycle is repeated. Seen with respiratory center depression caused by stroke or head injury, pneumonia in the elderly, congestive heart failure, or drug overdose.

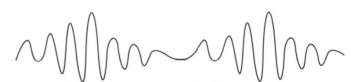

FIGURE 3-3   Cheyne-Stokes respirations.

B. Chest Inspection:
This should be performed with the patient seated and with clothing removed above the waist. If the patient is not able to sit in a chair, he or she should be placed in bed in Fowler position (i.e., head of bed elevated 45 degrees). **Inspection should include**

1. The rate, depth, and regularity of breathing compared with the norms for the patient's age and activity level.
2. Skin color, temperature, and condition, such as bruises or scars. Is the patient diaphoretic (perspiring)?

3. Chest symmetry: Compare one side of the chest with the other.
   a. Observe chest excursion while standing in front of the patient to determine whether both sides are expanding equally.
   b. Unequal expansion may indicate
      (1) Atelectasis
      (2) Pneumothorax
      (3) Chest deformities
      (4) Flail chest: **"Paradoxical"** respirations may be observed, in which the chest moves in on inspiration and out on expiration. Flail chest is the result of chest trauma, a fractured sternum, or fractured ribs.
4. Shape and size of chest: in comparison with norms
   a. Observe the AP diameter.
   b. An increased AP diameter is called a ***barrel chest* and is indicative of chronic lung disease.**
5. Work of breathing
   a. Should be evaluated to determine the level of breathing difficulty.
   b. While observing the patient's breathing process, determine the following factors:
      (1) Is the chest movement symmetric?
      (2) Are the accessory muscles being used?

The intercostal muscles and diaphragm are the major muscles for normal ventilation. The accessory muscles are the scalene and the sternomastoid muscles in the neck and the pectoralis major muscle in the anterior chest. When accessory muscles are used during ventilation, it is a sign of respiratory distress.

---

   (3) What is the shape of the chest?
   (4) What is the respiratory rate?
   (5) Is the breathing pattern regular or irregular?
   (6) Are there any bony deformities of the ribs, spine, or chest?
   (7) Is the patient's VT normal in relation to size and age?
   (8) Is expiration prolonged, shorter than inspiration, or equal to inspiration?
   (9) Are substernal, suprasternal, or intercostal retractions or nasal flaring observed? **These are all signs of respiratory distress.**

C. Inspection of the Extremities
   1. **Digital clubbing**

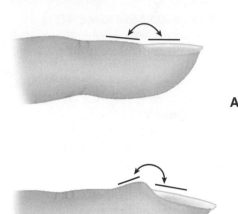

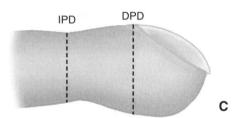

FIGURE 3-4   A, Normal digit configuration. **B,** Mild digital clubbing with increased hyponychial angle. **C,** Severe digital clubbing; the depth of finger at base of nail (DPD) is greater than the depth of the interphalangeal joint (IPD) with clubbing. From Wilkins RL, Stoller JK, Kacmarek R: *Egan's fundamentals of respiratory care,* ed 9, St Louis, 2009, Mosby.

   a. Digital clubbing is indicative of long-standing pulmonary disease: 75% to 85% of all clubbing is the result of pulmonary disease.
   b. Consists of enlargement of the distal phalanges of the fingers and, less commonly, the toes. There is a loss of the angle between the nail and dorsum of the terminal phalanx.
   c. It is the result of **chronic hypoxemia.**
   2. **Pedal edema**
      a. This refers to an accumulation of fluid in the subcutaneous tissues of the ankles.
      b. This symptom is commonly observed in patients with chronic pulmonary disease, in which their chronic hypoxemic state results in pulmonary vasoconstriction.

c. The right side of the heart works harder as it pumps blood through narrowed pulmonary vessels, which results in an increased workload on the right side of the heart, right ventricular hypertrophy, and, eventually, right-sided heart failure (cor pulmonale).

d. As right-sided heart pressures increase, venous blood flow returning to the heart is diminished, and the peripheral blood vessels become engorged. The ankles are most affected as a result of gravity. This is often accompanied by jugular venous distention (JVD). The jugular veins returning blood from the upper body also become engorged as a result of elevated pressure in the right side of the heart.

3. **Cyanosis**
   a. Refers to the bluish discoloration of the skin and nailbeds resulting from a **5 g/dL decrease in *oxygenated* Hb.** For example, a patient with an Hb level of 15 g/dL would have cyanosis if the oxygen saturation dropped to a level where only 10 g/dL was saturated with oxygen.
   b. Cyanosis may indicate decreased oxygenation or reduced peripheral circulation.
   c. Patients with decreased Hb levels (anemia) may not exhibit cyanosis even if tissue hypoxia is present. An anemic patient has a low oxygen-carrying capacity, which may result in tissue hypoxia but does not cause cyanosis unless 5 g/dL of unsaturated Hb is present. If there is not enough Hb in the blood to manifest it, cyanosis will not occur.
   d. Conversely, a patient with an increased level of Hb (polycythemia) has an increased capacity for carrying oxygen. This patient may have a level of 5 g/dL of unsaturated Hb and therefore may have cyanosis yet have enough saturated Hb to adequately oxygenate the tissues.

4. **Capillary refill**
   a. Perfusion to the extremities may be determined by assessing capillary refill.
   b. This is performed by compressing the patient's fingernail for a short time, then releasing it and observing the time it takes for blood flow to return to the nailbed.
   c. Normal refill time is less than 3 s.
   d. Patients with decreased cardiac output and poor digital perfusion have a longer refill time.

D. **Chest Deformities**

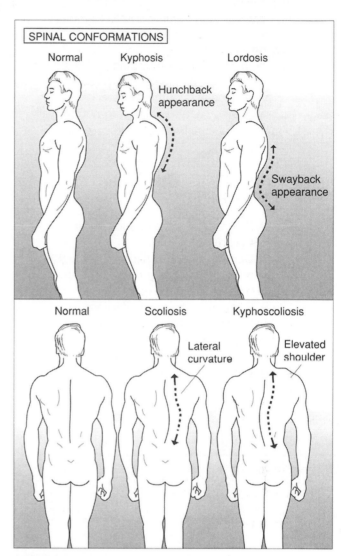

FIGURE 3-5

1. **Kyphosis**
   a. Concave curvature of the spine, resulting in a "hunchback" appearance. It is best assessed from an anterior view.
   b. Caused by degenerative bone disease or age or may be seen with COPD.
2. **Lordosis**
   a. Backward curvature of the lumbar spine, resulting in a "swayback" appearance.
   b. Usually not a cause of respiratory difficulties.
3. **Scoliosis**
   a. Lateral curvature of the thoracic spine, resulting in chest protrusion posteriorly and the anterior

ribs flattening out. Chest protrudes on right or left side.

b. Depending on severity, it may result in impaired lung movement.

4. **Kyphoscoliosis**
   a. Combination of kyphosis and scoliosis
   b. May be most adequately observed by noticing different heights of the shoulders.
   c. Cardiopulmonary problems do not normally present until patients reach their 40s or 50s.
   d. Pulmonary signs and symptoms of kyphoscoliosis
      (1) Dyspnea
      (2) Hypoxemia
      (3) Hypercapnia
      (4) Progressive respiratory insufficiency
      (5) Cardiac failure
      (6) Decreased lung capacity evidenced by results of pulmonary function tests **(restrictive disease)**
      (7) Frequent pulmonary infections
      (8) Uneven ventilation/perfusion ratio

5. **Pectus carinatum**

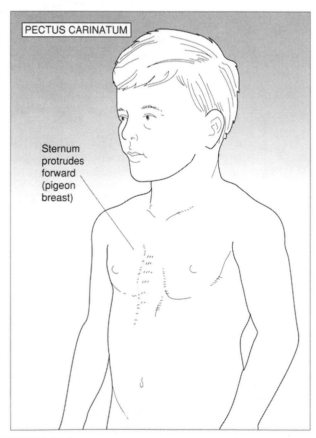

FIGURE 3-6

a. Also called *pigeon breast;* results in the forward projection of the xiphoid process and lower sternum.
b. Usually a congenital condition.
c. May cause dyspnea on exercise and more frequent respiratory infections as a result of interference with heart and lung movement.
d. In severe cases, surgical correction may be indicated.

6. **Pectus excavatum**

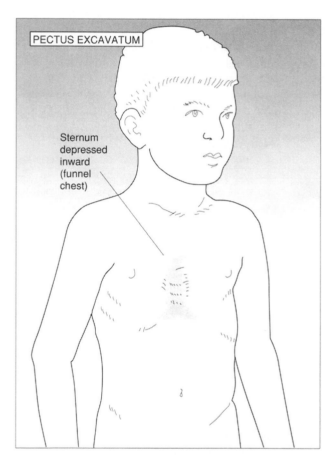

FIGURE 3-7

a. Also called *funnel chest;* results in a funnel-shaped depression over the lower sternum.
b. Usually a congenital condition.
c. May lead to dyspnea on exertion and more frequent respiratory infections.

7. **Barrel chest**

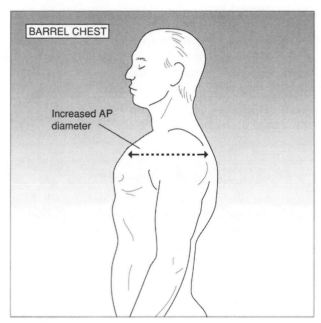

FIGURE 3-8

a. The natural recoil properties of the lungs are decreased because of air trapping and subsequent hyperinflation. This loss of lung elasticity causes the ribs to move more outward, which causes the barrel appearance.
b. The increased tone and development of the accessory muscles, which are used during breathing by patients with COPD, also contributes to the barrel appearance.
c. Seen almost exclusively in patients with chronic lung disease.
d. This hyperinflated state of the lungs pushes down on the diaphragm, which restricts its movement. The diaphragm is a dome-shaped muscle that is innervated by the phrenic nerve. Contraction of the muscle causes a decrease in pressure within the lungs below atmospheric levels, and air enters the airway. Hyperinflated lungs tend to flatten the diaphragm, diminishing its contracting ability. This decreases alveolar ventilation and chest excursion, which results in labored breathing.
e. Muscles normally used for ventilation are the **diaphragm and external intercostals,** but because the diaphragm of patients with COPD is flattened, they use their accessory muscles during normal ventilation.

E. **Palpation of the Chest**

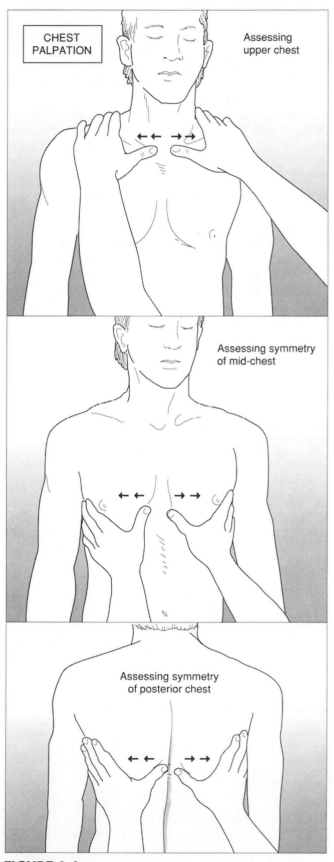

FIGURE 3-9

1. Use the sense of touch on the chest wall to assess physical signs.
2. Hands are placed on the chest to assess chest movement and vibration.
3. Vibrations felt on the chest wall as the patient speaks are called *tactile fremitus*. The vibrations originate at the vocal cords and are transmitted down the tracheobronchial tree, through the alveoli to the chest wall.
   a. The practitioner places his or her hands on the patient's chest and asks the patient to say certain words, such as "ninety-nine," as the practitioner palpates over different areas of the chest.
   b. Vibrations are **decreased** over pleural effusions, fluid, pneumothorax and in overly muscular or obese patients.
   c. Vibrations are **increased** over atelectasis, pneumonia, and lung masses.
4. For patients with suspected chest trauma or after thoracic surgery, assess for subcutaneous emphysema and crepitus. After chest trauma with pneumothorax or after thoracic surgery, air can leak into the subcutaneous tissues (subcutaneous emphysema). Palpating over subcutaneous air feels like crackling under the skin, which is referred to as *crepitus*.
5. Position of the trachea.

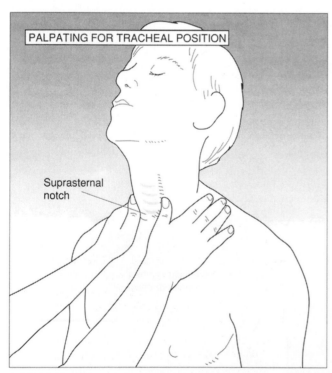

FIGURE 3-10

a. Assessed by placing both thumbs on each side of the suprasternal notch and gently pressing inward. Only soft tissue should be palpable. If the trachea is felt, it indicates that the trachea

has shifted and is no longer positioned midline, as it should be.
   b. A shift of the trachea's position may be the result of a tension pneumothorax or massive atelectasis.
   (1) Tension pneumothorax: **trachea shifts to the unaffected side (opposite side of pneumothorax)**
   (2) Atelectasis: **trachea shifts toward the affected side (same side as atelectasis)**
F. **Percussion of the Chest Wall**

 Exam Note

According to the most current NBRC exam content matrices for both the CRT and RRT exams, diagnostic chest percussion will no longer be covered. It is in the text here for general knowledge purposes.

1. This involves tapping on the chest directly with one finger or indirectly by placing one finger on a chest area and tapping on that finger over different areas of the chest.
2. There are five different sounds heard during percussion.
   a. **Hyperresonance**
   (1) A loud, low-pitched sound of long duration that is produced over areas that contain a greater proportion of air than tissue
   (2) Examples: air-filled stomach, emphysema (air trapping), pneumothorax
   b. **Resonance**
   (1) A low-pitched sound of long duration that is produced over areas with equal distribution of air and tissue
   (2) Example: normal lung tissue
   c. **Dullness**
   (1) A sound of medium intensity and pitch of short duration that is produced over areas that contain a higher proportion of tissue or fluid than air
   (2) Examples: atelectasis, consolidation, pleural effusion, pleural thickening, pulmonary edema
   d. **Flatness**
   (1) A sound of low amplitude and pitch that is produced over areas that contain a higher proportion of tissue than air
   (2) Examples: massive pleural effusion, massive atelectasis, pneumonectomy
   e. **Tympany**
   (1) A drumlike sound
   (2) Example: tension pneumothorax

G. Auscultation of Breath Sounds
1. **Normal breath sounds**
   a. **Vesicular**
      (1) Gentle rustling sound heard over the entire chest wall, except the right supraclavicular area. In a healthy person, vesicular sounds are often difficult to hear
      (2) Inspiration is longer than expiration, with no pause between
   b. **Bronchial**
      (1) Loud and generally high-pitched sound heard over the upper portion of the sternum, trachea, and both mainstem bronchi
      (2) Expiration is longer than inspiration, with a short pause between
      (3) If heard in other lung areas, it indicates atelectasis or consolidation
   c. **Bronchovesicular**
      (1) A combination of bronchial and vesicular breath sounds, normally heard over the sternum, between the scapulae, and over the right apex of the lung
      (2) Inspiration and expiration are of equal duration, with no pause between
   d. **Tracheal**
      (1) Harsh and high-pitched sound heard over the trachea
      (2) Expiration is slightly longer than inspiration
2. **Adventitious breath sounds**
   a. Abnormal breath sounds superimposed on normal breath sounds
   b. Classified as **crackles** (discontinuous sounds) and **wheezes** (continuous sounds).
      (1) **Crackles**
         (a) A bubbling or crackling sound that can be heard during inspiration or expiration and produced by air flowing through airways containing secretions or fluid.
         (b) Early inspiratory crackles, or crackles occurring in the early part of inspiration, are the result of larger proximal airways collapsing during expiration and are heard most commonly in patients with emphysema, chronic bronchitis, or asthma.
         (c) When peripheral alveoli and airways collapse during exhalation, late inspiratory crackles are heard as these airways pop open. Late inspiratory crackles are most commonly heard in patients with pulmonary edema, atelectasis, pneumonia, or restrictive lung disorders such as pulmonary fibrosis.

      (2) **Wheezes**
         (a) Breath sounds with a musical quality that are produced as air flows through constricted airways.
         (b) Airways may become constricted as a result of bronchospasm, mucosal edema, excessive sputum, or presence of foreign bodies.
         (c) May be heard on both inspiration and expiration.
         (d) Wheezes may be heard with asthma, bronchitis, congestive heart failure, and foreign body obstruction.
      (3) **Stridor**
         (a) Most commonly heard during inspiration and produced as air passes through a narrowed upper airway structure such as the glottis (glottic edema).
         (b) The diameter of the upper airway may be decreased as a result of infection, as in epiglottitis or croup, or with inflammation and swelling of the glottic area after extubation.
         (c) Stridor is a life-threatening sign that ventilation is compromised and immediate intervention is necessary. (See Chapter 4 on airway management.)
      (4) **Pleural friction rub**
         (a) A clicking or grating sound caused by friction that is produced as the parietal and visceral pleura rub against each other during the breathing process.
         (b) Most commonly associated with pleurisy. It is very painful.

H. Auscultation of Heart Sounds
1. **Normal heart sounds:** Heart sounds are thought to be produced as a result of sudden changes in blood flow through the heart that cause a vibration of the valves and chambers inside the heart. The normal heart sound is a "lubb-dub" sound.
   a. The first heart sound ("lubb") represents the closing of the atrioventricular (AV) valves.
      (1) The AV valves are the mitral valve (between the left atrium and left ventricle) and the tricuspid valve (between the right atrium and right ventricle).
      (2) The first heart sound is designated S_1.
   b. The second heart sound ("dub") represents the closing of the semilunar valves.
      (1) The semilunar valves consist of the pulmonic valve (between the right ventricle and the pulmonary artery) and the aortic valve (between the left ventricle and aorta).
      (2) The second heart sound is designated S_2.

c. A third and fourth heart sound **(S₃ and S₄)** may be heard, but they are more difficult to hear than S₁ and S₂ and are more easily heard in children.

   (1) **S₃** is thought to result from blood rushing into the ventricles during early ventricular diastole.

   (2) **S₄** is thought to result from atrial contraction.

2. **Abnormal heart sounds (murmurs)**

  a. Murmurs usually occur when blood flows in a turbulent fashion through heart structures that have a decreased cross-sectional area.

  b. Murmurs are described by the location of the sound, the part of the cardiac cycle in which they occur, and the intensity of the sound.

  c. **Conditions resulting in heart murmurs**

    (1) Aortic valve disease (e.g., stenosis, regurgitation)

    (2) Mitral valve disease (e.g., stenosis, regurgitation)

    (3) Pulmonic valve stenosis

    (4) Tricuspid valve insufficiency

✓ Exam Note

An abnormal sound heard over the heart, arteries, or veins that is caused by turbulent blood flow or an obstruction is referred to as a *bruit*.

I. **Chest X-ray Film Interpretation**

1. Useful terms when interpreting chest films:

  a. **Consolidation:** well-defined, solid-appearing lung that appears light on the film and is **caused by pneumonia**

  b. **Radiopaque:** white areas on the film that indicate fluids and solids (also referred to as *opacity* or *opacification*) and that are **caused by pneumonia and pleural effusion, for example**

  c. **Infiltrates:** scattered or patchy white areas on the film that are **caused by inflammatory processes** that indicate **atelectasis or disease**

  d. **Radiolucency:** dark areas on x-ray film **caused by the presence of air;** hyperlucency is characteristic of emphysema, asthma, or subcutaneous emphysema.

2. **Chest radiograph positions**

  a. Posteroanterior (PA)

    (1) This is the most commonly used position for chest films.

    (2) The patient is positioned upright, and the image is obtained during a maximal inspiration.

    (3) The x-ray passes through the chest from back (posterior) to front (anterior), and the film is anterior to the patient's chest.

  b. Anteroposterior (AP)

    (1) This position is often used for portable radiographs in the intensive care areas.

    (2) The x-ray passes through the chest from anterior to posterior.

    (3) The heart is more easily seen in this position, but the quality of the film is inferior to that of the PA film.

  c. Lateral

    (1) The image is obtained from the side with the patient upright while the x-ray passes through the chest laterally.

    (2) This position allows for visualization of the lung parenchyma behind the heart and the bases of the lungs.

  d. Oblique

    (1) This image is obtained with the patient turned 45 degrees to either the right or left.

    (2) This position is used to help differentiate a pulmonary or mediastinal lesion from structures that overlie it. This view is often used when bilateral lesions are present.

    (3) This position is also used for ventilation/perfusion scanning.

  e. Apical lordotic

    (1) In an upright position, the patient leans back at a 45 degree angle.

    (2) This position moves the shadow of the clavicles out of the way for better visualization of the upper lobes of the lungs.

  f. Lateral decubitus

    (1) The image is obtained with the patient lying on his or her side (side-lying position) with the film resting on the posterior surface of the chest.

    (2) This position is used to identify whether free fluid (pleural effusion or blood) is present in the chest. Fluid drains to the dependent area of the lung—the lung the patient is lying on—and creates a shadow. For example, if right-sided fluid is suspected, the patient should be placed on the right side.

    (3) This view is also helpful in determining the presence of a pneumothorax. Because air rises, the patient should be placed on the left side if a right pneumothorax is suspected.

 Chest radiographs are usually obtained with the patient at maximal inspiration, which should show the lungs well aerated and the diaphragm descended to about the level of the tenth rib. An image obtained on expiration may be beneficial in detecting a small pneumothorax that would otherwise be difficult to see on a routine inspiratory film. As the patient exhales, the lung volume is reduced while pleural air volume remains the same. The pneumothorax then occupies more of the thoracic volume and may be better visualized.

3. Evaluating conditions on chest x-ray film

> ⚠ Before viewing a patient's chest film, verify that the patient's name on the folder containing the film matches the patient's name on the upper corner of the film.

a. **Atelectasis**
   (1) Appears lighter than normal lung tissue.
   (2) May be indicated by elevated diaphragm, mediastinal shift (toward area of atelectasis), or increased density and decreased volume of a lung area.
b. **Pneumonia**
   (1) Appears white on x-ray film.
   (2) Consolidation of entire lobe or more may cause **mediastinal shift toward the consolidation.**
c. **Pneumothorax**
   (1) Air found in the pleural cavity appears dark with no vascular markings in the involved areas.
   (2) **Tension pneumothorax** may result in a mediastinal shift and a tracheal **shift away from the side of the pneumothorax.**
d. **ET tube placement**
   (1) The tube should rest about 2 to 5 cm above the carina. On an inspiratory film, the carina is located at the level of the fourth rib or fourth thoracic vertebra.
   (2) If the ET tube is inserted too far, it has a greater tendency to enter the **right mainstem bronchus.**
   (3) If the right mainstem is inadvertently intubated, diminished breath sounds are heard on the left and asymmetrical chest movement may be observed.
e. **Heart shadow**
   (1) Should appear white in the middle of the chest, and the left heart border should be easily determined.
   (2) A normal heart should be less than half the width of the chest at the level of the diaphragm. Increased heart size may indicate congestive heart failure (CHF).
f. **Diaphragm**
   (1) Should be rounded or dome shaped.
   (2) Appears white on x-ray film at the level of the tenth rib during a maximal inspiration.
   (3) Patients with hyperinflated lungs (i.e., as in COPD) have flattened diaphragms.
   (4) Both hemidiaphragms should be assessed for height and angle to the chest wall.
   (5) The dome of the right hemidiaphragm is normally 1 to 2 cm higher than the left because of space needed for the liver.
   (6) Elevation of one hemidiaphragm may be the result of gas in the stomach or of atelectasis.
g. **Determining proper exposure**
   (1) Determining the penetration of the x-ray is done by assessing the spinal processes in the center of the chest. They should be just barely distinguishable from each other. If the spinal processes are very distinct, with dark lines separating them, the film is overexposed.
   (2) An overexposed film appears darker and could be interpreted as "normal."
   (3) An underexposed film appears lighter and could result in an incorrect interpretation.
J. **Other Imaging Studies**
   1. **Computed tomography**
      a. CT is an imaging modality used to gain significant information of the thorax that a conventional chest radiograph cannot indicate.
      b. Scan times as fast as 0.4 s make it possible to scan the thorax in a single breath-hold.
      c. CT provides three-dimensional images of the thorax and is more accurate than ventilation/perfusion (V/Q) scanning in the diagnosis of pulmonary embolism. (See Chapter 12 on disorders of the respiratory system.)
      d. CT is used to detect the following:
         (1) Bony abnormalities
         (2) Soft tissue abnormalities
         (3) Pleural abnormalities
         (4) Parenchymal lung disease
         (5) Interstitial lung disease
         (6) Pulmonary embolism
         (7) Aortic dissection
   2. **Magnetic resonance imaging**
      a. MRI is another useful imaging technique of the thorax that provides accurate anatomic detail of the thorax.
      b. MRI is used to detect the following:
         (1) Soft tissue abnormality
         (2) Bone marrow pathology
         (3) Pleural disease
         (4) Diaphragmatic disease
         (5) Mediastinal abnormalities
         (6) Congenital heart disease
         (7) Cardiac abnormalities
         (8) Pulmonary embolism
         (9) Aortic dissection
         (10) Pelvic and lower extremity venous thrombosis
      c. Disadvantages of MRI:
         (1) Limited patient monitoring
         (2) Motion artifact caused by respiratory and cardiac motion, which can obscure images
         (3) Contraindicated in patients with pacemakers

(4) Because of the strength of the MRI magnets, most ventilators cannot be used near an MRI. Ventilators constructed of nonmagnetic materials have been developed. If these are not available, a ventilator-dependent patient must receive manual ventilation during the procedure.

3. **Positron emission tomography**
   a. PET is a relatively new imaging technique that detects pathologic processes, especially tumors of the thorax.
   b. PET can distinguish between benign and malignant thoracic tumors and often detects tumors that are not easily recognizable on CT.

K. **Pulse**
   1. Pulse is a direct indicator of the heart's action.
   2. Normal heart rate in an adult: 60 to 100 beats/min
   3. Normal heart rate in a child: 90 to 120 beats/min
   4. An abnormally low heart rate is called **bradycardia** and is caused by infection, hypothermia, heart abnormalities, and vagal stimulation.
   5. An abnormally high heart rate is called **tachycardia** and is caused by hypoxemia, fever, loss of blood volume, heart abnormalities, and anxiety.
   6. **Peripheral edema and venous engorgement** indicate inadequate pumping action of the heart, resulting from right-sided heart failure (cor pulmonale) or left-sided heart failure (CHF).
   7. **Paradoxical pulse** (pulsus paradoxus) is a pulse that becomes weaker on inspiration; it may be defined as a decrease in systolic pressure of more than 10 mm Hg during inspiration and may be seen in patients with severe COPD, including asthma, pericarditis, pulmonary embolism, CHF, and pericardial effusion. If paradoxical pulse is observed after chest trauma or cardiothoracic surgery, cardiac tamponade should be suspected. Cardiac tamponade is a life-threatening condition in which blood collects in the pericardial sac and causes pressure that prevents the heart from pumping adequately.
   8. **Pulsus alternans** is an alternating pattern of strong and weak pulses. The ventricle ejects more than the normal amount of blood with a contraction and then less than the normal amount of blood with the next contraction. This is commonly observed in patients with left ventricular failure (LVF) and usually indicates bigeminal premature ventricular contractions (PVCs). (See Chapter 9 on cardiac monitoring.)

L. **Blood Pressure**
   1. Blood pressure is measurement of the pressure within the arterial system.
   2. Normal range for adults: 100/60 mm Hg to 140/90 mm Hg

3. Normal range for children: 95/60 mm Hg to 110/65 mm Hg
4. Normal range for neonates: 60/30 mm Hg to 90/60 mm Hg
5. Systolic pressure (first or top number) is the pressure measured during ventricular contraction.
6. Diastolic pressure (last or bottom number) is the pressure measured while the ventricles are at rest.
7. The diastolic pressure is the most critical measurement because it is the lowest pressure that the heart and arterial system experience.
8. An abnormally low blood pressure is called **hypotension** and is usually caused by shock, high-volume blood loss, positioning, and central nervous system (CNS) depressant drugs.
9. An abnormally high blood pressure is called **hypertension** and is usually caused by cardiovascular imbalances, stimulant drugs, stress, and fluid retention resulting from renal failure.
10. Many factors affect blood pressure.
    a. Blood volume
    b. Blood viscosity
    c. Heart's pumping action
    d. Elasticity of blood vessels
    e. Resistance to blood flow through the vessels
11. Blood pressure is measured with a sphygmomanometer (blood pressure cuff).

M. **Body Temperature**
   1. Normal body temperature is 98.6° (37° C).
   2. Slightly higher temperature in children is normal as a result of a higher metabolic rate.
   3. An abnormally low body temperature is called **hypothermia** and is caused by sweating (diaphoresis), blood loss, exposure to cold temperatures, and abnormally high heat loss.
   4. An abnormally high body temperature is called **hyperthermia** and is caused by decreased heat loss, infection, or increased environmental temperature.

⚠️ A fever results in increased oxygen consumption, which leads to an increased work of breathing to meet the increased oxygen demands of the body.

---

   5. The term used to describe a person with normal body temperature is **afebrile;** the term used to describe a person with a fever is **febrile.**

N. **Assessing Mental Status**
   1. **Level of consciousness**
      a. Alert: Patient is awake and responds to stimuli.
      b. Obtunded and confused: Patient is awake but responds slowly to commands and may be disoriented.

c. Lethargic: Patient seems unconscious but, when stimulated, does awaken.

d. Coma: Patient is unconscious and, when stimulated, does not awaken.

2. **Orientation to time and place**

a. Ask patient the date.

b. Ask whether patient knows where he or she is.

3. **Ability to cooperate**

a. Ask patient to follow simple commands.

b. Patient cooperation is necessary for effective therapy, such as incentive spirometry or IPPB.

4. **Emotional state**

a. Ask patient to describe his or her feelings.

b. Note patient's emotional response while you are asking questions.

IV. **ASSESSMENT OF LABORATORY TEST RESULTS**
CRT Exam Content Matrix: IA3
RRT Exam Content Matrix: IA3, IC1, IIIE8

 Exam Note

Reviewing laboratory data such as electrolytes/chemistries, complete blood count (CBC), coagulation studies, and the like, is covered on the RRT exam only.

A. **Serum Electrolytes**

1. **Sodium** (Na^+)

a. Normal level: 135 to 145 mEq/L

b. Sodium is the major cation in the extracellular fluid, and its concentration is controlled by the kidneys by means of regulating the amount of water in the body.

c. **Hyponatremia** is an Na^+ level <135 mEq/L; causes include

(1) Renal failure

(2) CHF

(3) Excessive fever or sweating

(4) Long-term diuretic administration

(5) Inadequate sodium intake

(6) Excessive water ingestion

(7) Severe burns

(8) Gastrointestinal (GI) fluid losses (vomiting, diarrhea)

d. **Clinical symptoms of hyponatremia**

(1) Muscle weakness, **making ventilator weaning difficult**

(2) Confusion

(3) Muscle twitching progressing to convulsions

(4) Anxiety

(5) Alterations in level of consciousness

e. **Hypernatremia** is an Na^+ level >145 mEq/L; causes include

(1) Excessive water loss (sweating, diarrhea)

(2) Renal failure

(3) Inadequate water intake

(4) Mannitol diuresis

(5) Corticosteroid administration

f. **Clinical symptoms of hypernatremia**

(1) Confusion

(2) CNS dysfunction

(3) Seizure activity

(4) Coma

2. **Potassium** (K^+)

a. Normal value: 3.5 to 5.0 mEq/L

b. Potassium is the major intracellular cation.

c. **Hypokalemia** is a K^+ level <3.5 mEq/L; causes include

(1) Diuretic therapy

(2) Adrenocorticosteroid administration

(3) Vomiting, diarrhea

(4) Burns

(5) Severe trauma

d. **Clinical symptoms of hypokalemia**

(1) Muscle weakness leading to paralysis, respiratory failure, and hypotension

(2) Cardiac arrhythmias

(a) Premature atrial contractions and PVCs

(b) Atrial and ventricular tachycardia

(c) Asystole

(3) ST segment depression on electrocardiography (ECG)

(4) Decreased GI tract motility resulting in abdominal distention

e. **Hyperkalemia** is a K^+ level >5.0 mEq/L; causes include

(1) Acidosis

(2) Renal insufficiency

(3) Tissue necrosis

(4) Hemorrhage

f. **Clinical symptoms of hyperkalemia**

(1) Paralysis

(2) ECG abnormalities

(a) Shortened QT interval

(b) Widened QRS complex

(c) Prolonged PR interval

(d) Absence of P wave

(3) Cardiac arrhythmias

(a) Ventricular arrhythmias

(b) Nodal arrhythmias

3. **Chloride** (Cl^-)

a. Normal value: 95 to 105 mEq/L

b. Chloride is the major anion in the body; two thirds of chloride in the body is found in extracellular compartments. Because chloride is generally excreted with potassium as potassium chloride by the kidneys, decreased levels of one results in decreased levels of the other.

c. **Hypochloremia** is a Cl^- level <95 mEq/L; causes include

(1) Vomiting, diarrhea

(2) Furosemide (Lasix) diuresis

⚠ Hypochloremia may result in metabolic alkalosis.

  d. **Clinical symptoms of hypochloremia**
     (1) Muscle spasm
     (2) Coma (in severe hypochloremia)
  e. **Hyperchloremia** is a Cl⁻ level >105 mEq/L; causes include
     (1) Respiratory alkalosis
     (2) Metabolic acidosis
     (3) Dehydration
     (4) Administration of excessive amounts of NaCl⁻ and K⁺
  f. **Clinical symptoms of** hyperchloremia
     (1) Headache
     (2) Malaise
     (3) Weakness
     (4) Unconsciousness
     (5) Coma
4. **Calcium** (Ca)
  a. Normal value: 4.25 to 5.25 mEq/L
  b. Most of the body's calcium is contained in the bones; it plays a major role in neuromuscular function and cellular enzyme reactions.
  c. **Hypocalcemia** is a Ca level <4.25 mEq/L; causes include
     (1) Severe trauma
     (2) Renal failure
     (3) Severe pancreatitis
     (4) Vitamin D deficiency
     (5) Parathyroid hormone deficiency
  d. **Clinical symptoms of hypocalcemia**
     (1) Muscle spasm
     (2) Abdominal cramping
     (3) Convulsions (rare)
     (4) Prolonged QT interval on ECG
  e. **Hypercalcemia** is a Ca level >5.25 mEq/L; causes include
     (1) Hyperthyroidism
     (2) Vitamin A or D intoxication
     (3) Hyperparathyroidism
     (4) Sarcoidosis
     (5) Cancer metastasis to the bone
  f. **Clinical symptoms of hypercalcemia**
     (1) Muscle weakness, **making ventilator weaning difficult**
     (2) Fatigue
     (3) Mental depression
     (4) Anorexia
     (5) Nausea, vomiting
     (6) Coma (in severe cases)
5. **Bicarbonate** (HCO₃⁻) (See Chapter 10 on ABG interpretation.)
B. **Blood Urea Nitrogen**
  1. Urea is a substance produced in the liver; it is carried in the blood to the kidneys, where it is excreted in the urine.

2. If the kidneys fail to remove urea from the blood adequately, the blood urea concentration increases.
3. The normal blood urea nitrogen (BUN) level is 7 to 20 mg/dL.
4. **An elevated BUN level is indicative of renal failure.**
C. **Glucose**
  1. Normal serum level: 70 to 105 mg/dL
  2. Elevated levels observed in diabetic ketoacidosis; patient compensates with alveolar hyperventilation (Kussmaul respirations, as mentioned earlier in this chapter).
D. **Hematology Tests**
  1. **Red blood cells**
     a. The number of RBCs, also referred to as *erythrocytes,* determine the adequacy of oxygen transport.
     b. Normal level: 4 to 6 million/mm³ of blood
     c. A decreased RBC count (or anemia) indicates an inadequate oxygen-carrying capacity of the blood. Treatment is a blood transfusion.
  2. **Hemoglobin**
     a. Hb is the portion of the RBC that carries oxygen, so it is an indicator of the oxygen-carrying capacity of the blood.
     b. Normal level: 13.5 to 18.0 g/dL in males; 12 to 16 g/dL in females
     c. A subnormal Hb level indicates inadequate oxygen-carrying capacity in the blood. Treatment is a blood transfusion.
  3. **Hematocrit** (Hct)
     a. The Hct is the percentage of the total blood volume that is RBCs.
     b. Normal levels: 43% to 50% in males; 37% to 43% in females. Average levels: 35% to 45%
     c. A decreased Hct level indicates inadequate oxygen-carrying capacity in the blood. Treatment is a blood transfusion.
  4. **White blood cells**
     a. The WBC count determines the presence or absence of infection. WBCs are also referred to as *leukocytes.*
     b. Normal level: 5000 to 10,000/mm³ of blood
     c. An elevated WBC count indicates the presence of infection. The RCP should recommend a chest x-ray film and sputum culture to determine lung involvement.
E. **Coagulation Studies**
  1. Platelet count
     a. Normal level: 150,000 to 400,000/mm³ of blood
     b. Platelets are the smallest cells in the blood and are essential for coagulation (clotting).
     c. Decreased platelet count may be the result of bone marrow diseases or disseminated intravascular coagulation (DIC).

2. Prothrombin time (PT)
   a. A test used to determine the clotting ability of the blood
   b. Normal PT: 11.0 to 12.5 s
3. Partial thromboplastin time (PTT)
   a. Another test to determine the clotting ability of the blood
   b. Normal PTT: 60 to 85 s

 It is important for the respiratory therapist to assess these coagulation studies. Patients with decreased platelet counts or increased PT or PTT are at increased risk of hemorrhaging. This means great care must be taken during nasotracheal suctioning or arterial puncture. Nasotracheal suctioning should be minimized, and puncture sites should be compressed longer after an arterial stick than for other patients.

F. **Urinalysis** is a routine analysis that includes chemical analysis to detect protein (proteinuria), sugar (glucosuria), and ketones (ketonuria) and microscopic analysis to detect WBCs and RBCs.
   1. Proteinuria is usually a sign of kidney disease.
   2. Glucosuria is commonly found in patients with diabetes or in patients with kidney disorders.
   3. Ketonuria is observed in patients affected by starvation, diabetes, and alcohol intoxication. Ketones are formed as the body breaks down fat.
   4. Hematuria is defined as blood in the urine and is observed in patients with renal and genitourinary disorders.

☑ **Exam Note**

Normal urine output is 700 to 2000 mL/day.

V. **REVIEWING THE PATIENT CHART**
CRT Exam Content Matrix: IA1-8
RRT Exam Content Matrix: IA1-8
   A. Once the patient has been admitted and requires respiratory care, the chart should be reviewed for the following information.
   1. Patient history
   2. Physical examination on admission
   3. Current vital signs
      a. Heart rate
      b. Respiratory rate: If the rate remains elevated or there is little or no change in the patient's respiratory distress, the therapist should recommend modifications in the prescribed oxygen therapy (e.g., increasing the FiO_2, placing the patient on CPAP or bilevel positive airway pressure (Bi-PAP), or instituting mechanical ventilation). (See Chapter 11 on ventilator management.)
      c. Blood pressure: A decrease in blood pressure may indicate excessive positive end-expiratory pressure (PEEP) levels, requiring a decrease in

the prescribed level of PEEP. (See Chapter 11 on ventilator management.)
   4. Current respiratory care orders
      a. Oxygen delivery device
      b. Percentage or flow rate of oxygen
      c. Type of ventilator and prescribed variables
      d. Frequency and duration of prescribed treatments
      e. Medications ordered with the treatment
   5. Patient progress notes
   6. **ABG levels:** Abnormal values in PaO_2 or $PaCO_2$ indicate that changes in oxygen therapy or ventilatory variables are necessary. (See Chapters 10 and 11 on ABG interpretation and ventilator management.)
   7. Pulmonary function test results
      a. Determine severity of lung dysfunction.
      b. Determine obstructive or restrictive abnormalities.
      c. Determine recommendations for before and after bronchodilator studies to determine responsiveness to therapy.
   8. Laboratory data (See previous section.)

VI. **CLINICAL APPLICATION OF COMPUTERS**
CRT Exam Content Matrix: IIIA1-4
RRT Exam Content Matrix: IIIA1-2
   A. **Computerized Charting**
   1. Practitioners are now using handheld computers to chart information rather than recording in the patient chart manually.
   2. Patient orders, progress notes, treatment times, and ventilator settings are often charted through the computer. This information can be downloaded into a central workstation or may be printed for all practitioners to use. This can be very helpful when giving reports to the oncoming shift.
   3. Individual treatment monitoring should be done to include the frequency of therapy, date and time of therapy, positive and adverse effects of therapy, and medication administered. Breath sounds, secretion color and amount, and cough effort should also be monitored.

   B. **Computerized Monitoring**
   1. The most common types of computer monitoring of the patient are hemodynamic monitoring, ventilator monitoring, and ECG monitoring. Data collected can be stored so that an interpretation may be done at any time.
   2. Interpretations of ABG levels may be accomplished through computer software specifically designed for this purpose.
   3. Computer software provides for the calculation and interpretation of ventilation variables, such as static lung compliance, $P(A-a)O_2$, shunt calculations, and many other pulmonary and hemodynamic variables.

4. Computerized technology has been used for pulmonary function testing for several years. Interpretation of results is accomplished with program algorithms.
5. Computerized technology also helps document patient management and monitor therapist workload assignments.

VII. DEVELOPING RESPIRATORY CARE PLANS AND PROTOCOLS

CRT Exam Content Matrix: IIIH6-8
RRT Exam Content Matrix: IIIH6-8

A. Therapist-driven protocols (TDPs) are guidelines that are used to determine the appropriateness of respiratory care treatments; they include the correct delivery method, indications, and discontinuation protocols.
B. TDPs are written in either algorithm or outline form.
C. Advantages of TDPs
   1. Active involvement of the practitioner in determining therapy modifications as the patient's clinical status changes
   2. Improved treatment allocation
   3. Improved cost management

POSTCHAPTER STUDY QUESTIONS

1. What is yellow sputum indicative of?
2. What bacterial organism should be suspected if the patient's sputum is green and foul smelling?
3. List nine causes of dyspnea.
4. What does the term *orthopnea* mean and in which patients is it most commonly found?
5. Describe Kussmaul respirations and in which patients this breathing pattern is most often seen.
6. List three conditions in which asymmetrical chest movement may be observed.
7. Describe paradoxical respiration and name a condition in which it is most commonly observed.
8. Define pedal edema and what causes it.

9. Name a condition that results in the trachea shifting toward the side of the body that the condition is affecting.
10. Name a condition that results in the trachea shifting away from the affected side.
11. Which muscles are used for normal ventilation?
12. What causes the "barrel chest" appearance in patients with COPD?
13. Name two conditions in which a hyperresonant percussion note would be heard.
14. Name two conditions in which a dull percussion note would be heard.
15. List four conditions that result in heart murmurs.
16. List the normal values for the following electrolytes: sodium, potassium, and chloride.
17. Why would decreased sodium and potassium levels make weaning a patient from the ventilator more difficult?
18. What does an elevated BUN level indicate?
19. How does the respiratory system compensate when glucose levels increase in a diabetic patient?
20. List the normal levels for each of the following: RBC count, Hb level, Hct, and WBC count.
21. What do decreases in Hb level, Hct, and RBC count indicate?
22. Name two conditions that cause a decreased platelet count.
23. Patients with a decreased platelet count and increased PT are at a greater risk of what occurrence?

See answers at the back of the text.

BIBLIOGRAPHY

Farzan S: *A concise handbook of respiratory diseases*, ed 4, Stamford, CT, 1997, Appleton & Lange.
Hess D and others: *Respiratory care principles and practice*, ed 1, Philadelphia, 2002, Saunders.
Wilkins RL, Stoller JK, Kacmarek R: *Egan's fundamentals of respiratory care*, ed 9, St Louis, 2009, Mosby.
Wilkins R, Dexter JR, Heuer AJ: *Clinical assessment in respiratory care*, ed 7, St Louis, 2010, Mosby.
Wyka K, Matthews P, Clark W: *Foundations of respiratory care*, ed 1, Albany, 2002, Delmar.

MANAGEMENT OF THE AIRWAY

Answer the pretest questions before studying the chapter. This will help you determine your strong and weak areas in the material covered.

1. A patient has just been intubated, and the CO_2 detector placed on the proximal end of the ET tube reads 1.5%. The respiratory therapist should suspect which of the following?

   A. The tube is in the trachea.
   B. The tube is in the right mainstem bronchus and should be withdrawn 4 cm.
   C. The tube is in the esophagus.
   D. The tube is at the level of the carina and should be withdrawn 2 cm.

2. Opening the patient's airway using an oropharyngeal airway is most beneficial when which of the following causes the obstruction?

   A. Secretions
   B. Foreign body
   C. Edema
   D. Tongue

3. McGill forceps are used during which of the following procedures?

   A. Nasotracheal intubation
   B. Oral intubation
   C. Tracheotomy
   D. Insertion of an esophageal obturator airway (EOA)

4. The physician wants to begin weaning a patient from a tracheostomy tube. How may this best be accomplished?

   A. Deflate the cuff every 2 h.
   B. Change to a fenestrated tracheostomy tube.
   C. Keep the cuff inflated and remove the inner cannula.
   D. Change to a tracheostomy tube with a foam cuff.

5. You are called to a patient's room because a ventilator alarm is sounding. You hear an audible leak around the patient's ET tube during a ventilator breath and notice the exhaled volume reading is 150 mL less than the set VT. You check the cuff pressure and find that it is 12 mm Hg. Which of the following is the appropriate action to take?

   A. Maintain the current cuff pressure and increase the patient's VT to compensate for the leak.
   B. Instill enough air to maintain a cuff pressure of 30 mm Hg.
   C. While listening with a stethoscope at the larynx, instill air into the cuff until a slight leak is heard on inspiration.
   D. Instill enough air until only a slight audible leak is heard.

6. You want to pass a suction catheter into the patient's left lung to obtain a sputum specimen. What is the most appropriate method of accomplishing this?

   A. Have the patient turn his or her head to the left.
   B. Have the patient turn his or her head to the right.
   C. Use a coudé suction catheter.
   D. Use a catheter that is one half the internal diameter of the patient's airway.

See answers and rationales at the back of the text.

I. **UPPER AIRWAY OBSTRUCTION**
   CRT Exam Content Matrix: IB1a-b, 2b, 7d, IIIB1, III I1a-d
   RRT Exam Content Matrix: IB1a-b, 2b, 7d, IIIB1, III I1a-c
   A. **Main Causes of Upper Airway Obstruction**
      1. Tongue falling back against the posterior wall of the pharynx, which is caused by unconsciousness or CNS abnormality; patients with macroglossia (enlarged tongue) are at greater risk

2. Edema, or postextubation inflammation and swelling, of the glottic area
3. Bleeding
4. Secretions
5. Foreign substances
   a. Foreign bodies
   b. False teeth
   c. Vomitus
6. Laryngospasm

B. **Signs of Partial Upper Airway Obstruction**
   1. Crowing, gasping sounds on inspiration
   2. Inability to cough (with a slight obstruction, the patient may be able to cough)
   3. Increasing respiratory difficulty
   4. Good to poor air exchange (depending on the severity of the obstruction)
   5. Exaggerated chest and abdominal movement without comparable air movement
   6. Cyanosis (depending on the severity of the obstruction)

C. **Signs of Complete Upper Airway Obstruction**
   1. Inability to talk
   2. Increased respiratory difficulty with no air movement
   3. Cyanosis
   4. Sternal, intercostal, and epigastric retractions
   5. Use of accessory muscles of the neck and chest
   6. Extreme panic
   7. Unconsciousness and respiratory arrest if obstruction is not removed

D. **Treatment of Airway Obstruction**
   1. If the patient is conscious and has a partial airway obstruction, the patient should be monitored closely and allowed to try to relieve the obstruction on his or her own.
   2. If the patient is conscious and has a complete airway obstruction caused by food or a foreign object, abdominal thrusts must be performed until the object is dislodged. (See Chapter 6 on cardiopulmonary respiration [CPR].)
   3. If the patient is unconscious and has a partial or complete airway obstruction that is most likely caused by the tongue, the head tilt and chin lift maneuver will help relieve the obstruction by moving the tongue forward.

II. **ARTIFICIAL AIRWAYS**
   CRT Exam Content Matrix: IB1a-b, IB2b, IB4a, IB9c, IB10c, IC9, IIA7a-g, IIIB1-7, IIIE3d, IIIE4e, IIIE11, IIIF2g1, 5, IIIJ1,4

RRT Exam Content Matrix: IB1a-b, IB2b, IB4a, IB9c, IB10c, IC10, IIA3a-b, IIIB1-3d, IIIE3c, IIIE4b, IIIE9, IIIF2d1-2, IIIJ1, 4

A. **Oropharyngeal Airway**

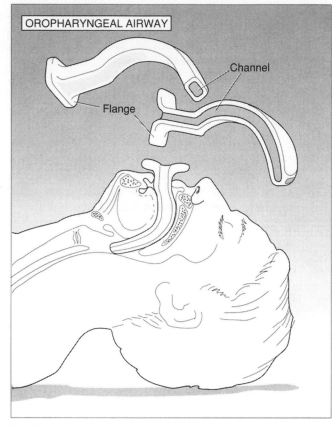

 OROPHARYNGEAL AIRWAY

Channel

Flange

FIGURE 4-1

1. This airway maintains a patent airway by lying between the base of the tongue and the posterior wall of the pharynx, preventing the tongue from falling back and occluding the airway.
2. This airway **must only be used on the unconscious patient** because a conscious patient would gag on the airway, which could potentially lead to aspiration.
3. This airway should **never** be taped in place because the airway must be easily removable to prevent vomiting and aspiration if the patient becomes conscious.

4. Proper insertion of the oropharyngeal airway
   a. Measure the airway from the corner of the lip to the angle of the jaw to ensure proper length.
   b. Remove foreign substances from the mouth.
   c. Hyperextend the neck.
   d. Using the cross-finger technique, open the patient's mouth and insert the airway with the tip pointing toward the roof of the mouth.
   e. Observe the airway passing the uvula, and rotate the airway 180 degrees.

5. **Hazards of oropharyngeal airways**
   a. The patient may gag or fight the airway; if this occurs, remove the airway immediately.
   b. If the airway is inserted improperly, the base of the tongue may be pushed into the back of the throat, obstructing the airway.
   c. If the airway is too large, the epiglottis may be pushed into the laryngeal area.
   d. If the airway is too small, it may be aspirated or ineffective in relieving obstruction.

6. **Important points concerning oropharyngeal airways**
   a. Oropharyngeal airways may be used in the unconscious, orally intubated patient to prevent the patient from biting the ET tube.
   b. Berman airways are made of hard plastic and have a groove down either side to guide a suction catheter to the glottic area.
   c. Guedel airways are made of a soft, pliable material, which has an opening through the middle to allow the passing of a suction catheter into the glottic area.

B. **Nasopharyngeal Airway**

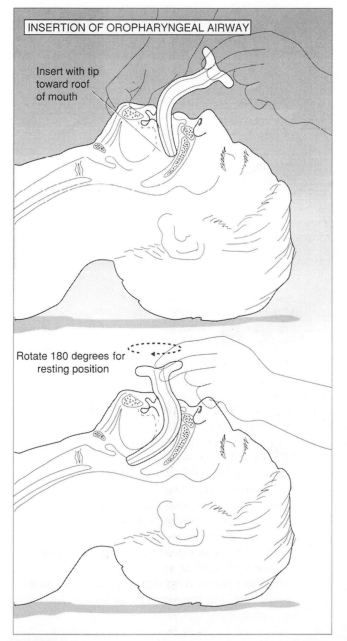

INSERTION OF OROPHARYNGEAL AIRWAY

Insert with tip toward roof of mouth

Rotate 180 degrees for resting position

FIGURE 4-2

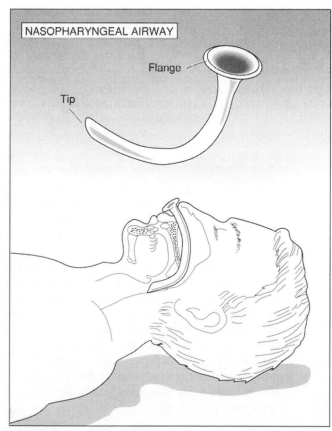

NASOPHARYNGEAL AIRWAY

Flange

Tip

FIGURE 4-3

1. This airway maintains a patent airway by lying between the base of the tongue and the posterior wall of the pharynx.
2. This airway is constructed of soft pliable rubber; it is inserted as follows:
   a. Select the proper size by measuring the airway from the tip of the nose to the earlobe. The outside diameter of the airway should be equal to the inside diameter of the patient's internal nares.
   b. Lubricate the airway with a water-soluble gel and insert into the patient's nostril.
   c. The flanged end should rest against the nose, and the distal tip should rest behind the uvula.
   d. Place tape around the flanged end to secure the airway in place. (A safety pin may be inserted through the flange and the pin taped to the face.)
3. This airway is tolerated by the conscious patient.
4. This airway is most commonly used to facilitate nasotracheal suctioning.
5. **Hazards of nasopharyngeal airways**
   a. An airway that is too small may be aspirated.
   b. Nasal irritation may result. To prevent nasal irritation, alternate nostrils daily.
C. **Laryngeal Mask Airway**

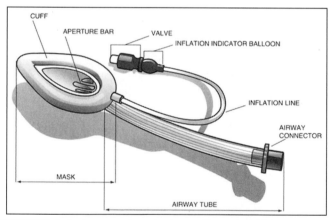

FIGURE 4-4   Laryngeal mask airway. Courtesy LMA North America, Inc.

1. The laryngeal mask airway (LMA) is designed to be used as an alternative to a face mask for achieving and maintaining control of the airway during surgery when tracheal intubation is not necessary or in emergencies when ET intubation cannot be accomplished after several attempts.
2. For the airway to be inserted successfully, the patient must be anesthetized so that the upper airway reflexes are obtunded; otherwise, laryngospasm may occur.

3. The LMA consists of a tube that is fused to an elliptical, spoon-shaped mask. When inserted, the tube protrudes from the patient's mouth and is connected to a manual resuscitator via a standard 15-mm adapter.
4. The mask resembles a miniature face mask and has an inflatable rim that is filled with air via a pilot valve–balloon system.
5. The tube opens into the middle of the mask through three vertical slits that prevent the tip of the epiglottis from falling back and blocking the lumen of the tube.
6. The LMA is inserted through the mouth and into the pharynx after being lubricated with a water-soluble gel. The device is advanced until resistance is met. Then the mask is inflated, providing a low-pressure seal around the laryngeal inlet. The posterior aspect of the tube is marked with a black line, which should be seen midline against the patient's upper lip when the airway is placed properly (see Figure 4-5).
7. LMAs are available in all sizes and can be used in patients of all ages, from neonates to adults.
8. **Indications for LMA**
   a. Difficult face mask fit
   b. Unsuccessful intubation and difficulty ventilating with bag-mask
   c. Unavailability of personnel trained in ET intubation
   d. Elective surgical procedures
9. **Contraindications for LMA**
   a. Health care provider not trained in the use of the LMA
   b. If risk of aspiration exists
10. **Advantages of the LMA**
    a. This airway can be quickly inserted to provide ventilation when bag-mask ventilation is not adequate and ET intubation cannot be accomplished.
    b. Tidal volume delivered may be greater when the LMA is used as opposed to bag-mask ventilation.
    c. There is less gastric insufflation than with bag-mask ventilation.
    d. The LMA ventilates equally as well as an ET tube.
    e. Training is simpler than for ET intubation.
    f. There is no risk of esophageal or bronchial intubation.
    g. There is less risk of trauma to the airway than with ET intubation.
    h. There is less coughing, laryngospasm, sore throat, and hoarseness than with ET intubation.

11. **Disadvantages of LMA**
    a. Does not provide protection against aspiration of gastric contents
    b. Cannot be used if the mouth cannot be opened more than 0.6 inches (1.5 cm)

    c. May not be effective when airway anatomy is abnormal
    d. May be difficult to provide adequate ventilation if high airway pressures are required

12. **Insertion technique**

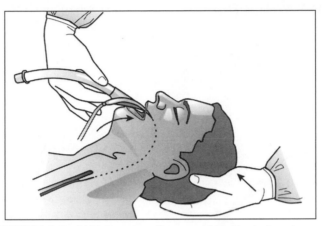

FIGURE 4-5   LMA Insertion. Courtesy LMA North America, Inc.

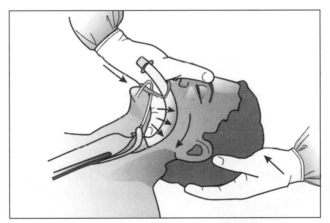

FIGURE 4-6   LMA Insertion. Courtesy LMA North America, Inc.

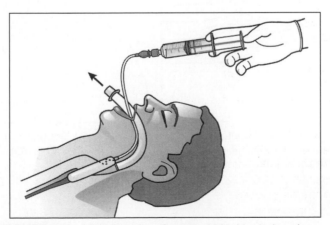

FIGURE 4-7   LMA Insertion. Courtesy LMA North America, Inc.

a. Using the index finger, advance the LMA until resistance is met. The tip of the LMA should rest against the upper esophageal sphincter in the hypopharynx. The cuff should be inflated until no leak is heard. To determine proper position, auscultate the lungs bilaterally. Capnography may also be used to confirm an adequate airway.

b. To determine whether mild laryngospasm is present as a result of light anesthesia, auscultate the anterolateral neck for the presence of wheezing.

c. Because the LMA does not protect the airway from regurgitation, the patient must not eat for several hours before insertion.

D. **Esophageal–Tracheal Combitube**

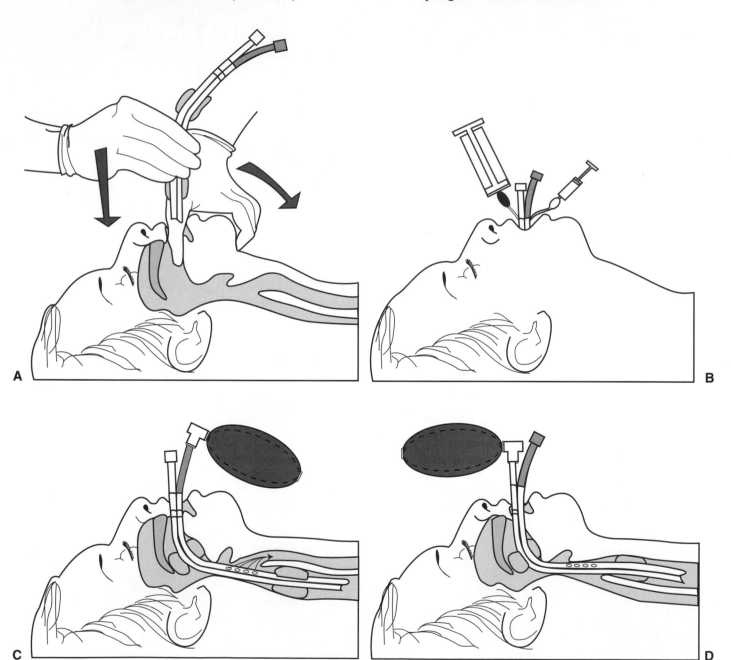

FIGURE 4-8   The Combitube is inserted with the head in the neutral position **(A)** and both cuffs inflated **(B).** The two possible locations of the distal lumen are the usual esophageal location **(C)**, in rare cases, the trachea **(D).** From Cairo J, Pilbeam S: *Mosby's respiratory care equipment,* ed 8, St Louis, 2010, Mosby.

1. The esophageal–tracheal combitube (ETC) is similar to an EOA but is a double-lumen tube. The tubes run parallel to each other.
2. Once the tube is inserted, a pharyngeal balloon that occludes the pharynx is inflated to prevent air from leaking out the nose or mouth. Because of this, a mask is not necessary. A cuff is located on the distal end of the tube.
3. Once the airway is advanced beyond the pharynx, it enters into either the trachea or the esophagus. It makes no difference which structure it enters.
4. A balloon at the distal end of the tube is inflated and will seal off either the trachea or the esophagus. If the tube rests in the trachea, that lumen is used to ventilate the patient just like an endotracheal tube. If the tube rests in the esophagus, the patient is ventilated through holes in the upper part of the tube below the pharyngeal cuff, like those on the EOA.
5. To determine which tube to ventilate through, attach the resuscitator bag to tube No. 1 (esophageal tube) and begin bagging. If the chest rises, breath sounds are auscultated over the lungs and no air is heard over the epigastric region; the ETC is in the esophagus, and ventilation is occurring through the holes above the distal cuff. The use of a CO_2 detector is very helpful in determining tube placement.
6. If the chest does not rise or sounds are only heard over the epigastrium, the resuscitator bag should be attached to the other tube (No. 2) and ventilation started. If the ETC is in the trachea, the chest should rise. Confirm the placement by auscultating over the epigastrium and the chest. The use of CO_2 detector is very helpful.
7. **Indications for the ETC**
   a. Difficult face mask fit
   b. Unsuccessful intubation and difficulty ventilating with bag-mask
   c. No one available that has been trained in endotracheal intubation
8. **Contraindications for the ETC**
   a. Patient with an intact gag reflex
   b. Patient with known or suspected esophageal disease
   c. Patient known to have ingested a caustic substance
   d. Suspected upper airway obstruction because of laryngeal foreign body or pathology
   e. Patient less than 4 feet tall
9. **Advantages of the ETC**
   a. Minimal training and retraining required
   b. Visualization of the upper airway or use of special equipment not required for insertion
   c. May be useful for patients with suspected neck injury because the head does not need to be hyperextended
   d. Face mask not needed because of the oropharyngeal balloon
   e. Can provide a patent airway with either tracheal or esophageal placement
   f. If placed in the esophagus, allows suctioning of gastric contents without interruption of ventilation
   g. Reduces the risk of aspiration of stomach contents
10. **Disadvantages of the ETC**
    a. Proximal port may be occluded with secretions
    b. Difficulty in determining proper tube location resulting in ventilation through wrong tube
    c. Soft tissue trauma because of rigidity of the tube
    d. Cannot suction the trachea if the tube is in the esophagus
    e. Esophageal trauma from poor insertion technique

E. **ET Tubes**
   1. **Indications for ET Tubes**
      a. Relief of upper airway obstruction resulting from laryngospasm, epiglottitis, or glottic edema
      b. Protection of the airway. The airway has four protective reflexes:
         (1) Pharyngeal reflex: gag and swallowing
         (2) Laryngeal reflex: laryngospasm
         (3) Tracheal reflex: coughing when trachea is irritated
         (4) Carinal reflex: coughing when carina is irritated

> When these reflexes are obtunded or knocked out, the airway must be protected with an ET tube. Paralysis, drugs, loss of consciousness, or neuromuscular disease may obtund these reflexes.

> As these reflexes become obtunded, they are lost in progression from the pharyngeal to the carinal. As they are recovered, they come back in progression from the carinal to the pharyngeal.

      c. Facilitation of tracheal suctioning
      d. Assistance in manual or mechanical ventilation
   2. **Hazards of ET tubes**
      a. Contamination of the tracheobronchial tree
      b. Cough mechanism reduced
      c. Damage to the vocal cords
      d. Laryngeal or tracheal edema
      e. Mucosal damage leading to tracheal stenosis
      f. Tube occlusion with inspissated secretions
      g. Loss of patient's dignity
      h. Loss of patient's ability to talk

3. **Steps to perform ET intubation**
   a. Select a laryngoscope with a **Miller (straight) blade** or a **McIntosh (curved) blade.** Make sure the lightbulb is tight because it will not light if it is loose. If the light source is dim or is yellowish in color, the batteries are weak and should be replaced.

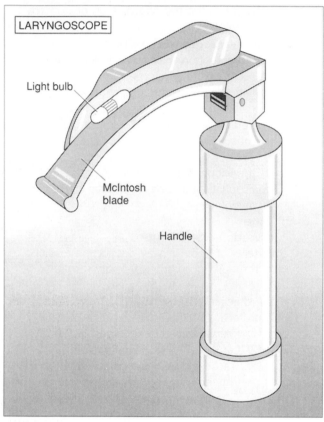

FIGURE 4-9

   b. Place the patient in the "sniffing position" (head above shoulder level).
   c. Select the proper size of ET tube, insert air into the cuff to make sure it holds air, and then deflate the cuff.
   d. Insert a stylet into the ET tube to make the tube more rigid for easier insertion. Make sure the stylet doesn't extend past the end of the tube.
   e. Insert the laryngoscope blade into the right side of the mouth and move the tongue to the left.

   f. Advance the blade forward.
      (1) The curved blade (McIntosh) should be inserted between the epiglottis and the base of the tongue (vallecula). With a forward and upward motion, raise the epiglottis to expose the glottis and vocal cords.
      (2) The straight blade (Miller) should be placed under the epiglottis and lifted upward and forward to expose the cords.

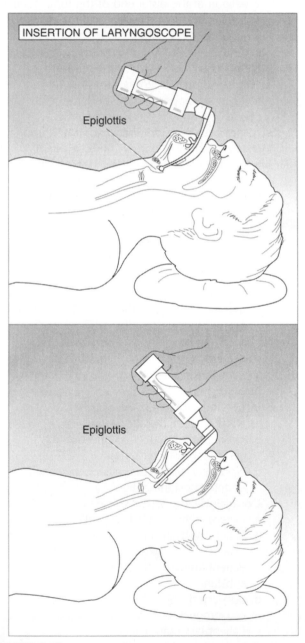

FIGURE 4-10

the right than the left, then the tube probably is in the right mainstem. Deflate the cuff and withdraw the tube until equal breath sounds are heard.

i. Another method to determine whether the tube is in the airway is by exhaled CO_2 analysis, or capnometry. **If the ET tube is in the airway, CO_2 levels begin to rise, as seen on the capnogram. End-tidal CO_2 levels are generally around 6%. If the tube is in the esophagus, the end-tidal CO_2 reading remains near zero.**

j. An easier and less expensive method of monitoring exhaled CO_2 levels is with the use of a disposable colorimetric CO_2 detector on the proximal end of the ET tube. The indicator on the detector changes colors when exposed to different CO_2 levels.

Exam Note

During resuscitative procedures when cardiac output and blood pressure are low, gas exchange is reduced and the CO_2 detector may read near zero even when the ET tube is in the trachea.

Exam Note

The average distance from the teeth to the carina is 27 cm. Note that the ET tube has markings in centimeters indicating the distance to the end of the tube from that point. Therefore, taping the tube at the 23- to 25-cm mark at the teeth will most likely place the tube in a proper position.

Table 4-1   Appropriate Endotracheal Tube Sizes

Newborns (by body weight)	
Less than 1 kg	2.5 mm
1 to 2 kg	3.0 mm
2 to 3 kg	3.5 mm
More than 3 kg	4.0 mm
Children (by age)	
6 mo	3.0-4.0 mm
18 mo	3.5-4.5 mm
2 yr	4.0-5.0 mm
3 to 5 yr	4.5-5.5 mm
6 yr	5.5-6.0 mm
8 yr	6.0-6.5 mm
12 yr	6.0-7.0 mm
16 yr	6.5-7.5 mm
Adults (by gender)	
Women	7.5-9.0 mm
Men	8.0-9.5 mm

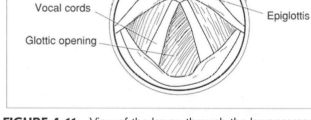

FIGURE 4-11   View of the larynx through the laryngoscope.

Vocal cords
Glottic opening
Epiglottis

Never exceed 15 to 20 s per intubation attempt. The blade and tube in the back of the throat may stimulate the vagus nerve, which may lead to bradycardia. Remove the blade and tube and use bag-mask ventilation until cardiac status has stabilized.

g. As the cords are observed, advance the ET tube **approximately 2 cm past the cords.**

h. Inflate the cuff and listen for equal and bilateral breath sounds. If louder sounds are heard on

Exam Note

If the tube is inserted too far, it will enter the right mainstem bronchus.

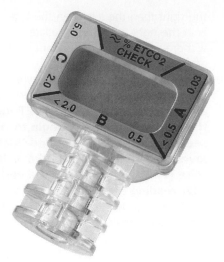

FIGURE 4-12 A Disposable colorimetric device for detecting the presence of CO_2 in expired gas. Courtesy Nellcor Puritan Bennett, Pleasanton, Calif. part of Covidien.

k. Tape the tube in place and obtain a stat chest x-ray film to ensure proper tube placement. The end of the tube should rest 2 to 5 cm above the carina. **The carina is seen on radiographs at the fourth rib or the fourth thoracic vertebra.**

4. **Parts of the ET tube**

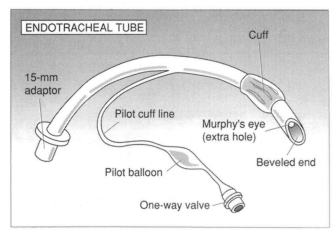

ENDOTRACHEAL TUBE

Cuff

15-mm adaptor

Pilot cuff line

Murphy's eye (extra hole)

Pilot balloon

Beveled end

One-way valve

FIGURE 4-13

5. **ET tube markings**
   a. IT (implantation tested): indicates the material in the tube is nontoxic and does not cause tissue reaction when implanted in rabbit tissue.

Polyvinylchoride is the most common material used in ET tubes.

   b. Z-79: the Z-79 Committee for Anesthesia Equipment for the American National Standards Institute. This committee ensures that the tube manufacturer is using material that is not toxic to tissues.
   c. ID: internal diameter of the tube in millimeters. This is how the tubes are designated by size.
   d. OD: outside diameter of the tube in millimeters. Also measured in French (Fr) units.
   e. Numbers and marks indicate the distance in centimeters from that mark to the distal tip of the tube.

6. **Complications of ET tubes**
   a. Poorly tolerated by conscious or semiconscious patients
   b. Difficult to stabilize because of the movement of the tube
   c. Stimulates oral secretions
   d. Gagging caused by tube irritation
   e. More difficult to pass suction catheter as a result of the curvature of the tube and poor stabilization
   f. Harder for the patient to communicate
   g. Harder to attach equipment to a poorly stabilized ET tube
   h. Patient may bite the tube, occluding air flow and setting off the ventilator high-pressure alarm, which ends inspiration prematurely.
   i. Erodes corners of patient's mouth

7. **Nasotracheal tubes**
   a. These are considered nonemergent tubes.
   b. **Nasotracheal intubation**
      (1) Nose should be anesthetized with lidocaine or cocaine spray. A vasoconstrictor, such as phenylephrine hydrochloride (Neo-Synephrine) drops, are used to shrink nasal mucosal blood vessels for easier tube insertion.
      (2) Lubricate the tube with water-soluble gel and insert through a patent nostril.
      (3) If the patient is alert and breathing spontaneously, try advancing the tube as the patient takes a deep breath or coughs. This is called "blind nasal intubation."
      (4) If the patient is not cooperative or is unconscious, visualize the tube in the mouth, grasp by **Magill forceps,** and guide through the vocal cords by means of direct visualization with a laryngoscope.
      (5) Tape the tube in place when proper placement is assured.

c. **Advantages of nasotracheal tubes (vs. oral tubes)**
   (1) Easier to stabilize
   (2) Better tolerated by the patient because gagging is not as likely
   (3) Less potential for inadvertent extubation
   (4) Easier to attach equipment
   (5) Easier to pass suction catheter
   (6) Easier for patient to eat or drink
d. **Complications of nasotracheal tubes**
   (1) Pressure necrosis of the nasal tissue
   (2) Sinus obstruction, leading to sinusitis
   (3) Obstruction of eustachian tube, resulting in middle-ear infections
   (4) Septal deviation
   (5) Bleeding during intubation or extubation
8. **High-Lo Evac Tube**
   a. This tube has a port to allow for continuous or intermittent suctioning of subglottic secretions. These secretions, if not removed, may drain down past the ET tube cuff to the lower airway, increasing the incidence of infection.
   b. These tubes are being used to help prevent ventilator-associated pneumonia (VAP).

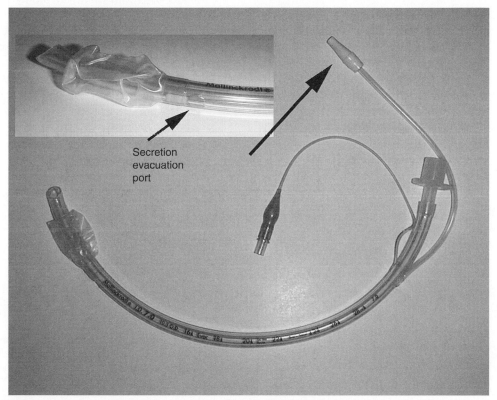

Secretion evacuation port

FIGURE 4-14   The Hi-Low Evac tube has a portal for suctioning subglottic secretions and is used as part of a program to reduce the incidence of ventilator-associated pneumonia in intubated patients. From Cairo J, Pilbeam S: *Mosby's respiratory care equipment,* ed 8, St Louis, 2010, Mosby.

F. **Tracheostomy Tubes**

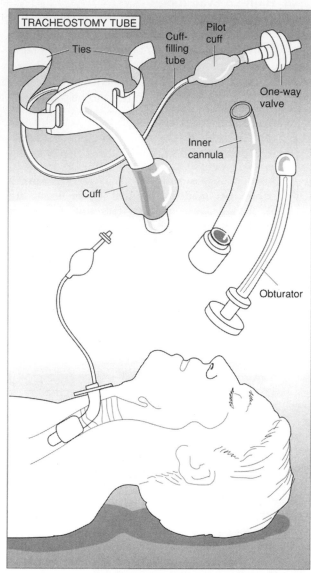

FIGURE 4-15

1. Insert tracheostomy tubes through an incision (stoma) made between the second and third tracheal rings.
2. Always insert the obturator into the outer cannula when advancing the tube into the stoma.
3. Once the tube is properly positioned, remove the obturator and insert the inner cannula.
4. Then inflate the cuff and secure the tube with tracheostomy ties.
5. Some tubes use foam cuffs (Mikity-Wilson Fome Cuff, Bivona Fome Cuf, and Kamen Fome Cuff), which are deflated during insertion; when the

tube is in place, the cuff is allowed to resume its normal foam shape, which provides an effective seal against the tracheal wall. (This type of cuff exerts about 20 mm Hg pressure on the tracheal wall.)

6. **Indications for tracheostomies**
   a. To bypass upper airway obstruction
   b. To prevent problems posed by oral or nasal ET tubes
   c. To allow patient to swallow and receive nourishment
   d. For long-term airway care (ET tubes should be left in no longer than 3 to 4 wk.)
7. **Immediate complications of tracheostomy tubes** occurring within the first 24 h and associated with the tracheotomy procedure:
   a. Pneumothorax
   b. Bleeding
   c. Air embolism from tearing of pleural vein
   d. Subcutaneous emphysema
8. **Late complications of tracheostomy tubes** occurring more than 2 days after the tracheotomy:
   a. Hemorrhage
   b. Infection
   c. Airway obstruction
   d. Tracheoesophageal fistula
   e. Interference with swallowing
   f. Rupture of innominate artery
   g. Stomal stenosis
   h. Tracheitis
9. **Tracheal Stoma Care**

Changing a tracheostomy tube within 48 h of the tracheotomy is not advisable and should only be done by a surgeon, if it is done at all, because the tracheal rings may recede when the tube is removed, making reintubation difficult.

a. Stoma care involves both the cleaning of the stoma site and the application of clean tracheostomy ties and dressing. This is a sterile procedure, so care must be taken to wear sterile gloves and perform the task as aseptically as possible.
b. The tracheostomy tube should be stabilized with one hand while the old dressing is removed. The old ties should be cut and then removed. Continuing to stabilize the tube at this point is essential to prevent accidental decannulation caused by coughing or sudden movement. Always have a spare tracheostomy tube at the bedside during this procedure.
c. The stoma area may be cleaned with 4- by 4-inch gauze pads soaked with hydrogen

peroxide. After cleaning, discard the pads in a dirty area away from the sterile field. The stoma should be assessed for swelling, redness, or pulsation of the tube.

d. Cotton-tipped applicators may be dipped in peroxide to do more detailed cleaning around the stoma site and flanges of the tracheostomy tube.

e. After the stoma site is cleansed, rinse the site using gauze pads dipped in sterile water. Gently dry the area by patting with sterile gauze pads.

f. Apply a sterile 4- by 4-inch gauze pad dressing supplied with the tracheostomy care kit. Never make a dressing by cutting the gauze pad to the proper size. Cotton filaments from the gauze pad may be absorbed into the stoma and may result in an abscess.

g. The new ties may then be applied. The ties should be cut to the proper size before beginning stoma care so that the tube may be stabilized throughout the procedure. Use a square knot to secure the tube. Never use a bow, which can be easily untied.

h. The chest should be auscultated immediately after the procedure to ensure that the tube has been maintained in the proper position. If the patient exhibits respiratory distress, determine whether ventilation is adequate. If there is doubt about proper tube placement, remove

the tube, cover the stoma with a sterile 4- by 4-inch gauze pad, and ventilate the patient's lungs by mouth or with bag-mask ventilation.

> ☑ **Exam Note**
>
> If after changing a tracheostomy tube, you observe subcutaneous emphysema and respiratory distress and can auscultate little or no air movement, the tube is malpositioned and must be removed immediately; ventilate the patient's lungs by bag-mask.

10. **Special tracheostomy tubes**
   a. **Fenestrated tracheostomy tube**
      (1) This tube is used to aid in weaning the patient from a tracheostomy tube and to allow the patient to talk.
      (2) With the inner cannula removed, air may pass through the hole (fenestration) in the outer cannula, which allows for weaning from the tracheostomy tube and enables speech.
      (3) The outer cannula may be plugged with the cap on the proximal end of the tube. With the cuff deflated, air flows through the tube, out the fenestration, and through the patient's upper airway.
      (4) If ventilation is necessary, the inner cannula may be reinserted and the cuff reinflated.

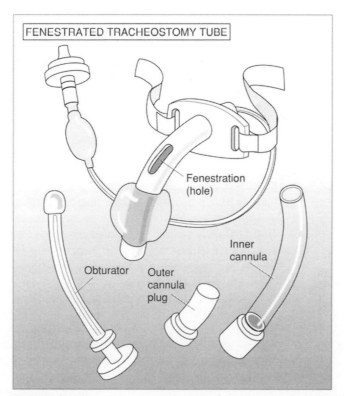

FENESTRATED TRACHEOSTOMY TUBE

Fenestration (hole)

Inner cannula

Obturator   Outer cannula plug

FIGURE 4-16

b. **Tracheostomy button**
   (1) This airway consists of a short, hollow tube that is used to replace the tracheostomy tube but can still maintain a patent stoma, in case problems arise.
   (2) The patient has complete use of the upper airway.

c. **Kistner tracheostomy tube**
   (1) This airway is used to wean patients from tracheostomy tubes while maintaining a patent stoma.
   (2) Kistner tubes are much like tracheostomy buttons, except they have a one-way valve on the proximal end of the tube.
   (3) Air enters through the one-way valve and the tube during inspiration. As the patient exhales, the valve closes and the air flows up through the vocal cords and out the nose and mouth.

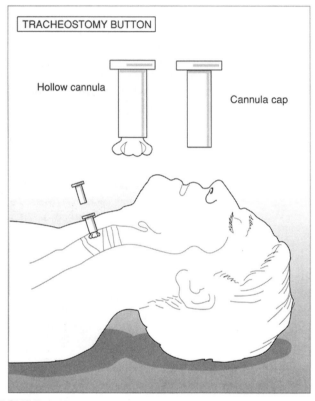

FIGURE 4-17

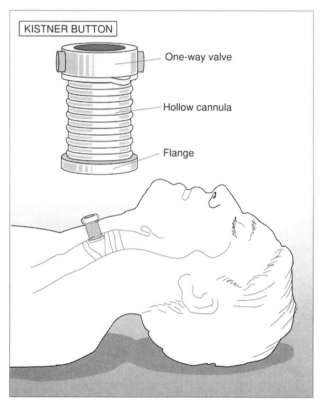

FIGURE 4-18

d. **Speaking tracheostomy tubes**
  (1) A constant gas flow is available above the cuff and around the vocal cords to allow speech.

  (2) The cuff remains inflated.
e. **Passy-Muir speaking valve**

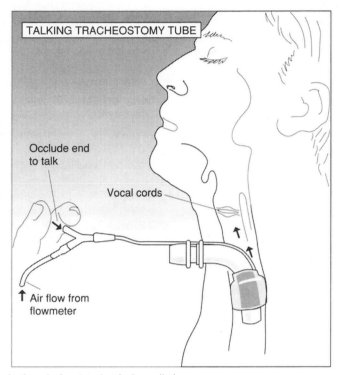

FIGURE 4-19   Passy-Muir valve in-line during mechanical ventilation.

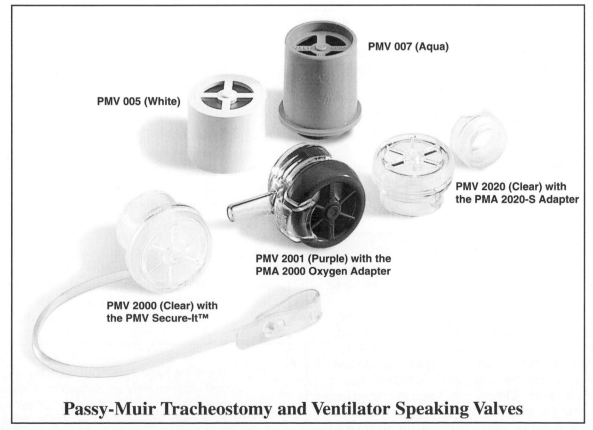

Passy-Muir Tracheostomy and Ventilator Speaking Valves

FIGURE 4-20   Passy-Muir speaking valves. Courtesy Passy-Muir, Irvine, Calif.

(1) The **Passy-Muir valve** is a commonly used tracheostomy speaking valve that is placed on the proximal end of the tracheostomy tube (15-mm adapter).

(2) **The cuff must be deflated**. The patient's inspired air passes through the valve, but on exhalation the valve closes and directs the air up through the upper airway and vocal cords to allow the patient to talk.

(3) The patient should be suctioned with the cuff deflated before the valve is attached so that secretions that have pooled above the cuff will not be aspirated into the airway.

(4) The valves may be used on spontaneously breathing patients or ventilator patients. If the valve is attached to a ventilator patient, the tidal volume must be increased to compensate for gas loss through the upper airway.

III. MAINTENANCE OF ARTIFICIAL AIRWAYS

CRT Exam Content Matrix: IB9p, IB10p, IIA8, IIA19, IIIB9, IIIC1b-c, IIIC2, IIIF2g3-4, IIIF2h1-4, IIIG1h
RRT Exam Content Matrix: IB9q, IB10q, IIIB4, IIIC1b-c, IIIC2, IIIG1h

A. Cuff Care

1. Tubes should employ **high-volume, low-pressure cuffs only** because less occlusion to tracheal blood flow occurs as a result of the application of less pressure. They are also called *floppy cuffs*. If excessive air is placed in the cuff, it acts as a **high-pressure cuff.**

2. To ensure that the cuff is exerting the least amount of pressure on the tracheal wall and is still providing an adequate seal, use the **minimal leak technique or minimal occluding volume technique.**

   a. **Minimal leak technique:** With the stethoscope beside the larynx, listen for airflow as the cuff is inflated. Inflate the cuff until no airflow is heard, then withdraw air slowly until a slight leak is heard.

   b. **Minimal occluding volume technique:** This is accomplished the same way as the minimal leak technique, except the cuff is slowly inflated just to the point where no leak is heard.

 Exam Note

If the peak inspiratory pressure (PIP) on the ventilator decreases after the minimal leak has been determined, the leak technique should be redone at the lower pressure. For example, the minimal leak test is done when the PIP is 40 cm H_2O, the patient is suctioned, and the PIP decreases to 30 cm H_2O. Because the cuff was inflated to create a slight leak at 40 cm H_2O and the PIP has decreased to 30 cm H_2O, there is now excessive air in the ET tube cuff. There should no longer be a leak at this lower PIP; therefore, the minimal leak technique should be determined again at 30 cm H_2O.

c. **Cuff pressures should be maintained between 20 and 25 mm Hg (25-34 cm H_2O)** to prevent tracheal wall damage. Tracheal mucosal capillary perfusion pressure is approximately 25 to 30 mm Hg. Pressures higher than this range will cut off blood flow to the mucosa, resulting in tracheal tissue damage. Always use the lowest cuff pressure—one that will produce only a slight leak when heard with a stethoscope at peak inspiration.

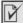 **Exam Note**

The exam questions regarding cuff pressure may indicate the pressure in either mm Hg or cm H_2O. Pay close attention to the units so that you do not select the wrong pressure. Remember, maximum cuff pressure is **25 mm Hg or 34 cm H_2O**.

d. If the cuff is inflated above 25 mm Hg (34 cm H_2O) and a leak is still heard, continue inflating the cuff using the minimal leak or occluding volume technique. It may be that the ET tube is too small and needs to take more air into the cuff to adequately seal the airway. In this case, the cuff pressure does not relate to the pressure on the tracheal wall. **To be safe, replace the ET tube with a larger one.**

B. Suctioning the Airway

1. **Technique of suctioning**

   a. Hyperoxygenate and hyperinflate the patient's lungs. This is done to help prevent hypoxemia, which may lead to tachycardia.

   b. Instill 3 to 5 mL of normal saline to help thin secretions; in infants, use 0.3 to 0.5 mL.

 Exam Note

Although studies indicate that instilling saline down the ET tube may result in higher incidences of oxygen desaturation and microorganisms being washed into the lower airway, the exam considers it an appropriate procedure to aid in the mobilization of secretions. Another alternative to saline lavage is to instill acetylcysteine (Mucomyst) or sodium bicarbonate (2%) down the airway. Although this may require a physician order, it appears to be more beneficial than the use of saline.

   c. Insert the catheter without applying suction and advance until an obstruction (the carina) is met. Do not jab with the catheter because this may cause carinal damage and bradycardia (vagal stimulation).

d. Withdraw the catheter approximately 1 to 2 cm and **apply suction** while rotating the catheter between the thumb and finger. **(This decreases mucosal damage.)**

e. Never leave the catheter in the airway for more than **15 s.**

f. On removal of the catheter, reoxygenate and hyperinflate the patient's lungs; wait 30 s to 1 min before entering the airway again.

> ⚠ Monitor the ECG and stop the procedure if complications occur; hyperoxygenate and ventilate the patient's lungs (if the patient is using a ventilator).

g. Repeat the steps until the secretions are removed by suctioning and the airway sounds clear.

h. Then suction the nasal and oral pharynx; remember to **never** reenter the ET tube with this catheter.

> ⚠ When performing nasotracheal suctioning, follow the above steps in addition to performing the subsequent techniques:
> (1) Lubricate the catheter with water-soluble gel.
> (2) Instruct the patient to take a deep breath or cough as the catheter advances to the oropharynx. This aids in inserting the catheter through the glottic opening.

2. **Selecting the proper size of catheter**

a. The suction catheter should not occupy more than **one half** of the internal diameter of the tube. (Suction catheters are sized by Fr units.)

☑ Exam Note

Using a catheter that occupies up to ⅔ the inside diameter of the ET tube may be acceptable, **but on the exam, never exceed ½ of the inside diameter.**

---

b. To estimate the proper catheter size, multiply the internal diameter of the ET tube by 2, then use the next smallest catheter size.

EXAMPLE:

What is the proper size of catheter to use when suctioning an 8.0-mm ET tube?

$$8.0 \times 2 = 16$$

The next smallest size catheter is 14 Fr. (Suction catheters come in the following sizes: 6½ Fr, 8 Fr, 10 Fr, 12 Fr, 14 Fr, 16 Fr.)

3. **Closed suction catheters**

a. A closed suction catheter system is a suction catheter enclosed inside a clear plastic sleeve attached to the patient's ET or tracheostomy tube; it allows for suctioning without removing the patient from the ventilator. This results in less potential for cardiac arrhythmias and desaturation during the suction procedure.

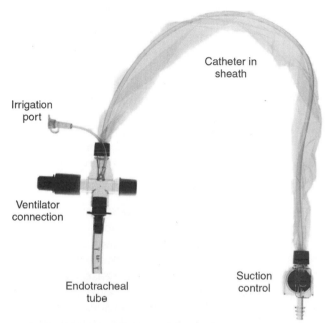

FIGURE 4-21   Closed suction catheter. From Hess DR: Managing the artificial airway. *Respir Care* 44:759, 1999.

b. Because the catheter remains sterile inside the sleeve and gloves are not necessary when this system is used, there is less risk of contaminating the patient's airway than when open suctioning with sterile gloves is used.

c. Potential problems with this system include the catheter being left in the ET tube after suctioning or the catheter migrating into the ET tube between suction procedures, which would result in increased airway resistance.

d. Although the manufacturers recommend changing the closed suction system daily, studies show that the system may be changed when the ventilator circuit is changed, about once per week.

4. **Other types of catheters**
   a. **Yankauer suction (tonsil):** used to suction the oropharynx

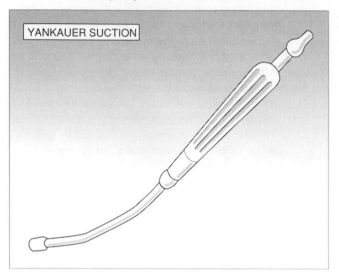

YANKAUER SUCTION

FIGURE 4-22

b. **Coudé suction catheter:** angled-tip catheter used to suction the left mainstem bronchus
5. **Indications for tracheal suctioning**
   a. To remove retained secretions that the patient cannot mobilize
   b. To maintain patency of artificial airways
   c. To obtain sputum for culture and sensitivity testing
6. **Hazards of tracheal suctioning**
   a. Hypoxemia: caused by inadequate oxygen level during suctioning; **increase FiO$_2$ to 1.0 before suctioning.** (Some advocate increasing FiO$_2$ only 10% to 15% on infants less than one month old to help prevent retinopathy of prematurity.)
   b. Arrhythmias: caused by hypoxemia and vagal nerve stimulation. The **vagus nerve** is stimulated as the catheter irritates the oral or nasal mucosa, tracheal mucosa, and carina, causing bradycardia.
   c. Hypotension: caused by bradycardia and prolonged coughing episodes.
   d. Atelectasis: caused by using a suction catheter that is too large or excessive suction pressure.
   e. Tissue trauma: caused by jabbing the catheter during insertion and improper lubrication during nasal suctioning.

> ☑ **Exam Note**
>
> Suctioning may suddenly stop as a result of a kinked suction catheter, a mucus plug lodged in the catheter, or a suction collection bottle that is full.

7. **Vacuum systems and collection bottles**
   a. The suction catheter is attached to a connecting tube, which attaches to the outlet of a collection bottle. This bottle attaches to a Diameter Index Safety System (DISS) connection on the suction or vacuum regulator, which is either a portable pump or a 50-psi vacuum wall outlet at the bedside.
   b. The vacuum regulator supplies the negative (subatmospheric) pressure necessary to suction the airway.
   c. The secretion collection bottle is generally equipped with a system that interrupts suction when the bottle becomes full of secretions.
   d. Most suction or vacuum systems provide up to −200 mm Hg pressure, but the desired vacuum level can be adjusted by occluding the suction regulator outlet and turning a vacuum control knob on the regulator. Most systems use locking mechanisms to prevent excessive suction pressures from being used.
   e. Appropriate suction levels
      Adults: −100 to −120 mm Hg
      Children: −80 to −100 mm Hg
      Infants: −60 to −80 mm Hg

IV. **ET TUBE EXTUBATION**
CRT Exam Content Matrix: IIIB9
RRT Exam Content Matrix: IIIB4
A. Procedure of Extubation
   1. Explain procedure to the patient.
   2. Increase the FiO$_2$ level.
   3. Suction down the ET tube.
   4. Suction the mouth and back of throat.
   5. Untape the ET tube, deflate the cuff, and instruct the patient to take a deep breath. **At peak inspiration, withdraw the tube.**
   6. Place on aerosol mask with appropriate level of oxygen. It is permissible to withdraw the tube while suctioning because this clears the airway while extubating.

> ⚠ A resuscitator bag may be used to deliver the deep breath and to better ensure that the tube is removed at peak inspiration.

B. **Complications of Extubation**
   1. **Laryngospasm**
      a. Spasm of the vocal cords caused by irritation of the tube, resulting in airway obstruction. This is detected by observing respiratory difficulty immediately after extubation.
      b. If laryngospasm occurs, administer a high FiO$_2$ concentration and, if it persists for more than 1 to 2 min, administer a bronchodilator via a handheld nebulizer.
   2. **Glottic edema** (discussed later)

> ⚠ Intubation equipment should be readily available at the bedside during extubation in case reintubation becomes necessary.

V. **LARYNGEAL AND TRACHEAL COMPLICATIONS OF ET TUBES**
CRT Exam Content Matrix: IIIF2g
RRT Exam Content Matrix: IIIF2d

A. **Sore Throat and Hoarseness**
   1. Are common results of tube irritation
   2. Usually subside within 2 to 3 days
   3. Are treated with cool aerosol

B. **Glottic Edema**
   1. **Inspiratory stridor** is the major clinical sign.
   2. Caused by
      a. Traumatic intubation
      b. Insertion with oversized ET tube
      c. Poor ET tube maintenance
      d. Allergic response to material in the ET tube
   3. Stridor should be treated with
      a. Cool aerosol to decrease swelling
      b. Vasoconstrictor, such as racemic epinephrine, via handheld nebulizer to constrict mucosal blood vessels and reduce swelling
      c. Corticosteroids, such as dexamethasone (Decadron), to reduce swelling

C. **Subglottic Edema**
   1. This edema occurs below the glottis at the level of the cricoid cartilage.
   2. This is a serious complication after extubation, which may lead to reintubation.
   3. If postextubation distress cannot be relieved, subglottic edema must be suspected.

D. **Vocal Cord Ulceration**
   1. Suspected if hoarseness continues for more than 1 wk
   2. Caused by
      a. Traumatic intubation
      b. Tight-fitting tube
      c. Allergic reaction to material in tube
      d. Excessive movement of the tube

E. **Tracheal Mucosal Ulceration**
   1. Is common after extubation
   2. Occurs at the area of the cuff site

F. **Vocal Cord Paralysis**
   1. Is caused by damage to the recurrent laryngeal nerve
   2. Usually occurs secondary to upper chest or neck surgery

G. **Laryngotracheal Web**
   1. Necrotic tissue at the glottic or subglottic level leads to fibrin formation, which combines with secretions and cellular debris to form a membrane, or web.
   2. Stridor and acute airway obstruction generally occur.

   3. The web should be suctioned from the airway immediately.
   4. The web often occurs several days after extubation.

H. **Tracheal Stenosis**
   1. This lesion is found at the cuff site or the level of the cricoid membrane.
   2. As the lesion heals, it constricts, leading to a narrowing of the airway.
   3. A narrowing of less than 50% of the diameter of the airway is not symptomatic.
   4. To help prevent tracheal stenosis, maintain cuff pressure by use of the **minimal leak technique.**

I. **Tracheal Malacia**
   1. Cartilaginous support of the trachea is lost.
   2. After extubation, the trachea collapses, leading to respiratory distress.

POSTCHAPTER STUDY QUESTIONS

1. To prevent venous congestion on the trachea wall, the ET tube cuff should be maintained below what level of pressure?
2. Inspiratory stridor is a major clinical sign of what airway condition?
3. What is the name of the speaking valve that may be attached to a ventilator patient's tracheostomy tube that allows the patient to talk?
4. Describe the purpose of an oropharyngeal airway.
5. What is the primary purpose of a fenestrated tracheostomy tube?
6. List the problems associated with the use of oral ET tubes.
7. How would you determine that an ET tube is resting in the right mainstem bronchus before a chest x-ray film is obtained?
8. What is a Yankauer suction device used for?
9. What is the maximum amount of suction pressure that may be used to suction an adult patient's airway?
10. When extubating a patient, the ET tube should be withdrawn at what point in the breathing cycle?

See answers at the back of the text.

BIBLIOGRAPHY

Aehlert B: *ACLS quick review study guide*, ed 3, St Louis, 2007, Mosby.

Branson RD, Hess DR, Chatburn RL: *Respiratory care equipment*, ed 2, Philadelphia, 1999, JB Lippincott.

Cairo J, Pilbeam S: *Mosby's respiratory care equipment*, ed 8, St Louis, 2010, Mosby.

Hess DR: Managing the artificial airway. *Respir Care* 44:759, 1999.

Hess DR et al: *Respiratory care principles and practice*, ed 1, Philadelphia, 2002, Saunders.

Wilkins JL, Stoller JK, Kacmarek R: *Egan's fundamentals of respiratory care*, ed 9, St Louis, 2009, Mosby.

White G: *Basic clinical lab competencies for respiratory care*, ed 4, Albany, 2003, Delmar.

Wyka K, Mathews P, Clark W: *Foundations of respiratory care*, ed 1, Albany, 2002, Delmar.

SPECIAL RESPIRATORY CARE PROCEDURES

PRETEST QUESTIONS

Answer the pretest questions before studying the chapter. This will help you determine your strong and weak areas in the material covered.

1. Which of the following are complications associated with bronchoscopy?

   1. **Pulmonary hemorrhage**
   2. **Pneumothorax**
   3. **Hypoxemia**

   A. 1 only
   B. 2 only
   C. 1 and 3 only
   D. 1, 2, and 3

2. While assisting with a bronchoscopy, you note that the physician is having difficulty entering the trachea. This may be the result of which of the following?

   A. Pneumothorax
   B. Hypoxemia
   C. Laryngospasm
   D. Pulmonary hemorrhage

3. After a bronchoscopy, the respiratory therapist notes that it is taking more ventilator pressure to ventilate the patient's lungs than before the procedure. This could be caused by which of the following?

   1. **Bronchospasm**
   2. **Pneumothorax**
   3. **Hypoxemia**
   4. **Pulmonary hemorrhage**

   A. 1 and 2 only
   B. 2 and 3 only
   C. 1, 2, and 4 only
   D. 2, 3, and 4 only

4. To aid in the evacuation of air from the pleural space, a chest tube should be inserted at what level?

   A. Supraclavicular space
   B. Second intercostal space anteriorly
   C. Sixth intercostal space anteriorly
   D. Eighth intercostal space anteriorly

5. The respiratory therapist notices on a patient's chest tube drainage system that there is fluctuation of the water level in the water-seal chamber with each patient breath and air bubbles seen only in the suction control chamber, which has a suction pressure of -15 cm H_2O. The most appropriate action is which of the following?

   A. Clamp the chest tube and check for leaks.
   B. Insert the chest tube farther, until bubbling stops in the vacuum chamber.
   C. Withdraw the chest tube until bubbling starts in the water-seal chamber.
   D. Recommend a chest radiograph to determine whether the pneumothorax has resolved.

6. The respiratory therapist observes that, during a patient's breathing cycle, there is no fluctuation in the water-seal chamber of the pleural drainage system. The most appropriate action is which of the following?

   A. Withdraw the tube until fluctuation is seen.
   B. "Strip" the chest tube to clear a possible obstruction.
   C. Increase the vacuum pressure.
   D. Clamp the chest tube and observe for leaks.

See answers and rationales at the back of the text.

REVIEW

I. **BRONCHOSCOPY**
   CRT Exam Content Matrix: IC2, IIA25, IIIJ2
   RRT Exam Content Matrix: IC3, IIA11, IIIJ2
   A. A technique for assessing and examining the bronchi by means of a bronchoscope, which is used for both therapeutic and diagnostic purposes

B. **Types of Bronchoscopes**
   1. Rigid bronchoscope

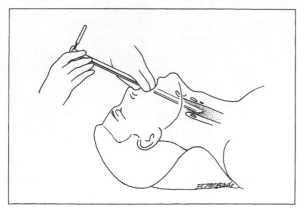

FIGURE 5-1 Rigid bronchoscope. From Scanlan CL, Simmons KF: Airway management. In Scanlan CL, Wilkins RL, Stoller JK: *Egan's fundamentals of respiratory care,* ed 7, St Louis, 1999, Mosby.

   a. Consists of a hollow metal tube with a light on its distal end.
   b. Tube is inserted orally, then passed between the vocal cords into the trachea.
   c. Is useful for removing aspirated foreign bodies and thick secretions from the lungs.
   2. Fiberoptic bronchoscope
   a. Consists of a collection of thin, threadlike glass strands called *fiberoptic filaments* with a light source projected to its distal end for visualization.

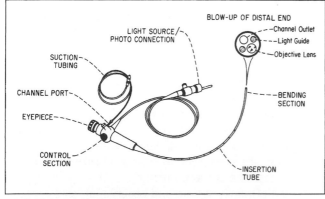

FIGURE 5-2 Fiberoptic bronchoscope. From Scanlan CL, Simmons KF: Airway management. In Wilkins RL, Stoller JK, Kacmarek R: *Egan's fundamentals of respiratory care,* ed 9, St Louis, 2009, Mosby.

   b. Is better tolerated by patients than the rigid bronchoscope because of its more flexible nature; it is therefore more commonly used.
   c. Preparatory regimen for fiberoptic bronchoscopy
      (1) Because bronchoscopy is uncomfortable, a mild sedative should be administered to the patient 1 to 2 h before the procedure. Commonly, **diazepam (Valium)** or **midazolam (Versed)** is used for this purpose. The level of sedation, referred to as **conscious sedation,** should be just enough to allow the patient to follow commands yet still be comfortable.
      (2) The airway must be dry during the procedure to aid in visualization, which is usually achieved by administering **atropine** 1 to 2 h before the procedure. Atropine may also decrease vagal tone, resulting in a decreased potential for bradycardia and hypotension, which can occur during the procedure.
      (3) The tube may be inserted orally, nasally, or through the ET tube. The bronchoscopic tube should be lubricated with a water-soluble jelly for easier nasal insertion. Often, **lidocaine (Xylocaine)** jelly is used both as a lubricant and for its anesthetic effects. In some cases, the RCP administers aerosolized lidocaine before the procedure.
      (4) Because of its flexibility, a fiberoptic bronchoscope can be advanced farther into the airway than a rigid one, thereby allowing more visualization of the conducting airways.
      (5) Biopsy forceps and brushes may be inserted through the bronchoscope to obtain tissue samples.
C. **Indications for Bronchoscopy**
   1. Removal of foreign bodies
   2. Removal of mucus plugs and thick secretions
      a. Is normally performed when secretions cannot be removed by routine suctioning techniques
      b. Once the site of the secretions is visualized, the area should be lavaged with saline before suctioning.
   3. Atelectasis that affects a lobe or an entire lung
   4. Pulmonary hemorrhage
      a. To locate the area of bleeding
      b. To control bleeding by instillation of epinephrine or iced saline lavage at the bleeding site
   5. When tracheal intubation is difficult as a result of upper airway trauma, obesity, tumors, or spinal deformity
      a. The ET tube is slipped over the fiberoptic bronchoscope; the scope should protrude well past the end of the ET tube.
      b. The vocal cords are visualized, and the scope is advanced through the cords to the midtracheal level, where the ET tube is then advanced over the scope to the proper position. The scope is then withdrawn.

6. Biopsy of suspected tumors
7. When sputum is needed for culture and sensitivity studies

D. **Complications of Bronchoscopy**
1. Hypoxemia
   a. Monitor oxygen saturation during procedure.
   b. Increase oxygen percentage during procedure.
2. Laryngospasm
   a. Makes advancing the tube more difficult.
   b. Bronchodilator should be readily available.
3. Bronchospasm
   a. Results from irritation of the airway.
   b. Bronchodilator should be readily available.
4. Arrhythmias
   a. Result from vagal stimulation.
   b. Monitor ECG and remove bronchoscope until cardiac status is stabilized.
5. Hemorrhage
   a. May occur during insertion.
   b. May occur after biopsy.
6. Respiratory depression
   a. Results from sedatives given before the procedure.
   b. Monitor respiratory status closely.
7. Hypotension
   a. Results from vagal nerve stimulation.
   b. May result from sedatives given before the procedure.
8. Pneumothorax
   a. Results from inadvertent puncture of the lung.
   b. Monitor respiratory status closely.

E. **Respiratory Therapist's Responsibilities during Bronchoscopy**

> Responsibilities of the RCP vary according to the institution's protocols. Those listed below are among the most common responsibilities.

1. Prepare the patient and explain the procedure.
2. Administer aerosolized local anesthetic to the patient's upper airway.
3. Conduct patient monitoring throughout the procedure.
   a. Pulse and blood pressure
   b. Respiratory rate
   c. ECG
   d. Oxygen saturation
   e. Level of consciousness

4. Collect sputum and tissue samples that the physician has obtained and prepare them for laboratory analysis.
5. Clean the bronchoscope properly after the procedure. The Centers for Disease Control and Prevention recommends that bronchoscopes be sterilized by immersion in glutaraldehyde (Cidex) for 3 to 10 h.

II. **CHEST TUBE INSERTION AND MONITORING**
CRT Exam Content Matrix: IIIJ5
RRT Exam Content Matrix: IIIJ5
A. Chest tubes are used to drain substances that accumulate in the pleural space.
B. Substances that may accumulate in the pleural space and their diagnoses include:
1. Air: pneumothorax
2. Blood: hemothorax
3. Lymph: chylothorax
4. Serous fluid: pleural effusion
5. Pus: pyothorax or empyema

> The term *hydrothorax* is often used to refer to lymph, serum, or plasma in the pleural space.

C. To help evacuate air (pneumothorax) from the pleural space, the chest tube is usually inserted in the second, third, or fourth intercostal space. To remove fluids, the tube is placed lower, usually in the sixth or seventh intercostal space.
D. Chest tube insertion is done under local anesthesia; for large tubes, regional anesthesia with an intercostal block is used.
E. Chest tubes are sutured in, and the insertion distance should be monitored daily to ensure the tube is not migrating outward. If the proximal hole on the chest tube slips out of the chest, air enters the tube, resulting in bubbling in the system, which appears to be a persistent leak in the lung.

> Once the air is evacuated from the pleural space, spontaneous healing or sealing of the leak in the lung usually occurs.

F. **Chest Tube Drainage Systems**
1. **One-bottle system**
   a. Fluid or air drains from the pleural space through the chest tube and enters the drainage bottle through a glass tube, which is submerged under water. This forms a seal that acts like a one-way valve to prevent air from entering the pleural cavity.
   b. Air entering the bottle is then vented out the short tube in the top of the bottle.
   c. The one-bottle setup is both a water-seal container and a collection container.

2. **Two-bottle system**
   a. In this system, a second bottle is added to collect air exiting the pleural space. Liquid drains into the first bottle.
   b. The purpose of this system is to better control the amount of suction applied. A suction source may be connected to the vent of the water-seal bottle.

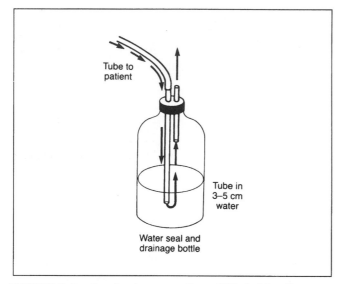

FIGURE 5-3 One-bottle system. From O'Toole M, editor: *Miller-Keane encyclopedia and dictionary of medicine, nursing, and allied health,* revised revision, Philadelphia, 2005, Saunders.

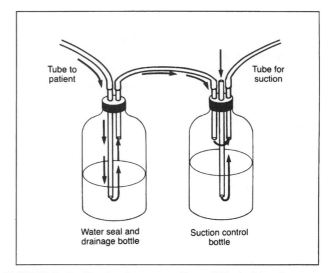

FIGURE 5-4 Two-bottle system. From O'Toole M, editor: *Miller-Keane encyclopedia and dictionary of medicine, nursing, and allied health,* RR, Philadelphia, 2005, Saunders.

3. **Three-bottle system**
   a. A third bottle may be added to determine the amount of subatmospheric pressure in the water-seal bottle.

b. The amount of suction is determined by how far under the water the tube is submerged.
c. A suction source may be attached to the third bottle's vent to maintain a desired constant subatmospheric pressure.

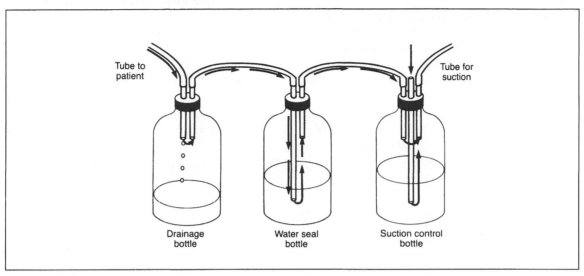

FIGURE 5-5 Three-bottle system. From O'Toole M, editor: *Miller-Keane encyclopedia and dictionary of medicine, nursing, and allied health,* RR, Philadelphia, 2005, Saunders.

d. The most common chest tube drainage system is a plastic three-chambered system (Pleur-Evac).

Pleur-Evac System

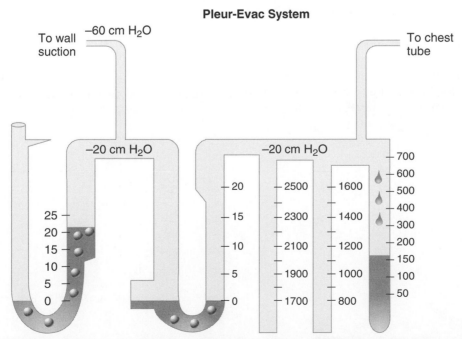

FIGURE 5-6 From Wilkins RL, Stoller JK, Kacmarek R: *Egan's fundamentals of respiratory care,* ed 9, St Louis, 2009, Mosby.

G. Important Points Concerning Chest Tube Drainage

1. The water level in the water-seal bottle fluctuates with changes in pleural pressure that occur with normal breathing. **If no fluctuation is occurring in the water-seal bottle, obstruction of the tube should be suspected.**
2. Chest tubes may become obstructed as a result of blood clots or kinks in the tube itself. **Obstructed chest tubes may result in a tension pneumothorax.**
3. To ensure adequate drainage and tube patency, "strip" or "milk" the tube every 1 to 2 h. Accomplish this by compressing and releasing the tubing, which will create a sudden gush of suction, thereby clearing the tube of an obstruction caused by a clot.
4. Occasional bubbling in the water-seal bottle is normal as air enters from the pleural space. Excessive or persistent bubbling may indicate air leaks in the system. The absence of bubbling indicates that no air is being removed from the pleural space, which is a sign of the patient's improvement.
5. If an air leak is suspected, the chest tube should be clamped to identify the source of the leak.
6. Clamping of the tube is required when changing drainage bottles but must be done with caution in patients with pleural air leaks because a tension pneumothorax may result.
7. The drainage and collection bottles must be kept at a level below the chest to prevent backflow.
8. The drainage and collection system must be kept airtight; there can be no leaks around the connections. The glass tube **must always** be kept submerged under the water.
9. If a suction source is connected to the vent tube in the suction bottle, a negative pressure (not to exceed −15 cm H_2O) is usually necessary.
10. After the lung reexpands, the chest tube should remain in place for another 1 to 2 days. After the tube is removed, the wound should be covered with a sterile petroleum jelly dressing to prevent air from entering the pleural space.

POSTCHAPTER STUDY QUESTIONS

1. List five indications for bronchoscopy.
2. List eight complications of bronchoscopy.
3. Name one medication that is commonly used to achieve conscious sedation before bronchoscopy.
4. What is the purpose of administering atropine before bronchoscopy?
5. How should the bronchoscope be cleaned after the procedure?
6. What is the purpose of inserting a chest tube?
7. If the water in the water-seal bottle is not fluctuating, what should be suspected?
8. If a chest tube becomes obstructed, what may occur?
9. If an air leak from a chest tube is suspected, what should be done first?
10. How much negative pressure is generally required to help evacuate fluid or air from the pleural space?

See answers at the back of the text.

BIBLIOGRAPHY

Des Jardins T: *Cardiopulmonary anatomy and physiology: essentials for respiratory care*, ed 4, Albany, 2002, Delmar.
Hess D and others: *Respiratory care principles and practice*, ed 1, Philadelphia, 2002, Saunders.
O'Toole M, editor: *Miller-Keane encyclopedia and dictionary of medicine, nursing, and allied health*, RR, Philadelphia, 2005, Saunders.
Scanlan CL, Simmons KF: Airway management. In Scanlan CL, Wilkins RL, Stoller JK: *Egan's fundamentals of respiratory care*, ed 7, St Louis, 1999, Mosby.
Scanlan CL, Simmons KF: Airway management. In Wilkins RL, Stoller JK, Kacmarek R: *Egan's fundamentals of respiratory care*, ed 9, St Louis, 2009, Mosby.
Wilkins RL, Stoller JK, Kacmarek R: *Egan's fundamentals of respiratory care*, ed 9, St Louis, 2009, Mosby.

PRETEST QUESTIONS

Answer the pretest questions before studying the chapter. This will help you determine your strong and weak areas in the material covered.

1. You enter a patient's room to give a treatment and observe the patient is unconscious and not breathing. After calling for help, your **first** action should be which of the following?

   A. Deliver two breaths.
   B. Begin chest compressions.
   C. Perform abdominal thrusts.
   D. Open the airway.

2. After 10 min of CPR, an infant's pulse returns but no ventilatory effort is present. The respiratory therapist should do which of the following?

   A. Continue compressions and rescue breathing at a ratio of 15 : 2.
   B. Stop compressions and deliver one breath every 6 s.
   C. Deliver five back blows, until breathing resumes.
   D. Stop compressions and deliver one breath every 3 s.

3. A patient has been intubated, and CPR is being performed. The patient's ECG strip indicates asystole, and the physician is unable to start an intravenous (IV) line. The respiratory therapist should recommend which of the following immediately?

   A. Instill sodium bicarbonate directly down the ET tube.
   B. Continue to attempt to start an IV in a peripheral vein.
   C. Instill epinephrine directly down the ET tube.
   D. Inject epinephrine directly into the myocardium.

4. Which of the following drugs is used to treat ventricular fibrillation during CPR?

   1. **Epinephrine**
   2. **Lidocaine**
   3. **Atropine sulfate**

   A. 1 only
   B. 2 only
   C. 1 and 2 only
   D. 2 and 3 only

5. During CPR, the patient's ECG strip indicates ventricular fibrillation. The patient has been defibrillated with 200 J using a biphasic defibrillator with no change in the ECG reading. The respiratory therapist should recommend which of the following?

   A. Repeat defibrillation with 300 J.
   B. Repeat defibrillation with 450 J.
   C. Instill sodium bicarbonate directly down the ET tube.
   D. Continue two-rescuer CPR with a compression/ventilation ratio of 5 : 2.

6. A patient's ECG strip indicates atrial fibrillation and cardioversion should be attempted. The defibrillator should be set at what level to return the heart to normal function?

   A. 50 J
   B. 150 J
   C. 250 J
   D. 400 J

See answers and rationales at the back of the text.

REVIEW

I. **CARDIOPULMONARY RESUSCITATION**
   CRT Exam Content Matrix: IB2a, IIIG4d, III I1a-d
   RRT Exam Content Matrix: IB2a, IIIG4a, III I1a-c
   A. **Obstructed Airway (in a Conscious Adult)**
      1. Determine whether there is an airway obstruction by asking the patient if he or she is choking and if he or she can speak or cough.
      2. Perform **abdominal thrusts** until the foreign body is expelled or the patient loses consciousness.
      3. If the patient loses consciousness, place the patient on his or her back and call for help.
      4. Use the tongue/jaw lift to open the mouth. If an object is visible perform a finger sweep with the patient's head turned to the side.
      5. Open the airway by using the head tilt/chin lift method.
      6. Give two breaths.
      7. If the ventilation attempts fail (determined by observing the chest not rising or difficulty in expelling air into the patient), reposition the

airway and perform ventilation again. If there is still no air movement, straddle the patient's thighs and perform up to five abdominal thrusts. (Perform chest thrusts in pregnant or obese victims.)

8. Again, perform a finger sweep, if an object is visible, and reattempt ventilations.
9. Repeat this sequence until the airway is cleared.

B. **Obstructed Airway (in an Unconscious Adult)**
1. Determine unresponsiveness.
2. Activate emergency medical service (EMS) or code team.
3. Position the patient on his or her back.
4. Open the airway using the head tilt/chin lift method.
5. **Determine breathlessness:** place ear over the patient's mouth, then **look, listen, and feel for air movement.**
6. Attempt ventilation.
7. If there is no air movement, reposition the airway and reattempt ventilation.
8. If there is still no air movement, straddle the patient's thighs and perform up to five abdominal thrusts.
9. Perform a finger sweep, if an object is visible, with the patient's head turned to the side.
10. Attempt ventilation.
11. Repeat the sequence until the airway is cleared.

C. **One-Rescuer CPR (Adult Patient)**
1. Determine unresponsiveness.
2. Call for help. Activate EMS.
3. Position patient on his or her back.
4. Open the airway using the head tilt/chin lift method.
5. Determine breathlessness: place ear over the patient's mouth, then look, listen, and feel for air movement.
6. Give two breaths while observing chest rise. (Allow lungs to deflate between breaths.)
7. Determine pulselessness by palpating the **carotid artery.** (Palpate **brachial artery** in an **infant.**)
8. Begin chest compressions at a rate of 100/min (30 compressions to two breaths).
9. Continue until patient responds, help arrives, or you can physically no longer continue.

D. **Two-Rescuer CPR (Adult Patient)**
1. When a second rescuer arrives, he or she should take over as the new compressor, while the first rescuer gets into position to be the breather. Palpate for a spontaneous pulse at this time.
2. If no pulse is present, continue CPR at a compression/ventilation ratio of 30:2.
3. The compressor should pause briefly after the fifteenth compression so the breather can administer a breath.

4. Intubate the patient as soon as possible to provide a more effective airway and to prevent air from entering the stomach during ventilation.

E. **Neonatal Resuscitation (Immediately after Delivery)**
1. Dry and warm the infant.
2. Suction the nose and mouth with a bulb syringe or DeLee suction catheter.
3. If meconium is seen, intubate the infant and suction the trachea.
4. Provide tactile stimulation to stimulate breathing.
5. If the infant is not breathing or the heart rate is less than 100 beats/min, begin positive pressure ventilation with 100% oxygen with a bag-mask.
   a. The initial ventilation rate should be 40/min.
   b. The initial ventilation pressure should be 30 to 40 cm H_2O, and all the breaths thereafter should be at 15 to 20 cm H_2O. (When resuscitating an infant hours after delivery that has respiratory problems resulting in decreased lung compliance, you may need higher pressures for ventilation.)

> The manual resuscitator should have a manometer attached to measure peak inspiratory pressure.

6. After performing ventilation for 15 to 30 s, reassess the pulse; if the heart rate is less than 60 beats/min, then continue ventilation and start chest compressions.
   a. The compression rate should be approximately 120/min.
   b. Once the heart rate is 60 beats/min or higher, discontinue compressions while maintaining manual ventilation.
   c. If the heart rate stays below 60 beats/min, intubate the infant. Continue positive pressure ventilation and chest compressions, and reassess the infant periodically.
7. Drugs used during neonatal resuscitation
   a. **Epinephrine** is a cardiac stimulant that should be administered either via IV drip or **directly down an ET tube** when the following occurs
      (1) If the heart rate remains less than 60 beats/min after 30 s of chest compressions and manual ventilation
      (2) If a heart rate cannot be detected
      (3) See section on pharmacologic intervention during CPR on p. 80.
   b. **Volume expanders** are administered to increase vascular fluid volume to reverse relative hypovolemia. They include

(1) Whole blood (type O-negative blood cross-matched with mother's blood)

(2) Normal saline solution

(3) Saline solution with 5% albumin

(4) Ringer's lactate solution

c. **Sodium bicarbonate** is indicated in the presence of documented metabolic acidosis, which is caused by increased lactic acid production as a result of prolonged asphyxia.

d. **Naloxone hydrochloride (Narcan)** is a narcotic antagonist that reverses narcotic-induced respiratory depression. In infants, this most commonly occurs when narcotics are administered to the mother within 4 h of delivery. **Naloxone hydrochloride administration is indicated when severe respiratory depression is present and the mother is known to have had narcotics in the past 4 h.**

> Naloxone hydrochloride may be administered intravenously, intramuscularly, subcutaneously, or instilled down the ET tube.

II. **ADULT, CHILD, AND INFANT CPR MODIFICATIONS**
CRT Exam Content Matrix: III I1a-d
RRT Exam Content Matrix: III I1a-c
A. **Compression/Ventilation Ratios (for One Rescuer)**
1. Adult: compression/ventilation ratio is 30:2; 100 compressions/min
2. Child: compression/ventilation ratio is 30:2; 100 compressions/min
3. Infant: compression/ventilation ratio is 30:2; at least 100 compressions/min

B. **Compression/Ventilation Ratios (for Two Rescuers)**
1. Adult: compression/ventilation ratio is 30:2
2. Child: compression/ventilation ratio is 15:2
3. Infant: compression/ventilation ratio is 15:2

> The adult's cardiopulmonary status should be reassessed after five cycles, and the infant or child's status should be reassessed after 20 cycles.

C. **Rescue Breathing for Patients with a Pulse**
1. Adult: one breath every 5 to 6 s (10 to 12 breaths/min)
2. Child: one breath every 3 to 5 s (12 to 20 breaths/min)
3. Infant: one breath every 3 s (20 breaths/min)

D. **Compression Depth**
1. Adult: **1½ to 2 inches** with two hands stacked and the heel of one hand on the lower half of the patient's sternum
2. Child: **⅓ to ½ the AP diameter of the chest** with one hand on the lower half of the patient's sternum
3. Infant: **⅓ to ½ the AP diameter of the chest** with two or three fingers a finger's breadth below the nipple line.

III. **CPR: SPECIAL CONSIDERATIONS**
CRT Exam Content Matrix: III I1a-d
RRT Exam Content Matrix: III I1a-c
A. **Do not** hyperextend the neck of an infant to open the airway because this may close off the airway.
B. If a manual resuscitator bag-mask is not available for rescue breathing, **use a mask with a one-way valve to prevent contamination from the patient's exhaled air.** Mouth-to-mouth ventilation is used only if no other means is available.
C. Manual compressions achieve only about **25% to 35% of normal cardiac output.**
D. On entering a room wherein one-rescuer CPR is being performed, the first step to take before changing to two-rescuer CPR is to establish the presence or absence of a pulse.
E. The best indicator of adequate cerebral blood flow while performing chest compressions is pupillary reaction.
F. Patients with suspected **neck injuries** should have their airways opened by the **jaw-thrust maneuver without head tilt**.
G. **Hazards of CPR**
1. Rib fractures (especially in infants and elderly persons) may lead to pneumothorax or lacerated liver.
2. Fat embolism may result from microfractures of the ribs or sternum. Fat leaks from bone marrow and enters the venous circulation.
3. Gastric distention results from air entering the stomach from rescue breathing. This air should be removed from the stomach with a nasogastric (NG) tube because a distended abdomen interferes with lung expansion.

IV. **MANUAL RESUSCITATORS**
CRT Exam Content Matrix: IIA5
RRT Exam Content Matrix: None listed
A. **Uses of Manual Resuscitators**
1. Rescue breathing
2. Hyperinflation of lungs before tracheal suctioning
3. During transport of patient who requires artificial ventilation

B. Manual Resuscitator

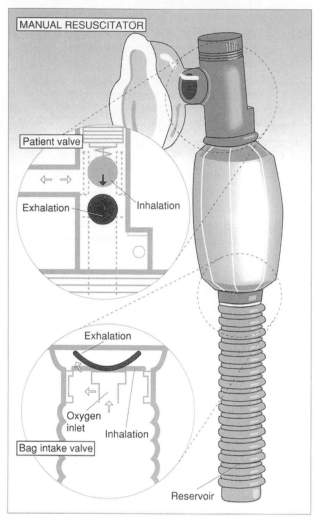

FIGURE 6-1

C. **Design of Resuscitators:** all are basically the same
1. A non-rebreathing valve with a standard universal adapter consists of a 22-mm OD that fits standard resuscitation masks and a 15-mm ID that connects to standard ET or tracheostomy tubes.
2. The non-rebreathing valve also houses the exhalation valve and ports, which prevent the rebreathing of exhaled air.
3. The resuscitators use **self-inflating bags** by means of a bag intake valve. **(The bag may still be used to ventilate, even without gas flowing to it.)**

4. A reservoir attachment should be connected to the bag intake valve so that, as the bag reinflates, it fills with supplemental oxygen instead of room air. This ensures that higher oxygen levels (approaching 100%) will be delivered to the patient.
5. Most resuscitator bags have pressure-relief devices that open to the atmosphere at a pressure of 40 cm H_2O so that excessive pressures are not delivered to the patient's lungs.
6. Some resuscitators come equipped with PEEP valves for patients who are being manually ventilated. This is very beneficial because it has been shown that stopping PEEP in patients who need a bag-mask causes drastic reductions in their PaO_2 if they receive ventilation without PEEP.
7. **To achieve the highest delivered O_2 levels possible, use the following criteria**
   a. Always use a reservoir attachment, if available.
   b. Use the highest flow rate available (10 to 15 L/min).
   c. Use the longest possible bag refill time (meaning a slower ventilation rate). Allow the bag to fully refill before the next breath. A faster ventilation rate decreases the percentage of delivered O_2.
   d. Do not use large stroke volumes (i.e., the volume squeezed from the bag), if possible. High volumes delivered from the bag result in more room air being entrained, thus lowering levels of O_2. **(This is not significant if a reservoir attachment is used.)**

D. **Hazards of Using Manual Resuscitators**
1. Leaks during inspiration caused by improperly fitted face mask or inadequately filled ET tube cuff
2. Equipment malfunction caused by sticking valves, missing parts, improper assembly, or dirty valve mechanisms
3. Poor ventilation technique

 Exam Note

If little or no resistance is met and the chest does not rise adequately when the bag is squeezed, suspect a leak around the exhalation valve, O_2 intake valve, or ET tube cuff or a poor-fitting mask.

E. **Gas-Powered Resuscitators**

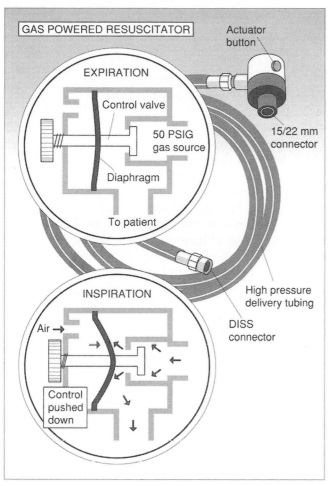

FIGURE 6-2

F. **Mouth-to-Valve Mask Ventilation**

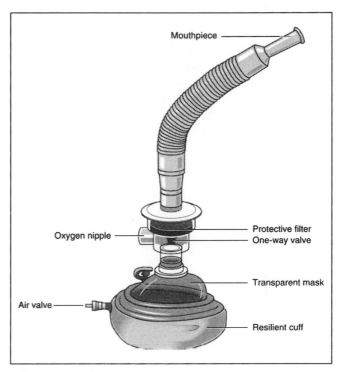

FIGURE 6-3 One-way valve system.

1. These are usually pressure-limited devices.
2. Some use demand valves, which open and deliver gas if the patient creates a negative pressure.
3. They usually have manual control buttons to initiate inspiration if the patient has apnea.
4. They are capable of delivering 100% O_2.
5. Volume delivery decreases if the pressure needed to ventilate the patient's lungs is higher than the capacity of the unit.
6. The unit is powered from a 50-psi O_2 wall outlet. If the diaphragm in the unit breaks, the patient's airway could be exposed to this high pressure.
7. These units have pressure-relief devices that vent pressures above 50 cm H_2O.

1. This method of ventilation provides an option to mouth-to-mouth ventilation, which should be avoided unless there is no other means of ventilating the patient's lungs.
2. Mouth-to-valve mask rescue breathing involves placing one end of the one-way valve on a mask. The other end has a mouthpiece attached. The rescue breather may manually ventilate the patient's lungs through the mouthpiece; the patient's exhaled air passes around the exhalation ports to the outside.
3. This one-way valve system for rescue breathing protects the breather from cross-contamination from the patient's exhaled air.

V. **PHARMACOLOGIC INTERVENTION DURING CPR**
CRT Exam Content Matrix: IIID5c, IIIG4d, III I1a-d, III I3d
RRT Exam Content Matrix: IIID5c, IIIG4a, III I1a-c, III I3d

A. **Routes of Administration**
   1. A central venous line (central line) is the ideal route, if available. It is inserted into the vena cava from the subclavian, jugular, or femoral vein.

2. A peripheral IV line is the best route when central venous line is not available.

3. Intraosseous infusion (IO) may be used when IV cannulation is unsuccessful or is taking too long. IO infusion is the infusion of medications, blood products, and fluids into the bone marrow cavity; from there, the infusion will then be delivered to the venous circulation. Any drug given IV may be administered IO.

4. **ET tube:** drugs such **lidocaine, epinephrine, atropine, vasopressin, and naloxone hydrochloride** may be instilled directly into the tracheobronchial tree via the ET tube for rapid absorption.

   To more easily recall CPR drugs that can be administered through the ET tube, remember the acronym *NAVEL*.

   N—Naloxone hydrochloride
   A—atropine
   V—vasopressin
   E—epinephrine
   L—lidocaine

> The instilling of these drugs through the ET tube may be permissible if the IV or IO route is not available, but it is not preferred. Recent studies indicate that giving resuscitation drugs through the ET tube results in lower blood concentrations than if the same dose is given IV. The recommended dose of drugs that are administered endotracheally are generally two to three times the IV dose, but the optimal endotracheal drug dose of most drugs is not known.

5. **Intracardiac:** Epinephrine is the only drug that may be injected directly into the heart but only when the ET tube or IV route is not available or when administration via those routes has failed to elicit a response.

B. **Drugs Commonly Administered during CPR**
   1. **Epinephrine**
      a. Indications
         (1) Asystole
         (2) Sinus arrest
         (3) Ventricular fibrillation
      b. Route of administration
         (1) IV bolus
         (2) **ET tube**
         (3) Intracardiac
      c. Dosage is one of the following
         (1) 1 mg IV every 5 minutes
         (2) 2 to 2.5 times the IV dose down ET tube

      d. Pharmacologic actions
         (1) Increased heart rate
         (2) Increased force of contraction of the heart
         (3) Increased coronary perfusion pressure
         (4) Vasoconstriction
   2. **Lidocaine**
      a. Indications
         (1) Ventricular fibrillation
         (2) Ventricular tachycardia
      b. Route of administration
         (1) IV bolus
         (2) IV drip
         (3) **ET tube**
      c. Dosage: 1-mg/kg IV bolus followed by additional boluses of 0.5 to 1.5 mg/kg every 3 to 5 min, up to a total of 3 mg/kg, or 2 to 3 mg/kg through the ET tube. Continuous infusion (drip) may be started at a rate of 2.0 to 4.0 mg/min when perfusion is restored after ventricular fibrillation.
      d. Pharmacologic actions: decreases ventricular activity
   3. **Atropine sulfate**
      a. Indications
         (1) Sinus bradycardia
         (2) Asystole
         (3) Nodal bradycardia
      b. Route of administration
         (1) IV bolus
         (2) **ET tube**
      c. Dosage
         (1) 1.0 mg IV every 5 min for asystole
         (2) 0.5 mg IV every 5 min (to a 2.0-mg maximum) for bradycardia
      d. Pharmacologic actions
         (1) Increased heart rate
         (2) Increased force of contraction of the heart
   4. **Procainamide**
      a. Indications
         (1) Ventricular tachycardia
         (2) Ventricular fibrillation
         (3) PVCs
      b. Route of administration
         (1) IV bolus
         (2) IV drip
      c. Dosage
         (1) 50-mg IV bolus every 5 min
         (2) 1- to 4-mg/min IV drip of a 100-mg/mL preparation
      d. Pharmacologic actions
         (1) May cause hypotension
         (2) Increases electrical stimulation threshold
         (3) Decreases electrical activity of the ventricles
   5. **Propranolol hydrochloride**
      a. Indications
         (1) Myocardial infarction (MI)
         (2) Angina pectoris

(3) Supraventricular arrhythmias

(4) Ventricular tachycardia

b. Route of administration: IV bolus

c. Dosage: 1 to 5 mg (to a maximum of 1 mg/min) of a 1-mg/mL preparation

d. Pharmacologic actions

(1) Decreased heart rate

(2) Decreased stroke volume

(3) Increased left ventricular end-diastolic pressure (LVEDP)

6. **Dobutamine hydrochloride**

a. Indications: depressed myocardial contractility

b. Route of administration: IV drip

c. Dosage: 2.5 to 10 μg/kg/min

d. Pharmacologic actions

(1) Increased cardiac output

(2) Enhanced atrioventricular conduction

7. **Isoproterenol hydrochloride**

a. Indications

(1) Bradycardia

(2) Heart block

(3) Hypotension

b. Route of administration: IV drip

c. Dosage: 1 mg/500 mL of 5% dextrose (2 μg/mL)

d. Pharmacologic actions

(1) Increased heart rate

(2) Increased force of contraction of the heart

8. **Dopamine hydrochloride**

a. Indications: hypotension

b. Route of administration: IV drip

c. Dosage: 2 to 30 μg/kg/min

d. Pharmacologic actions

(1) Increased cardiac output

(2) Increased blood pressure

9. **Sodium nitroprusside (Nipride)**

a. Indications: hypertension

b. Route of administration: IV drip

c. Dosage: 0.5 to 8.0 μg/kg/min

d. Pharmacologic actions

(1) Peripheral vasodilation

(2) Decreased blood pressure

10. **Calcium chloride**

a. Indications

(1) Hypocalcemia

(2) Hyperkalemia

b. Route of administration: IV (do not mix with other medications)

c. Dosage: 0.2 mL/kg

d. Pharmacologic actions: increased force of contraction of the heart

11. **Vasopressin**

a. Indications

(1) Cardiac arrest

b. Route of administration: IV

c. Dosage: 40 units IV push (one-time dose); may be used in place of first or second dose of epinephrine in cardiac arrest

d. Pharmacologic actions: vasoconstriction of peripheral, pulmonary, cerebral, and coronary blood vessels

---

The use of sodium bicarbonate ($NaHCO_3$) is no longer recommended during CPR. It has been found to cause adverse effects, including a shift of the HbO_2 curve to the left (decreased release of O_2 by Hb), depression of cerebral and myocardial function, and deactivation of catecholamines (e.g., isoproterenol and epinephrine) used during the resuscitative effort.

A rapid response team (RRT), also called the medical emergency team (MET) is often activated when a critically ill patient is deteriorating. The team is called to help prevent the development of a cardiac arrest and improve the patient's medical outcome. The team generally comprises a physician, nurse, and respiratory therapist with critical care training who are available at all times. The team will be notified by other hospital staff based on well-defined guidelines for activation of the team.

VI. **DEFIBRILLATION AND CARDIOVERSION**
CRT Exam Content Matrix: IIIJ7
RRT Exam Content Matrix: IIIJ8

A. **Defibrillation**

1. Defibrillation is a nonsynchronized current of electricity delivered to the heart during ventricular fibrillation.

2. It is administered by means of paddles placed on specific areas of the chest. After conducting gel is applied to the paddles, one paddle is placed below the clavicle and to the right of the upper part of the sternum. The other paddle is placed on the midaxillary line just to the left of the left nipple.

3. The initial electric current delivered should be **200 J (W/s) for adults using a biphasic defibrillator** and **360 J for a monophasic defibrillator** and 2 J/kg of body weight in infants and children. If this level is not effective in restoring normal ventricular activity, it may be increased to **no more than 360 J for adults** or 4 J/kg in infants and children.

4. This high charge of electricity delivered to the myocardium is intended to reverse life-threatening ventricular arrhythmias by causing complete depolarization of the cardiac muscle, thereby disrupting the electrical circuits in the heart that are causing the ventricular fibrillation.

5. Lidocaine and epinephrine may be administered because they improve the success of defibrillation.

6. It is essential that appropriate levels of electric current be used to prevent myocardial damage and cardiac arrhythmias.
7. The **precordial thump,** a sharp, quick blow delivered to the midportion of the sternum by the fleshy part of the fist, is recommended for a witnessed cardiac arrest when a defibrillator is not available.

B. **Cardioversion**
1. Cardioversion is a synchronized current of electricity delivered to the heart during ventricular depolarization (QRS complex).
2. Cardioversion is used to terminate the following arrhythmias
   a. Atrial flutter
   b. Atrial fibrillation
   c. Ventricular tachycardia
   d. Paroxysmal supraventricular tachycardia
   e. Ventricular fibrillation (defibrillation is usually indicated)
3. Cardioversion delivers a lower energy level than does defibrillation. Normal levels for cardioversion are a charge of 25 to 100 J to restore normal cardiac rhythm in adults and 0.2 to 1.0 J/kg in infants and children.
4. The respiratory therapist's duties in assisting with this procedure should include the following.
   a. Monitor heart rate and respiratory rate
   b. Monitor O_2 saturation
   c. Have O_2 delivery device readily available
   d. Have manual resuscitator and intubation equipment readily available (See Chapter 9 on cardiac monitoring for further information on ECGs and specific arrhythmias).

VII. **ADVANCE DIRECTIVES**
CRT Exam Content Matrix: IA1, IB5f
RRT Exam Content Matrix: IA1, IB5e
A. An **advance directive** is a written document stating a person's decisions regarding medical treatment that is to be initiated (or not initiated) should the person not have the physical or mental capacities to communicate their wishes.
B. A **living will** is a type of advance directive that patients put in writing regarding their wishes about medical treatment if they become terminally ill and not capable of making decisions about their medical care. A living will directs physicians to either withhold or withdraw "death-delaying" treatments. This does not include hydration and nutrition. The directives in a living will apply only to patients who have a terminal illness.
C. A **durable power of attorney** for health care is another type of advance directive in which a legal guardian is appointed to make the medical decisions for a patient who cannot make those decisions on their own. The withdrawal of

hydration and nutrition by feeding tube is permissible with this type of directive.
D. Do-not-resuscitate (DNR) protocols are often part of the advance directive. If no documentation for DNR protocols is present, resuscitation is generally begun while, at the same time, attempting to obtain orders from the physician.
E. DNR protocols may vary from state to state, but generally if the patient is in full cardiac or respiratory arrest, EMS personnel will follow these protocols
   1. Do not initiate CPR.
   2. Do not insert an oropharyngeal airway or endotracheal tube.
   3. Do not provide any kind of ventilatory assistance.
   4. Do not initiate chest compressions.
   5. Do not administer cardiac resuscitation drugs.
   6. Do not defibrillate.
F. If the patient is not in full respiratory or cardiac arrest but the patient's breathing and pulse rate is inadequate, resuscitation should not be administered; however, the following is generally allowed
   1. Oxygen administration
   2. Airway suctioning
   3. Use of a cardiac monitor
   4. Emotional support
   5. Control of bleeding
   6. Initiation of an IV line

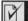 As mentioned previously, protocols vary from state to state. The above protocols are offered only as an example. Health care professionals should be familiar with the protocols in their area.

VIII. **TRANSPORTING THE CRITICALLY ILL PATIENT**
CRT Exam Content Matrix: III I3a-b
RRT Exam Content Matrix: III I3a-b

☑ **Exam Note**

Questions relating to transporting patients via land or air appear on the RRT examination only.

A. **Patients may be transported by either land or air.**
   1. **Important Points Concerning the Transport of Patients by Land or Air**
      a. Unstable patients must be transported with great care to avoid worsening of their condition.
      b. The practitioner should hold the ET tube with one hand and the bag with the other. This better stabilizes the tube and helps avoid inadvertent extubation.

c. Sudden changes in speed or direction may cause a drop in the patient's blood pressure.

d. Special attention must be given to monitoring lines that could become dislodged during transport.

e. Ventilators used for transport should have demand valves to conserve gas.

f. Patients should be adequately sedated to help prevent anxiety and allow safer transport.

g. During transport in an unpressurized aircraft, rapid increases in altitude result in decreased atmospheric pressure and PO_2. This may be managed by increasing delivered O_2 concentrations.

h. Higher altitudes (lower atmospheric pressure) may increase the size of an untreated pneumothorax and increase ET tube cuff pressure, which may decrease capillary perfusion to the trachea.

i. Lightweight equipment (e.g., transport ventilators) is necessary for air transportation.

j. Patient monitoring is more difficult in aircraft, especially helicopters.

k. Heated humidity or aerosol for ventilators or masks during transport is not necessary for such short-term use.

B. **Respiratory Care Equipment Needed during Transport**

1. O_2 system (tanks or liquid)
2. Portable suction machine and catheters
3. Portable ventilator
4. Portable ECG unit
5. Arterial pressure monitor
6. Pulse oximeter
7. Intubation equipment
8. Manual resuscitator

IX. **PARTICIPATING IN DISASTER MANAGEMENT**
CRT Exam Content Matrix: III I3c
RRT Exam Content Matrix: III I3c

A. No one will ever forget the tragedy that took place in New York City on September 11, 2001. After that terrible event, anthrax mailings occurred throughout the country. Even more recently, the threat of influenza in pandemic proportions has been a real concern.

B. Because of the potential for an event resulting in mass casualties, the U.S. medical community has taken steps to ensure that mechanical ventilators are available for the possibly thousands of individuals who may require life support.

C. To make sure an adequate number of ventilators are available should a mass disaster occur, the U.S. Centers for Disease Control and Prevention's Strategic National Stockpile program has more than 6000 ventilators at their disposal.

D. Planning at the local level for such an event is essential. Because respiratory therapists are responsible for setting up and maintaining mechanical ventilators, they must be actively involved in disaster management planning, training, and implementation.

E. A reliable triage system must be implemented during a mass casualty event so that patients who require ventilator support can be identified.

F. Because critical care respiratory therapists may be in short supply, noncritical care therapists who have been trained in critical care situations such as this will be called on to assist in patient care.

G. Because infants and children will also be victims, the ventilators must also be capable of maintaining this age group.

H. Routine training programs must be implemented to train all caregivers for a mass disaster.

I. The respiratory therapist must play a key role in training caregivers in the use of the mechanical ventilator.

POSTCHAPTER STUDY QUESTIONS

1. List three medications that are commonly instilled directly down the ET tube.
2. What is the major indication for the administration of dopamine?
3. List two indications for lidocaine.
4. Sodium nitroprusside (Nipride) is indicated for the treatment of what condition?
5. Describe the proper airway management of a postterm neonate in whom meconium aspiration is suspected.
6. When resuscitating a neonate immediately after delivery, what is the proper ventilation rate and peak inspiratory pressure for manual ventilation?
7. List four criteria that aid in delivering the highest O_2 concentration with a manual resuscitator.
8. What is the initial current delivered during defibrillation of an adult with a monophasic defibrillator? With a biphasic defibrillator?
9. What is the maximum current used to defibrillate an adult?
10. List two drugs that may be administered to improve the success of defibrillation.
11. List five arrhythmias that cardioversion is used to terminate.
12. How many joules are delivered to the patient during cardioversion?
13. List three potential consequences that could affect a patient during an air transport at high altitude.

See answers at the back of the text.

BIBLIOGRAPHY

Aehlert B: *ACLS quick review study guide*, ed 3, St Louis, 2007, Mosby.

American Heart Association: *CPR guidelines*, Dallas, 2005.

Hess DR and others: *Respiratory care principles and practice*, ed 1, Philadelphia, 2002, Saunders.

Wilkins RL, Stoller JK, Kacmarek R: *Egan's fundamentals of respiratory care*, ed 9, St Louis, 2009, Mosby.

HYPERINFLATION THERAPY

PRETEST QUESTIONS

Answer the pretest questions before studying the chapter. This will help you determine your strong and weak areas in the material covered.

1. Which of the following increases the delivered VT to a patient taking an IPPB treatment with the Bird Mark 7 IPPB machine?

   1. **Increasing flow rate**
   2. **Increasing inspiratory pressure**
   3. **Decreasing sensitivity**
   4. **Decreasing flow rate**

   A. 1 and 2 only
   B. 1 and 3 only
   C. 2 and 4 only
   D. 1, 2, and 3 only

2. During an IPPB treatment, the patient suddenly complains of chest pain and becomes short of breath. On assessing the patient, you auscultate the chest and hear decreased breath sounds on the left. These findings are consistent with which of the following?

   A. Atelectasis
   B. Left-sided pneumothorax
   C. Pulmonary embolism
   D. Pleural effusion

3. The respiratory therapist is administering IPPB, and the patient complains of feeling light-headed and dizzy. What should the therapist do to correct this?

   A. Instruct the patient to pause longer between breaths.
   B. Instruct the patient to take deeper breaths.
   C. Increase the inspiratory pressure.
   D. Decrease the inspiratory flow.

4. While the respiratory therapist is administering IPPB, the patient begins coughing up large amounts of blood. The therapist should

   A. Continue the treatment and notify the physician that a chest radiograph is needed.
   B. Decrease the inspiratory pressure.
   C. Stop the treatment briefly and resume it when the patient is feeling better.
   D. Stop the treatment and notify the physician.

5. Which of the following are hazards of IPPB therapy?

   1. **Excessive ventilation**
   2. **Increased cardiac output**
   3. **Decreased ICP**

   A. 1 only
   B. 2 only
   C. 1 and 3 only
   D. 2 and 3 only

6. The respiratory therapist has received an order to deliver IPPB to a patient with head trauma. What modifications in therapy may benefit this patient?

   1. **Use a higher flow rate.**
   2. **Use lower peak pressures.**
   3. **Set the sensitivity to −5 cm H$_2$O.**

   A. 1 only
   B. 2 only
   C. 1 and 2 only
   D. 2 and 3 only

7. Incentive spirometry is ordered for a patient after abdominal surgery. Which of the following statements by the respiratory care practitioner would be most appropriate in the initial explanation of the therapy to the patient?

   A. "You may experience pain and light-headedness from this therapy."
   B. "We are trying to improve your inspiratory capacity."
   C. "This therapy will help you take deep breaths and expand your lungs."
   D. "Your doctor has ordered this therapy to prevent atelectasis."

8. Sustained maximal inspiratory maneuvers performed with an incentive spirometer would be MOST effective in the

   A. Treatment of pneumonia.
   B. Prevention of pneumonia.
   C. Treatment of preexisting atelectasis.
   D. Prevention of atelectasis.

9. The initial inspiratory goal for a patient receiving incentive spirometry should be

   A. Twice the patient's measured tidal volume.
   B. Equal to the patient's measured tidal volume.
   C. At least 1500 mL.
   D. 5 mL/kg of body weight.

See answers and rationales at the back of the text.

REVIEW

I. **INTRODUCTION TO IPPB THERAPY**
   CRT Exam Content Matrix: IIA6a, IIA11b, IIB5, IIIA1a-b, IIID2a, IIIF1, IIIF2a
   RRT Exam Content Matrix: IIA2a, IIIA1a-b, IIID2a, IIIF1, IIIF2a

   A. IPPB is defined as a short-term (10 to 15 min) breathing treatment in which pressures above atmospheric pressure are delivered to the patient's lungs via a pressure-limited ventilator.
   B. Effective IPPB depends on four factors
      1. A respiratory therapist who has been well trained and has a knowledge of the equipment, medications used, reasons for therapy, and side effects and goals of therapy
      2. A relaxed, informed, and cooperative patient
      3. A pressure-limited IPPB machine with a means of measuring VT
      4. Proper instruction of the patient on breathing patterns and cough techniques by the respiratory therapist

II. **PHYSIOLOGIC EFFECTS OF IPPB**
   A. **Increased Mean Airway Pressure**
      1. During normal spontaneous inspiration, airway pressure drops below atmospheric pressure (-2 cm H_2O), thereby setting up a pressure gradient between the atmosphere (at nose and mouth) and the airways. Air flows into the airways, gradually building pressure back up to atmospheric level. Air flow stops, and passive exhalation occurs as a result of the natural recoil properties of lung tissue. The lung is never subjected to significant positive pressure.
      2. During an IPPB machine breath, positive pressure is applied to the airways to improve the ventilation status of the lung. This is what is meant by "increased mean airway pressure"; it is the average (mean) pressure in the airways during one breathing cycle.

   B. **Increased VT**
      1. IPPB should deliver a VT of 12 to 15 mL/kg of ideal body weight.
      2. Delivered VT depends on the patient's lung status (e.g., compliance and airway resistance).
         a. Decreased compliance results in a decreased delivered VT.
         b. Increased compliance results in an increased delivered VT.
         c. Decreased airway resistance results in an increased delivered VT.
         d. Increased airway resistance results in a decreased delivered VT.
      3. Delivered VT may be measured with a respirometer or gas-collection bag on the exhalation port.
      4. The inspiratory pressure control adjusts the delivered VT.
         a. Increase pressure to increase delivered VT.
         b. Decrease pressure to decrease delivered VT.

   C. **Decreased Work of Breathing**
      1. A patient experiencing acute hypoventilation may avoid intubation and use of a mechanical ventilator (possibly only temporarily) by administration of frequent IPPB treatments.
      2. The practitioner must encourage the patient to relax and allow the IPPB unit to do all the work for the patient's work of breathing to decrease.
      3. IPPB may increase the patient's work of breathing if
         a. The machine sensitivity (triggering mechanism) is set too low, making it difficult for the patient to cycle the machine into inspiration. **The patient should be required to pull no more than -2 cm H_2O of pressure to initiate inspiration.**
         b. The flow rate is inadequate to meet the patient's inspiratory flow demands. Increase the flow rate if inspiratory time is prolonged and if the manometer needle is **rising slowly or lagging** to peak pressure. Another indication that the flow is inadequate is if the manometer needle remains near zero throughout most of the inspiration and then rises quickly to peak pressure.
         c. The delivered VT is inadequate. Monitor the VT and listen to basilar breath sounds to ensure adequate volumes are being delivered.
         d. Adequate time is not allowed for passive exhalation to occur. The machine **sensitivity** (triggering mechanism) may be set **too high, which may result in self-cycling.**

D. **Alteration of the Inspiratory and Expiratory Time**

1. When a patient with respiratory difficulties receives IPPB, the alveolar ventilation should be improved, thereby making the patient more comfortable, less "air hungry," and returning the inspiration:expiration (I:E) ratio and respiratory rate to normal.
2. The normal I:E ratio for an adult is 1 : 2.

E. **Mechanical Bronchodilation**

1. A patient with respiratory disease experiences an **increased resistance to air flow** as the diameter of the airways decreases as a result of **bronchospasm, secretions,** and other factors.
2. When positive pressure is applied to constricted airways, dilation of these airways can occur to a greater degree than with spontaneous breathing.

⚠ Some studies show that higher flow rates and pressures may cause a bronchoconstrictive reflex in the airways. This may be counteracted by administering bronchodilating agents.

F. **Cerebral Blood Flow Alteration**

1. A patient receiving IPPB may experience light-headedness, dizziness, or faintness from reduced $PaCO_2$ levels and the resultant alkalemia. **Decreased $PaCO_2$ levels result in cerebral vasoconstriction, thus decreasing cerebral blood flow.**
2. To prevent reduced $PaCO_2$ levels, encourage the patient to breathe slowly and to pause between breaths.
3. A 50-mL flex tube should be connected between the mouthpiece and manifold, allowing a slight rebreathing of CO_2 and preventing decreased $PaCO_2$ levels.

III. **INDICATIONS FOR IPPB THERAPY**

A. Increased work of breathing
B. Hypoventilation
C. Need for delivery of medications to a patient who cannot take a deep breath (10 to 15 mL/kg of ideal body weight)
D. Inadequate cough
E. Increased airway resistance
F. Atelectasis, especially in sedated postoperative patients and patients recovering from chest or abdominal surgery who are reluctant to breathe deeply
G. Pulmonary edema
H. Need for aid in weaning from continuous mechanical ventilation

IV. **HAZARDS OF IPPB THERAPY**

A. **Excessive Ventilation**

1. Leads to decreased $PaCO_2$ levels, causing cerebral vasoconstriction and resulting in dizziness
2. Patient should be instructed not to stand or walk immediately after the treatment.

B. **Excessive Oxygenation**

1. Patients with severe COPD may breathe by the "hypoxic drive" mechanism. If the IPPB treatment is given with O_2, it may elevate the PaO_2 above the normal level (50 to 65 mm Hg), which may knock out the patient's drive to breathe.

☑ **Exam Note**

Although the "hypoxic drive" theory is highly debated and its validity is often questioned, the exam may still ask questions dealing with this subject.

2. Hypoxic drive potential is indicated by the following ABG levels: pH, 7.35 to 7.40 (compensated); $PaCO_2$, more than 50 mm Hg; PaO_2, less than 65 mm Hg.

C. **Decreased Cardiac Output**

1. Positive pressure applied to the airways is likewise exerted on blood vessels returning blood to the heart. This restricts venous blood return to the heart, which in turn decreases cardiac output from the left ventricle.
2. Avoiding high inspiratory pressures and long inspiratory times minimizes this hazard.
3. If there is a decreased venous return during the therapy, the patient may experience **tachycardia** and a **decrease in systemic blood pressure,** which is caused by decreased left ventricular filling pressure.

D. **Increased ICP**

1. Blood flow from the head is restricted as positive pressure is exerted on the superior vena cava, which is returning blood to the heart from the upper body. This keeps more blood in the cerebral vessels, which elevates ICP levels.
2. Normal ICP is less than 10 mm Hg.
3. Using lower pressures and shorter inspiratory times (increased flows) and having the patient positioned in the Fowler position or sitting on the edge of the bed minimizes this hazard.
4. This is not a common hazard, except in patients with closed head injuries or CNS disease.

E. **Pneumothorax**

1. Most common in patients with COPD with bullous disease or emphysema with bleb formation.

2. Patients who complain of sudden chest pain, shortness of breath, or other breathing difficulties and who have tachycardia during IPPB must be suspected of having a pneumothorax.
3. Listen with a stethoscope for bilateral breath sounds and observe for asymmetric chest movement.
4. If pneumothorax is suspected, the treatment must be stopped immediately.

F. **Hemoptysis**
1. The coughing up of blood during or after IPPB may not be caused by IPPB itself but may be related to a strong cough accompanying the treatment.
2. The treatment must be stopped immediately because air could be forced into a blood vessel, resulting in an air embolism.

G. **Gastric Distention**
1. Caused by swallowing air during the treatment.
2. May cause the patient to complain of nausea during or after the treatment.

H. **Nosocomial Infection**
1. Circuits should be changed every 24 h.
2. Appropriate filters should be used on the IPPB unit to prevent machine contamination.
3. Practitioners should wash their hands before and after every treatment.

V. **CONTRAINDICATIONS TO IPPB THERAPY**
A. **Untreated Pneumothorax: Absolute Contraindication**
1. IPPB should not be administered under any circumstances with this condition because it only worsens the problem.
2. IPPB is safe for patients with a pneumothorax who have a chest tube in place.

B. **Pulmonary Hemorrhage: Absolute Contraindication**
1. If IPPB is administered in this situation, air may enter a blood vessel, resulting in an air embolism.

C. **Relative Contraindications** (under certain circumstances IPPB may be administered or the therapy may be modified)
1. **Tuberculosis**
a. May lead to the spread of the disease, if the patient is not receiving antituberculosis medications.
b. IPPB is safe if the patient is receiving such drugs.
2. **Subcutaneous emphysema**
a. Indicates an air leak from the lung, and further positive pressure would worsen the condition.
b. This condition is not a danger in itself, but it may be an indication of a more severe condition, such as pneumothorax or pneumomediastinum.

3. **Hemoptysis**
a. This condition indicates an open pulmonary blood vessel, which could lead to an air embolism.
b. The origin of the bleeding must be determined.
4. **Closed head injury**
a. IPPB may increase ICP; therefore ICP must be monitored closely during IPPB in these patients.
b. To lessen the potential of increasing ICP, use **higher flow rates (decreased inspiratory time) and lower peak pressures.**
5. **Bullous disease**
a. Patients with bullae or bleb formation, such as those with COPD, are more susceptible to a pneumothorax. Bullae and blebs constitute weak air spaces and rupture easily.
b. Lower peak inspiratory pressures help alleviate this problem.
c. Rupturing of blebs or bullae may result from a strong cough effort during the treatment. These patients must be monitored closely.
6. **Cardiac insufficiency**
a. Patients with decreased blood pressure, decreased cardiac output, or other such cardiac problems must be monitored closely for further cardiac side effects.
b. Further cardiac problems may result from
(1) Positive pressure causing decreased venous return
(2) Cardiac side effects of bronchodilating agents
7. **COPD patient with air trapping**
a. IPPB may lead to an increase in air trapping in these patients, causing an inadvertent PEEP, which may decrease cardiac output.
b. These patients already have hyperinflated lungs, and IPPB may worsen this condition.
8. **Uncooperative patient**
a. Patient must be cooperative for treatment to be effective.
b. Alternative therapy should be considered.

VI. **POSITIVE EFFECTS OF IPPB IN THE TREATMENT OF PULMONARY EDEMA**
A. Decreases venous return.
B. Increases VT to improve ventilation and oxygenation, which results in improved cardiac activity.
C. Improves oxygenation by increasing the diameter of the fluid-filled alveoli so that more surface area is available for gas exchange.
D. Delivers aerosolized ethanol (40% to 50% concentration in water), which results in the dissipation of foamy edematous fluid.

E. Increases oxygenation because the treatment is delivered with 100% oxygen.

VII. **PROPER ADMINISTRATION OF IPPB**
A. Assemble all equipment and check machine for leaks.
B. Affirm physician order: If there is a question about the order, such as medication dosage, contact the physician for clarification.
C. Briefly review the patient chart for the following
1. Last treatment given
2. Latest chest film interpretation
3. Latest ABG results
D. Wash hands.
E. Identify patient by wristband, introduce yourself, and explain the reasons for administering the treatment.
F. Connect the circuit to the IPPB unit and plug into gas source.
G. Place medications in nebulizer.
H. Auscultate breath sounds to locate problem areas (e.g., atelectasis, secretions).
I. Determine heart rate and respiratory rate.
J. Assist the patient to an upright position because this allows better ventilation.
K. Place the mouthpiece in the patient's mouth and encourage the patient to keep his or her lips sealed tight and to breathe only through the mouth. (Use nose clips if the patient has difficulty.)
L. Instruct the patient to "sip" on the mouthpiece and allow the machine to fill the lungs until it cycles off. **Tell the patient to hold his or her breath for a count of three before exhaling** to better distribute medications and improve gas exchange. **Tell the patient to pause before the next breath.**
M. Set machine variables.
1. Inspiratory pressure: Start at lower than the desired pressure and gradually increase as treatment continues. (Increase the flow rate as pressure is increased to maintain the same inspiratory time.)
2. Flow rate
3. Nebulization
4. Sensitivity
N. Check vital signs halfway through the treatment. Allow a brief rest period.

O. After 10 min or when the medication is completely nebulized, encourage the patient to cough.
P. Check vital signs again.
Q. Encourage the patient to cough periodically for the next 30 min to 2 h as the effect of the medications peaks.
R. Wash hands.
S. Record vital signs, tolerance to treatment, cough effort, sputum characteristics (i.e., color, amount, consistency), and measured exhaled IPPB VT in the patient's chart.

VIII. **CHARACTERISTICS OF SPECIFIC IPPB UNITS**
How IPPB machines operate are not generally covered on the exams. The following information is stated to gain a better understanding of the machines which could indirectly help with specific IPPB questions.
A. **Bird Mark 7**
1. The Bird Mark 7 is a pneumatically powered and controlled ventilator. It is designed to operate with oxygen or air at a pressure of 50 psig. It is pressure-cycled, and its settings include a patient cycle, a time cycle, or a manual cycle.

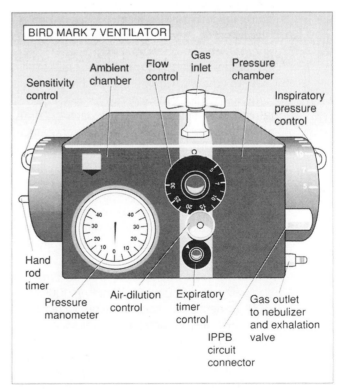

FIGURE 7-1

2. **Gas flow through the Bird Mark 7**
a. Gas enters the unit from the 50-psig wall outlet through a brass filter.
b. The first control that the gas travels to is the **flow rate control,** which is a simple needle valve.
c. From the flow rate control, gas travels to the **ceramic switch,** which is positioned

between the ambient chamber and pressure chamber of the unit. Depending on the position of the ceramic switch, flow is either blocked or is allowed to pass through.

d. For the patient to trigger the unit into inspiration, he or she must create enough negative pressure to separate a metal clutch plate from a magnet in the ambient chamber. This pulls the ceramic switch to the right, allowing gas flow to continue through the unit.

e. As gas flows past the ceramic switch, the gas splits: part of the flow supplies the expiratory drive line and nebulizer and the other part flows into the ambient chamber through a Venturi tube, which entrains ambient air. This increases flow and decreases the percentage of O_2.

f. The "mixed" gas then travels through the Venturi gate and into the pressure chamber, where the patient circuit is connected and flow continues on to the patient. The gate contains a spring with a tension of 2 cm H_2O that closes toward the end of inspiration. This blocks "mixed" gas from entering the pressure chamber, which results in only source gas (O_2) going to the chamber and the FiO_2 increasing to approximately 90% during the last portion of the inspiratory cycle.

g. Inspiration ends as gas in the patient's lungs builds up to a pressure that overcomes the magnetic force between another magnet and metal clutch plate located in the pressure chamber.

3. **Bird Mark 7 Controls**
   a. **Flow control**
      (1) The scale is made up of reference numbers and does not represent liters per minute.
      (2) Flow rates available are 0 to 80 L/min on air mix and 0 to 50 L/min on 100% O_2.
      (3) To decrease inspiratory time, increase flow rate; to increase inspiratory time, decrease flow rate.

(4) Flow wave patterns on Bird Mark 7
   (a) Square wave (constant flow) on 100% O_2
   (b) Tapered wave (decelerating flow) on air mix

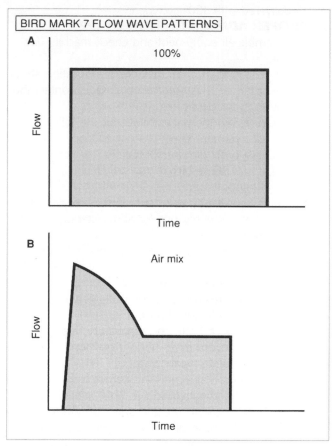

FIGURE 7-2

b. **Air mix control**
   (1) When pulled out, it allows flow into the ambient chamber and then through a Venturi tube, which results in air entrainment and delivery of 40% to 90% O_2.

(2) When pushed in, it blocks flow to the ambient chamber, not allowing for air entrainment, and therefore delivering 100% O_2.

(3) The air-mix setting creates a higher flow rate; 100% O_2 creates a lower flow rate.

c. **Inspiratory pressure control**

(1) Adjusts the position of the magnet in the pressure chamber closer to or farther away from the metal clutch plate.

(2) The closer the magnet is to the metal clutch plate, the higher the inspiratory pressure required to move the clutch plate and to end inspiration.

(3) Increasing pressure increases VT; decreasing pressure decreases VT

d. **Sensitivity control**

(1) Adjusts the position of the magnet in the ambient chamber closer to or farther away from the metal clutch plate.

(2) The closer the magnet is to the metal clutch plate, the more negative pressure is required by the patient to cycle the machine into inspiration (and vice versa).

(3) The position of the magnet should be such that the patient is required to generate a pressure of no more than −2 cm H_2O to initiate inspiration.

e. **Expiratory timing device**

(1) This is a needle valve that controls a leak from the expiratory timer cartridge and is used to automatically cycle the unit.

(2) It should always be turned off while administering IPPB, or the unit will self-cycle.

f. **Hand timer rod**

(1) Located on the left side of the unit (ambient pressure side) and used to manually cycle the unit off or on.

B. **Bennett PR-2 Ventilator**

1. The PR-2 is a pneumatically powered, pressure-limited ventilator that may be patient- or time-triggered and flow- or time-cycled.

2. **Diluter regulator**

a. This is an adjustable reducing valve that controls the pressure generated in the patient circuit.

b. It is adjustable from 0 to 50 cm H_2O.

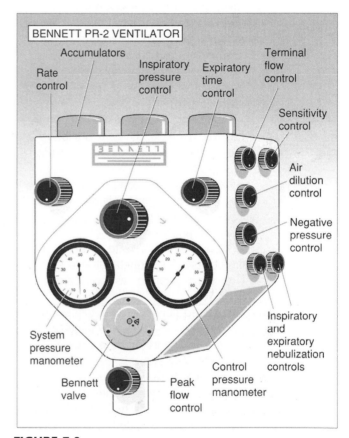

FIGURE 7-3

3. **Bennett valve**
   a. This is the heart of the PR-2. Gas comes from the diluter regulator to this valve and rotates it to the opened position. Gas then travels on to the patient via the circuit. The valve also opens in response to the patient's negative pressure.
   b. As inspiratory pressure increases, the flow begins to decrease (resulting from a decrease in the pressure gradient), rotating the Bennett valve to the closed position, stopping gas flow, and ending inspiration.
4. **PR-2 controls**
   a. **Inspiratory pressure control**
      (1) Adjusts the peak inspiratory pressure
      (2) Adjustable from approximately 0 to 50 cm H_2O
   b. **Dilution control**
      (1) When the dilution control knob is pushed in, air entrainment is allowed and the percentage of delivered O_2 varies from 40% to 90%.
      (2) When the dilution control knob is pulled out, no air entrainment is allowed and 100% O_2 is delivered.
   c. **Terminal flow control**
      (1) Adds an additional 12 to 15 L/min of flow below the Bennett valve to help cycle the unit off in case leaks are present.
      (2) This added flow goes to a Venturi tube, which decreases the percentage of O_2 (especially important if the patient is receiving 100% O_2).
   d. **Sensitivity control**
      (1) Turning this control counterclockwise increases the sensitivity, making it easier for the patient to cycle the unit into inspiration (and vice versa).
      (2) When the sensitivity control is turned off, the unit is factory-set for the patient to initiate inspiration by generating a pressure of –0.5 cm H_2O.
   e. **Peak flow control**
      (1) In its fully open position (all the way to the left), the flow rate is approximately 90 to 100 L/min with air dilution and 20 cm H_2O of pressure.
      (2) In the fully closed position (all the way to the right), the flow is approximately 15 L/min.
   f. **Nebulization control**
      (1) Separate controls for inspiratory or expiratory nebulization.
      (2) Gas that is sent to the nebulizer is source gas (100% O_2 if the unit is plugged into an O_2 outlet); therefore, the percentage

of O_2 increases when the nebulizer is used for medications.
   g. **Rate control and expiratory time**
      (1) Used to automatically trigger the unit on.
      (2) Turning the rate control to the right sets the rate (adjustable from 0 to 50 breaths/min).
      (3) The expiratory time control lengthens the expiratory time.
      (4) These controls should be turned off during the administration of IPPB; otherwise, the unit self-cycles.
C. **Bennett AP-5**
   Recently the exam has asked questions regarding this machine as the one to be used in the home setting because it runs on electricity.

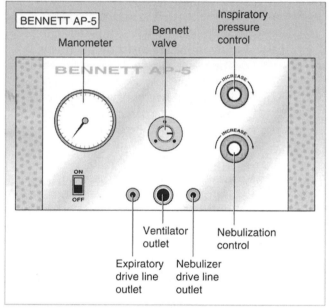

FIGURE 7-4

1. This IPPB unit is **electrically powered,** and inspiratory flow is powered by a compressor.
2. Compressed gas is not necessary for the functioning of this IPPB machine; therefore, it is a popular model for use in the home.
3. It is pressure-limited and patient-cycled and has a continuous flow for nebulization that comes from the compressor to the jet of the nebulizer.
4. Maximum peak pressure is approximately 30 cm H_2O.
IX. **FACTORS TO CONSIDER WHEN USING A PRESSURE-LIMITED IPPB MACHINE**
   A. **Effects on delivered VT**
      1. Increased airway resistance results in decreased VT.
      2. Decreased airway resistance results in increased VT.
      3. Increased lung compliance results in increased VT.
      4. Decreased lung compliance results in decreased VT.

5. Increased inspiratory pressure results in increased VT.
6. Decreased inspiratory pressure results in decreased VT.
7. Increased flow results in decreased VT.
8. Decreased flow results in increased VT.

B. **Effects on inspiratory time**
1. Increased flow results in decreased inspiratory time.
2. Decreased flow results in increased inspiratory time.
3. Increased lung compliance results in increased inspiratory time.
4. Decreased lung compliance results in decreased inspiratory time.
5. Increased airway resistance results in decreased inspiratory time.
6. Decreased airway resistance results in increased inspiratory time.

X. **PROBLEMS WITH IPPB AND CORRECTIVE ACTIONS**
A. The patient is having difficulty cycling the IPPB machine into the inspiratory phase. **Corrective actions**
1. Adjust the sensitivity so that the patient has to generate a pressure of −0.5 to −2 cm H₂O to start inspiration.
2. Make sure the machine is plugged into the wall gas outlet.
3. Ensure machine tubing connections are all tight.
4. Ensure the patient has lips sealed tightly around the mouthpiece or, if a mask is used, that there are no leaks around it.
5. If the Bird Mark 7 is used, ensure the flow control is turned on.

B. The patient complains of dizziness and tingling in the extremities during the treatment but has no appreciable increase in heart rate. **Corrective action:** Instruct the patient to breathe slower and to pause longer between breaths.

C. The patient's heart rate increases more than 20 beats/min during treatment. **Corrective action:** Stop treatment immediately and notify the physician. This is most likely the result of the nebulized bronchodilating agent stimulating the heart.

D. The patient cannot cycle the IPPB machine off. **Corrective actions**
1. Tighten all tubing connections.
2. Ensure that there are no leaks around the mouthpiece or mask.
3. Ensure that the ET tube or tracheostomy-tube cuff is inflated adequately.
4. If using the Bennett PR-2, check to make sure that the Bennett valve is not stuck.
5. If using the PR-2, turn on the terminal flow control to help compensate for leaks.
6. Check the expiratory valve function.

E. As the patient inhales, there is no nebulization of the medication. **Corrective actions**
1. Ensure that the capillary tube of the nebulizer is connected.
2. If using the Bennett PR-2, ensure that the nebulization control is turned on.
3. Ensure that the nebulizer drive line is connected.
4. Ensure that there is medication in the nebulizer.
5. Ensure that the nebulizer is positioned in an upright position.

F. During inspiration, the manometer needle stays in the negative area for the first half of the breath and then rises to the positive area during the last half. **Corrective action:** Increase the machine flow rate.

G. The IPPB machine repeatedly cycles on shortly after the patient has begun the expiratory phase. **Corrective actions**
1. Decrease the machine sensitivity.
2. If using the Bird Mark 7, ensure that the expiratory time for apnea control is turned off.
3. If using the Bennett PR-2, ensure that the rate control is turned off.

XI. **INCENTIVE SPIROMETRY (SUSTAINED MAXIMAL INSPIRATORY THERAPY)**
CRT Exam Content Matrix: IIA13, IIID1a-b, IIIF2b
RRT Exam Content Matrix: IIID1, IIIF2b
A. **Goals of Incentive Spirometry**
1. To prevent postoperative atelectasis.
2. To treat preexisting atelectasis.
3. To improve the cough mechanism.
4. To maintain the airway during the preoperative period.
   a. Strengthens lung muscles before surgery
   b. Improves mobilization of secretions
5. To provide early detection of atelectasis or pneumonia by observing decreasing inspiratory capacity levels.

B. **Hazards of Incentive Spirometry**
1. Hyperventilation.
2. Pneumothorax (unlikely but higher incidence in COPD patients).
3. Increased intrapleural pressure and stimulation of the vagal reflex, causing bradycardia if the sustained maximal inspiratory pause is performed against a closed glottis (Valsalva maneuver).

C. **Requirements for Effective Incentive Spirometry**
1. Cooperative patient.
2. Motivated patient.
3. Patient's respiratory rate should be less than 25 breaths/min.
4. Patient's vital capacity (VC) should be more than 10 mL/kg of body weight; **IPPB may be indicated if VC is less than 10 mL/kg.**

D. **Steps in Performing Incentive Spirometry**

1. Explain in understandable terms the importance of deep breathing and coughing. (Avoid terms such as atelectasis, inspiratory capacity, and the like; rather, use terms that the average nonmedical person can easily understand.)

2. Determine the patient's initial inspiratory goal. A good starting point is twice the patient's tidal volume. Some incentive spirometers come with a nomogram based on the patient's gender, age, and height to determine the normal inspiratory capacity.

3. Place the patient in a semi-Fowler or Fowler position. Always place the patient in a sitting position to allow for a better inspiratory effort.

4. Instruct the postoperative patient to splint the incision site when inhaling. Assist the patient when necessary.

5. Then instruct the patient in the following steps for therapy

   a. Hold the spirometer in an upright position or place on a flat surface.

   b. Place the mouthpiece in the mouth and keep lips sealed tight.

   c. After a normal exhalation, inhale slowly and as deeply as possible (inspiratory capacity). Hold the breath for 3 to 5 s, then remove the mouthpiece and exhale normally.

   d. Rest and breathe normally for approximately 30 s.

   e. Repeat the maneuver 8 to 10 times per waking hour.

6. Document the procedure and the patient response to therapy in the patient chart.

7. Evaluate the patient periodically to ensure that a proper breathing technique is being used.

E. **Incentive Spirometry Devices**

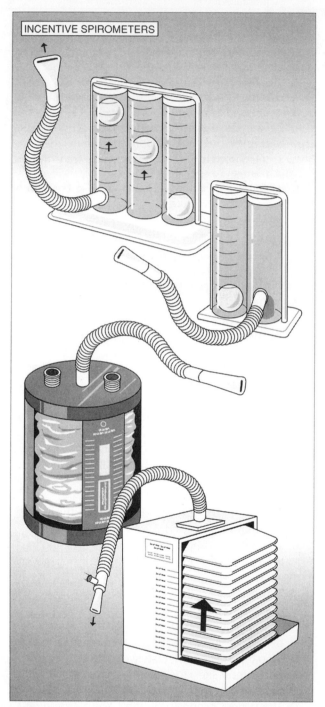

FIGURE 7-5

POSTCHAPTER STUDY QUESTIONS

1. List five physiologic effects of IPPB.
2. List seven indications for IPPB.
3. List eight hazards of IPPB.
4. List two absolute contraindications to IPPB.
5. The pulse rate must not exceed how many beats/min before the treatment must be terminated?
6. What effect does an increased airway resistance have on delivered VT on a pressure-limited IPPB machine?
7. What effect does an increased lung compliance have on the delivered VT on a pressure-limited IPPB machine?
8. How does a decreased lung compliance affect inspiratory time?
9. List ways to help correct a situation in which the patient has difficulty cycling the IPPB machine into the expiratory phase.
10. How should an IPPB treatment be modified for a patient with a closed head injury?
11. Incentive spirometry is indicated if a patient can obtain a vital capacity of what level?
12. What is another term used for incentive spirometry?
13. List three requirements necessary for incentive spirometry to be effective.

See answers at the back of the text.

BIBLIOGRAPHY

Cairo JM, Pilbeam S: *Mosby's respiratory care equipment*, ed 8, St Louis, 2009, Mosby.

Hess D et al.: *Respiratory care principles and practice*, ed 1, Philadelphia, 2002, Saunders.

Wilkins RL, Stoller JK, Kacmarek R: *Egan's fundamentals of respiratory care*, ed 9, St Louis, 2009, Mosby.

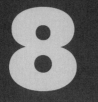
BRONCHOPULMONARY HYGIENE TECHNIQUES

PRETEST QUESTIONS

Answer the pretest questions before studying the chapter. This will help you determine your strong and weak areas in the material covered.

1. Postural drainage and percussion are not indicated in which of the following conditions?

    A. Bronchiectasis
    B. Cystic fibrosis
    C. Pulmonary edema
    D. Acute atelectasis

2. In which of the following airway clearance techniques is the patient instructed to alter VT in three phases before a cough effort?

    A. Intrapulmonary percussive ventilation
    B. Autogenic lung drainage
    C. Positive expiratory pressure (PEP) therapy
    D. Chest percussion or vibration

3. The respiratory care practitioner receives an order for postural drainage on a patient to mobilize secretions from the anterior segment of the right upper lobe of the lung. How should the patient be positioned for the lung to drain most effectively?

    A. Patient lying supine with pillows under the knees
    B. Patient lying on right side in Trendelenburg position
    C. Patient lying on stomach in Trendelenburg position
    D. Patient lying on left side, rotated back 25 degrees, with the bed flat

4. A 34-year-old patient using a 40% aerosol mask has right lower lobe pneumonia. He becomes short of breath and his SpO$_2$ decreases from 96% to 89% when lying on his right side. What should the respiratory therapist recommend?

    A. Increase the O$_2$ to 80%
    B. Place the patient on his left side
    C. Have the patient begin using CPAP
    D. Suction the patient

See answers and rationales at the back of the text

REVIEW

I. **CHEST PHYSICAL THERAPY**
   CRT Exam Content Matrix: IIA14a, IIIA1a-b, IIIC1a, IIIC4, IIIF1, IIIF2f1-2
   RRT Exam Content Matrix: IIIA1a-b, IIIC1a, IIIF1

   A. Chest physical therapy (CPT) is a variety of techniques aimed at the mobilization of pulmonary secretions and promotion of greater use of the respiratory muscles, which should result in an increase in the distribution of ventilation.
      Techniques included in CPT are
      1. Postural drainage
      2. Chest percussion
      3. Chest vibration
      4. Cough techniques
      5. Breathing exercises (see Chapter 15 on respiratory home care)

   B. **Goals of CPT**
      1. To prevent the accumulation of pulmonary secretions
      2. To improve the mobilization of retained secretions
      3. To improve the distribution of ventilation
      4. To decrease airway resistance

   C. **Indications for CPT**
      1. Lung conditions that cause increased difficulty in mobilizing pulmonary secretions
         a. Bronchiectasis
         b. Cystic fibrosis

> ☑ **Exam Note**
>
> CPT is indicated for patients who produce more than **30 mL of secretions per day** and have difficulty clearing them from the airway.

---

   2. Acute respiratory failure with retained pulmonary secretions
   3. Acute atelectasis
   4. Ventilation and perfusion abnormalities resulting from retained pulmonary secretions
   5. Inefficient breathing patterns in patients with COPD

6. Prevention of postoperative respiratory complications

D. **Contraindications for CPT**
1. Patients with ICP greater than 20 mm Hg
2. Recent spinal surgery or injury
3. Head and neck injury (until stabilized)
4. Active hemoptysis
5. Empyema
6. Bronchopleural fistula
7. Rib fractures
8. Pulmonary edema associated with congestive heart failure
9. Large pleural effusions
10. Tube feeding or recent meal
11. Subcutaneous emphysema
12. Pulmonary tuberculosis
13. Lung contusion
14. Osteoporosis

E. **Postural Drainage Positions**

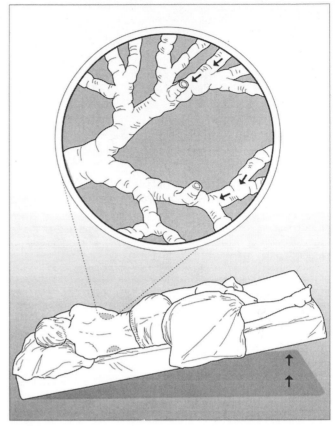

FIGURE 8-2   Position to drain the lateral basal segment of the lower lobe of the lung.

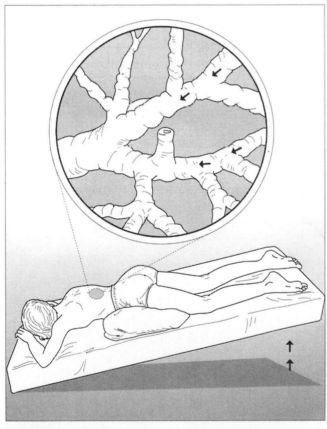

FIGURE 8-1   Position to drain the posterior basal segment of the lower lobe of the lung.

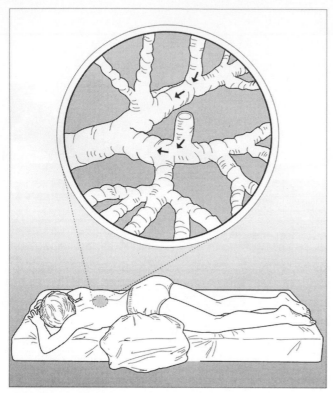

FIGURE 8-3 Position to drain the superior segment of the lower lobe of the lung.

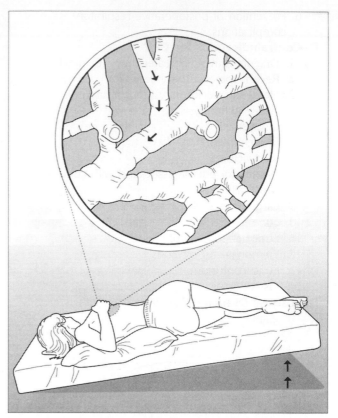

FIGURE 8-5 Position to drain the lateral and medial segments of the right middle lobe of the lung.

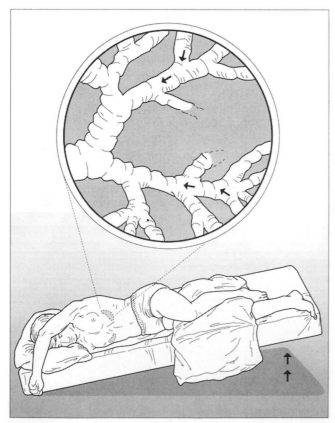

FIGURE 8-4 Position to drain the anterior basal segment of the lower lobe of the lung.

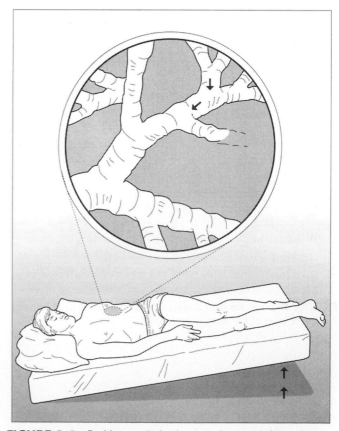

FIGURE 8-6 Position to drain the superior and inferior lingular segments of the left lung.

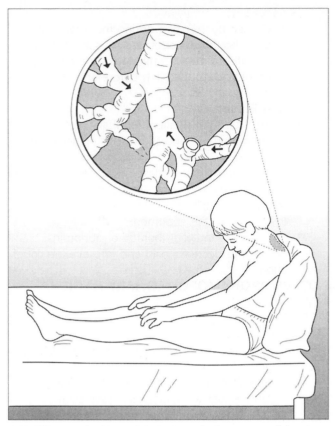

FIGURE 8-7   Position to drain the apical segment of the upper lobe of the lung.

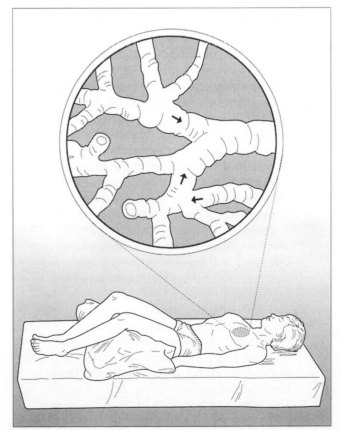

FIGURE 8-8   Position to drain the anterior segment of the upper lobe of the lung.

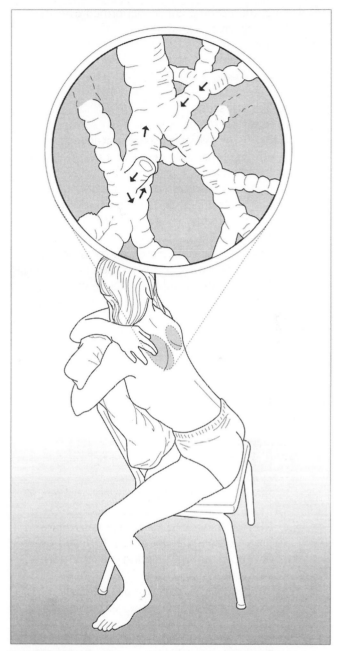

FIGURE 8-9   Position to drain the posterior segment of the upper lobe of the lung.

F. **Percussion**
   1. A means of improving the mobilization of pulmonary secretions by manually striking the chest wall with a cupped hand or placing a mechanical percussor on the chest wall. Both of these techniques are generally performed with the patient in postural drainage positions.
   2. Mechanical percussors operate on either compressed air or electricity and are thought to be more effective than manual hand percussion.
   3. Percussion should be performed over each specified area for 2 to 5 min.

4. Percussion should not be performed over the following areas
   a. Spine
   b. Sternum
   c. Scapulae
   d. Clavicles
   e. Surgical sites
   f. Areas of trauma
   g. Bare skin: Although some practitioners advocate manually percussing over bare skin, the energy wave produced by the air trapped under the hand is not significantly reduced by a light covering, such as a hospital gown.
   h. Female breasts

G. **Vibration**
   1. For manual vibration, place one hand on top of the other over a specified lung segment, and with a vibrating motion, apply moderate pressure.
   2. Instruct the patient to take a deep breath, and apply vibration during exhalation.
   3. Mechanical vibrators may be used; place the vibrator attachment over specified areas. Do not apply the vibrator to one area for more than 45 to 60 s at a time.
   4. Vibration helps to mobilize retained pulmonary secretions.

H. **Complications of CPT**
   1. Hypoxemia
      a. Especially in patients with COPD or cardiac disease or in obese patients.
      b. Modification of drainage position makes CPT more tolerable for these patients.
      c. May be minimized by administration of a bronchodilating agent before CPT and delivery of supplemental O_2 during the treatment.
   2. Rib fractures
      a. Caused from overly vigorous percussion.
      b. Most common in neonates and elderly patients.
   3. Increased airway resistance
      a. Patient should be instructed to cough periodically throughout the treatment.
      b. Suction equipment should be readily available for patients having difficulty expectorating secretions.
   4. Increased ICP
      a. Patients with head trauma should not be placed in the Trendelenburg (head down) position.
      b. Increased ICP may result from prolonged coughing during CPT.
   5. Hemorrhage
   6. Decreased cardiac output
      a. Often the result of positional hypotension.
      b. Check heart rate periodically during the treatment.

7. Aspiration
   a. Caused by vomiting during the treatment.
   b. CPT should be performed no sooner than 1 h after a meal. Continuous tube feedings should be stopped 1 h before and during treatment.

I. **Cough Technique**
   1. Instruct the sitting patient to inhale deeply through the nose and to hold his or her breath for 3 to 5 s.
   2. Instruct the patient to clasp his or her arms across the abdomen and produce two to three sharp coughs without taking a breath, while pressing the arms into the abdomen.
   3. Use a pillow to splint thoracic or abdominal incisions to decrease pain and improve the cough effort.

II. **OTHER BRONCHOPULMONARY HYGIENE TECHNIQUES**
CRT Exam Content Matrix: IIA14b-c, IIIA1a-b, IIIC1d, IIIC4, IIIF2f1-2
RRT Exam Content Matrix: IIIA1a-b, IIIC1d, IIIC14

A. **Autogenic Drainage**
   1. Autogenic drainage is a modified coughing technique that is comparable in secretion clearance to postural drainage and percussion techniques.
   2. Place the patient in a sitting position and instruct him or her to use a breathing pattern that varies lung volume and expiratory flow in three different phases.
      a. Phase 1: From the resting expiratory level, the patient takes the deepest breath possible (inspiratory capacity maneuver) followed by breathing at low lung volumes for several breaths.
      b. Phase 2: The patient increases VT to low to middle volumes for several breaths. (These breaths are slightly larger the than normal VT.)
      c. Phase 3: The patient then increases VT to moderate volumes for several breaths. After this phase is completed, instruct the patient to cough.
   3. This type of breathing pattern helps loosen secretions and moves them into larger airways so that they may be mobilized with an effective cough.
   4. This technique has shown some promise in patients with cystic fibrosis. It appears to mobilize secretions in a way comparable to postural drainage and percussion but without the degree of O_2 desaturation, and it is tolerated better in these patients.
   5. This technique is difficult to teach the patient, which can pose a problem because it is taught for the patient's independent use.

B. **Intrapulmonary Percussive Ventilation**
 1. This airway clearance technique uses a pneumatic ventilator to deliver a series of small VTs at high frequency (110 to 225 cycles/min).
 2. The length of each percussive cycle is controlled by either the practitioner or the patient using a thumb control button.
 3. These pressurized bursts of gas are delivered to the patient via a mouthpiece. Bronchodilating or mucolytic agents may be administered through a pneumatic nebulizer during this 15- to 20-min treatment.
 4. The pulsed gas flow is as effective in breaking up secretions for easier mobilization as postural drainage and percussion are in patients with cystic fibrosis.
 5. This procedure has an advantage over conventional CPT in that fatigue and practitioner technique are not a factor.

C. **High-Frequency Chest Wall Oscillation**
 1. High-frequency chest wall oscillation (HFCWO) is a technique to improve sputum clearance from the airways.
 2. An inflatable vest is wrapped around the patient's chest and is attached to an air-pulse generator, which intermittently injects small volumes of air into the vest and then ejects them out at a high rate. This creates oscillatory movement that helps mobilize secretions.
 3. The duration of therapy is usually about 30 min, and an oscillation frequency of between 5 and 25 Hz (300 to 1500 cycles/min) is used.
 4. This technique has not yet been proven to be as effective as postural drainage or percussion in patients with cystic fibrosis.

D. **PEP Therapy**
 1. PEP is a bronchial hygiene therapy used in the management of airway secretions and postoperative atelectasis.
 2. It is becoming increasingly popular as an alternative to CPT and incentive spirometry, especially in pediatric patients with cystic fibrosis and bronchiectasis.
 3. It is also effective in preventing postoperative atelectasis by opening airways and improving gas exchange.
 4. PEP is achieved by having the patient exhale through a mask or mouthpiece with a resistance valve. The valve creates back pressure into the patient's airway. Different sizes of resistors or adjustable resistors are used to increase or decrease the amount of PEP. **Generally, PEP levels of 10 to 20 cm H₂O are used.**

5. **Therapeutic effects of PEP**
 a. Improved distribution of inspired volume in the lung by means of collateral air channels (pores of Kohn).
 b. Prevention of expiratory airway collapse.
 c. Generation of pressure on exhalation in an area distal to the site of mucus obstruction.

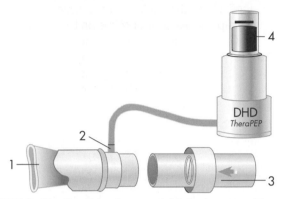

FIGURE 8-10 Example of commercial single-use positive expiratory pressure (PEP) device (DHD TheraPEP). *1*, Mouthpiece; *2*, pressure tap; *3*, one-way inlet valve; *4*, pressure generator. From Wilkins RL, Stoller JK, Kacmarek R, et al: *Egan's fundamentals of respiratory care,* ed 9, St Louis, 2009, Mosby.

6. **Contraindications to PEP**
 a. Acute sinusitis
 b. Middle ear infection
 c. Epistaxis (nose bleed)
 d. Recent facial, oral, or skull injury or surgery
 e. Active hemoptysis

7. **Steps in performing PEP mask therapy**
 a. Assemble equipment and select appropriate expiratory resistor (10 to 20 cm H₂O)
 b. Position the patient sitting up with elbows resting on the table; apply the mask tightly (to prevent leaks) over the nose and mouth.
 c. Instruct the patient to inhale a larger-than-normal volume but not quite as deep as possible and then actively exhale but not forcefully; expiration should last two to three times longer than inspiration.
 d. The patient should perform 10 to 20 of these PEP breaths, and then remove the mask and perform two to three "huff" coughs, also referred to as the forced expiratory technique (FET), which requires forceful exhaling from a middle to low lung volume with an open glottis. This is very effective for secretion clearance.
 e. The patient should cough normally to mobilize secretions.
 f. The procedure is repeated four to six times per session.

8. PEP therapy may be an effective alternative to postural drainage and percussion and has the added benefit that the patient can perform this

simple task independently with fewer side effects.

9. PEP therapy may also be combined with aerosolized bronchodilator therapy if a nebulizer or an inhaler is attached to the one-way inspiratory valve of the PEP device.

10. If the pressure being used appears to be ineffective while assessing the patient during therapy, increase the PEP level by 3 to 5 cm H_2O and continue to monitor.

E. Flutter Valve

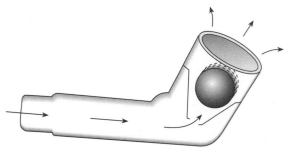

FIGURE 8-11 Flutter valve. From Wilkins RL, Stoller JK, Kacmarek R: *Egan's fundamentals of respiratory care,* ed 9, St Louis, 2009, Mosby.

1. The flutter valve is a pipe-shaped oscillatory PEP device (see diagram) through which the patient exhales to produce a PEP of between 10 and 25 cm H_2O. The angle at which this device is held will determine the PEP. The more upright the flutter is held, the higher the PEP generated back down the airway.

2. Instruct the patient to inhale slowly, just a bit more than a normal breath (not totally filling the lungs), and hold the breath for 2 to 3 s. The patient should then exhale reasonably fast, but not forcefully, through the flutter device, which causes a stainless steel ball to be pushed up into the angled portion of the device to produce PEP. The angle causes the ball to oscillate, or "flutter," up and down. The oscillations are transmitted down the respiratory tract, creating vibrations that result in mobilization of secretions.

3. This technique should be repeated 5 to 10 times to help loosen secretions and should be followed by coughing to aid in the removal of sputum. The treatment should last 5 to 15 min.

4. The effectiveness of the device is controversial, but some studies have shown improved secretion clearance in patients with cystic fibrosis.

5. The flutter valve may be disassembled after each use and rinsed in tap water and dried before reassembly. In the home, the device should be cleaned every 2 days in a soap solution and disinfected at regular intervals; it should be soaked in a 1:3 solution of white vinegar and water for 15 min, dried, and reassembled for future use.

F. Acapella Oscillatory PEP Device

1. The acapella combines the characteristics of a PEP valve and a flutter valve.

2. It uses a counterweighted plug and magnet that directs the patient's exhaled air through a pivoting cone to generate vibrations down the tracheobronchial tree. The PEP level and vibration frequency may be adjusted to meet the patient's clinical needs.

☑ Exam Note

Autogenic drainage, intrapulmonary percussive ventilation, HFCWO, PEP therapy, and flutter valve therapy should all be considered as effective alternatives to chest percussion and postural drainage for patients with secretion management problems caused by cystic fibrosis or bronchiectasis. These therapies may also be beneficial for patients who cannot tolerate postural drainage and percussion.

POSTCHAPTER STUDY QUESTIONS

1. What is the most appropriate pressure range for PEP therapy?
2. What is the range of pressure used for flutter valve therapy?
3. What types of patients seem to benefit the most from intrapulmonary percussive ventilation?
4. Intrapulmonary percussive ventilation, flutter valve therapy, and PEP therapy may be alternatives for what other popular therapy?
5. List five complications of CPT.
6. To drain the posterior basal segment of the lower lobe of the lung, how should the respiratory care practitioner position the patient? *prone head down*
7. List four contraindications to PEP therapy.

See answers at the back of the text.

BIBLIOGRAPHY

Cairo JM, Pilbeam S, *Mosby's respiratory care equipment,* ed 7, St Louis, 2004, Mosby.

Hess D et al, *Respiratory care principles and practice,* ed 1, Philadelphia, 2002, Saunders.

Wilkins RL, Stoller JK, Kacmarek R, et al: *Egan's fundamentals of respiratory care,* ed 9, St Louis, 2009, Mosby.

CARDIAC MONITORING

Answer the pretest questions before studying the chapter. This will help you determine your strong and weak areas in the material covered.

1. Which statement about the P wave on an ECG is *FALSE?*

   A. It represents atrial depolarization.
   B. It is a positive wave on the graph.
   C. Normal duration time is 0.06 to 0.10 s.
   D. It represents ventricular repolarization.

2. Artifacts found on an ECG may be caused by which of the following?

   1. **Electrical interference at the bedside.**
   2. **Poor electrode contact with the skin.**
   3. **Excessive movement of the patient.**

   A. 1 only
   B. 2 only
   C. 1 and 3 only
   D. 1, 2, and 3

3. In which of the following cardiac arrhythmias is the QRS complex abnormally shaped as well as wider than normal?

   A. Sinus tachycardia
   B. Premature ventricular contractions (PVCs)
   C. Atrial fibrillation
   D. Premature atrial contractions (PACs)

4. A patient with a blood pressure of 110/50 mm Hg and a pulse rate of 75 beats/min has which of the following pulse pressures?

   A. 40 mm Hg
   B. 50 mm Hg
   C. 60 mm Hg
   D. 70 mm Hg

5. A weak pulse is detected distal to the arterial catheter in a patient. This is indicative of which of the following?

   A. Infection
   B. Hemorrhage
   C. Thrombosis
   D. Tachycardia

6. Which of the following conditions results in a decreased central venous pressure (CVP) reading?

   1. **Hypovolemia**
   2. **Vasoconstriction**
   3. **Air bubbles in the CVP line**

   A. 1 only
   B. 2 only
   C. 1 and 2 only
   D. 1 and 3 only

See answers and rationales at the back of the text.

I. **ELECTROCARDIOGRAPHY**
   CRT Exam Content Matrix: IA8a, IB9a, IB10a, IIA17-18
   RRT Exam Content Matrix: IA8a, IB9a, IB10a
   A. **Electrical Conduction of the Heart**
      1. The sinoatrial (SA) node is the pacemaker of the heart; it usually initiates about 75 impulses/min.
      2. Once an impulse has been initiated by the SA node, the impulse travels down to the AV node.
      3. From the AV node, the impulse travels on to the bundle of His, located in the interventricular septum.
      4. The bundle of His divides into the right and left bundle branches, which deliver the impulses to the right and left sides of the heart.
      5. The bundle branches divide even further into the Purkinje fibers, which send the impulse to individual muscle fibers of the ventricles, which causes ventricular contraction.
      6. Once the SA node sends an impulse, the conduction system depolarizes, sending the impulse through the conduction system to the heart muscle, which depolarizes and contracts. After contraction, repolarization occurs, and the

heart is in a resting state, called **_diastole._** The term used for the heart in contraction is **_systole._**

B. **ECG Leads.** Through the use of various numbers of electrodes (leads) placed on the patient's body, the electrical activity of the heart can be monitored. The device to which the electrodes are attached is the **electrocardiograph**. The electrical activity of the heart recorded on graph paper is called the **electrocardiogram** and may be displayed continuously on an ECG monitor, called an **oscilloscope.**

C. **Standard 12-Lead ECG Has Three-Lead Systems**
1. Standard limb leads (three leads) (+, positive pole; −, negative pole)
   a. The leads are placed on the right arm, left arm, and left leg.
   b. **Limb lead I** measures the electrical potential between the right arm (−) and left arm (+).
   c. **Limb lead II** measures the electrical potential between the right arm (−) and left leg (+).
   d. **Limb lead III** measures the electrical potential between the left arm (−) and the left leg (+).
   e. A ground is placed on the right leg.
2. Augmented leads (three leads)
   a. The same electrodes used in the standard leads are used for augmented lead composition but in different combinations.
   b. **Lead aVR:** Leads are connected to right arm (+), left arm, and left leg. The right arm is the positive electrode and records electrical activity from the direction of the right arm.
   c. **Lead aVL:** Leads are connected to left arm (+), right arm, and left leg. The left arm is the positive electrode and views the electrical activity from the direction of the left arm.
   d. **Lead aVF:** Leads are connected to left leg (+), right arm, and left arm. The left leg is the positive electrode and views the electrical activity from the direction of the bottom of the heart.
3. Precordial (chest) leads (six leads)
   a. **Lead 1 (V_1):** positioned at the **fourth** intercostal space at the **right** border of the sternum
   b. **Lead 2 (V_2):** positioned at the **fourth** intercostal space at the **left** border of the sternum
   c. **Lead 3 (V_3):** positioned in a straight line between lead 2 and lead 4
   d. **Lead 4 (V_4):** positioned at the midclavicular line and at the **fifth** intercostal space
   e. **Lead 5 (V_5):** positioned at the anterior axillary line, level with lead 4 horizontally
   f. **Lead 6 (V_6):** positioned at the midaxillary line, level with lead 4 and 5 horizontally

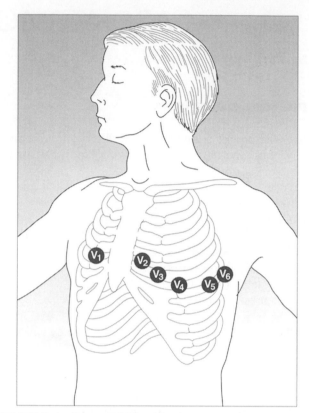

FIGURE 9-1 Precordial (chest) leads.

> ☑ **Exam Note**
>
> The 12-lead ECG is not normally used for long-term ECG monitoring, such as that seen in the intensive care unit (ICU) or coronary care unit (CCU).

D. **Long-Term ECG Monitoring**
1. Lead placements (three leads)
   a. The first electrode is placed on the upper right side of the chest (−).
   b. The second electrode is placed on the lower left side of the chest (+).
   c. The third electrode is used as a ground and may be attached to any location that is convenient.
2. To obtain a clear ECG reading, there must be good skin contact with the electrode; otherwise, artifacts will appear. An electrode gel is used to improve conduction. Hair should be shaved from the chest if an electrode is to be attached in that area. Other causes of artifacts are electrical interference and excessive movement of the patient.

E. ECG Graph Paper

1. The ECG paper is made up of very small squares, which represent 0.04 s horizontally and 0.5 mV vertically (voltage axis).
2. So that counting time is easier, there is a darkened line at every fifth small square; from one darkened line to the next is 0.20 s (0.04 s × 5 squares).
3. Most ECG paper has short vertical lines at the top to designate 3-s intervals, which makes it easier to calculate the heart rate.

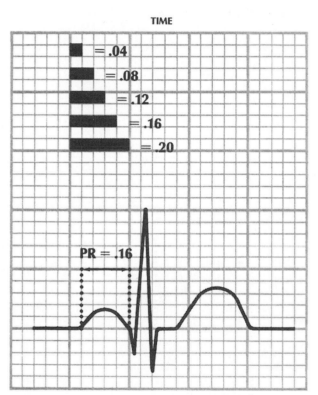

FIGURE 9-2 Normal electrocardiographic (ECG) pattern. From Davis D: *Differential diagnosis of arrhythmias,* ed 2, Philadelphia, 1997, Saunders.

F. Normal ECG Pattern: The ECG strip shows a baseline and positive and negative deflections from it.

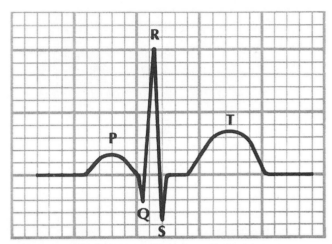

FIGURE 9-3 One cardiac cycle. From Davis D: *Differential diagnosis of arrhythmias,* ed 2, Philadelphia, 1997, Saunders.

G. **ECG Waves:** One cardiac cycle consists of a series of waves, represented by the letters P, Q, R, S, and T.

1. **P wave**
   a. Positive wave
   b. **Represents atrial depolarization (contraction)**
   c. Duration: 0.06 to 0.10 s
2. **Q wave**
   a. Negative wave that follows the P wave
   b. May be absent even in healthy people
3. **R wave**
   a. Positive wave that follows the Q wave
4. **S wave**
   a. Negative wave that follows the R wave
5. **QRS complex**
   a. **Represents ventricular depolarization (contraction).** Atrial repolarization occurs during the QRS complex and therefore is not seen on the ECG.
   b. Duration: 0.06 to 0.12 s

c. **Widened QRS seen in right bundle-branch block**

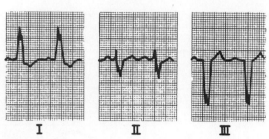

I   II   III

FIGURE 9-4 Electrocardiographic (ECG) tracing showing the widened QRS complex. From Levitsky MG, Cairo JN, Hall SM: *Introduction to respiratory care,* Philadelphia, 1990, Saunders.

6. **T wave**
   a. Positive wave
   b. Represents ventricular repolarization
   c. **Inverted (negative wave) T waves** indicate the presence of coronary artery disease.

7. **PR interval**
   a. Measured from the beginning of the P wave to the beginning of the Q wave.
   b. Represents the time it takes for the impulse to travel from the SA node through the AV node.
   c. Duration: 0.12 to 0.20 s
   d. May be prolonged in first- and second-degree heart block

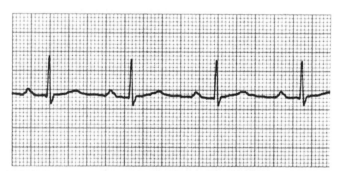

FIGURE 9-5 Electrocardiographic (ECG) tracing showing a prolonged PR interval. From Davis D: *Differential diagnosis of arrhythmias,* ed 2, Philadelphia, 1997, Saunders.

8. **ST segment**
   a. Measured from the end of the S wave to the beginning of the T wave
   b. Measures the time that is required for ventricular repolarization to begin
   c. The ST segment may be elevated above the baseline or depressed below the baseline. This is an indication of **cardiac ischemia.** Cardiac ischemia results from a decreased amount of oxygenated blood delivered to the left ventricle because of narrowed coronary arteries. If the blood supply is not restored, ventricular muscle

may die; this is called **infarction. ST segment elevation or depression is a sign of coronary artery disease.**

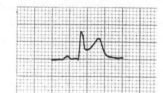

FIGURE 9-6 Electrocardiographic (ECG) tracing showing ST segment depression. From Davis D: *Differential diagnosis of arrhythmias,* ed 2, Philadelphia, 1997, Saunders.

H. **Normal Heart Rhythm**

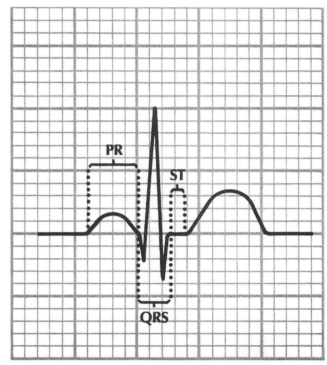

FIGURE 9-7 Normal heart rhythm. From Davis D: *Differential diagnosis of arrhythmias,* ed 2, Philadelphia, 1997, Saunders.

1. Atrial depolarization (contraction) is represented on the ECG as the P wave.

Blood supply to the heart is supplied by two main arteries: the right and left coronary arteries, which originate from the aorta. The right coronary artery extends down to feed the right ventricle and then separates into several branches. The left coronary artery divides into two major branches: the circumflex branch, which feeds the upper lateral wall of the left atrium and left ventricle, and the left anterior descending branch (anterior interventricular artery), which feeds the anterior portion of the heart.

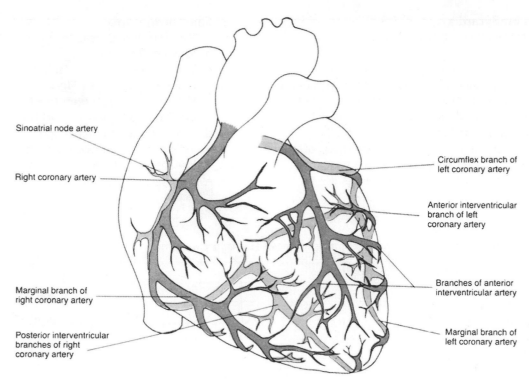

Sinoatrial node artery

Right coronary artery

Marginal branch of
right coronary artery

Posterior interventricular
branches of right
coronary artery

Circumflex branch of
left coronary artery

Anterior interventricular
branch of left
coronary artery

Branches of anterior
interventricular artery

Marginal branch of
left coronary artery

FIGURE 9-8   Primary and secondary arteries in the heart. From O'Toole M, editor: *Miller-Keane encyclopedia and dictionary of medicine, nursing, and allied health,* revised revision, Philadelphia, 2005, Saunders.

2. Cardiac impulse travels to the AV node, bundle of His, and the Purkinje fibers, which are represented on the ECG as the PR interval.
3. Cardiac impulse reaches muscles in the ventricles, causing ventricular depolarization (contraction), which is represented on the ECG as the QRS complex.
4. Ventricular repolarization is represented on the ECG as the ST segment and T wave.
I. **Basic Steps to ECG Interpretation**
1. **Calculate heart rate**
   a. As mentioned, most ECG paper has 3-s intervals marked off at the top of the paper. **Count the number of R waves in a 6-s period and multiply by 10 to obtain the number of beats/minute.**
   b. Normal rate: 60 to 100 beats/min
   c. Bradycardia: less than 60 beats/min
   d. Tachycardia: more than 100 beats/min
2. **Determine regularity of the rhythm**
   a. Using calipers, measure the distance between a pair of R waves. Leave the calipers at that distance, and measure the next pair of R waves to determine whether the distance is the same.
   b. Continue measuring the distance between successive pairs of R waves to determine

whether it is constant. If the distances remain constant, the rhythm is regular.
3. **Observe P waves and PR interval**
   a. Make sure that there is a P wave before every QRS complex and that they are of the same shape.
   b. Using calipers, measure several PR intervals to determine whether they are consistent.
   c. As stated earlier, the normal PR interval is 0.12 to 0.20 s. If the PR interval is longer than 0.20 s, first-degree heart block is present.
4. **Determine length of the QRS complex**
   a. Remember, the QRS complex represents the time it takes for ventricular depolarization to occur. The normal QRS complex takes 0.06 to 0.12 s; any longer duration would indicate heart block.

☑ **Exam Note**

If all the above observations are within normal limits, the ECG shows normal sinus rhythm.

J. **Cardiac Arrhythmias:** most often encountered by RCPs

1. **Sinus bradycardia**
   a. Rate: less than 60 beats/min
   b. Rhythm: regular
   c. Wave pattern abnormalities: none
   d. Cause: stimulation of vagus nerve (e.g., during tracheal suctioning), hypothermia, increased ICP; sinus bradycardia may be normal in well-conditioned athletes.
   e. Treatment: If accompanied by shortness of breath, hypotension, or abnormal beats, atropine is used; a pacemaker may also be indicated.

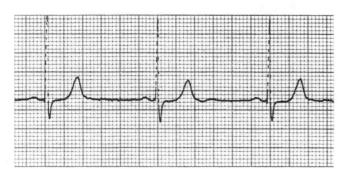

FIGURE 9-9 Sinus bradycardia. From Davis D: *Differential diagnosis of arrhythmias,* ed 2, Philadelphia, 1997, Saunders.

2. **Sinus tachycardia**
   a. Rate: 100 to 160 beats/min
   b. Rhythm: regular
   c. Wave pattern abnormalities: none
   d. Cause: hypoxemia, increased sympathetic nervous system stimulation (e.g., fear, anxiety), medication
   e. Treatment: stop underlying cause; administration of digitalis or beta blockers

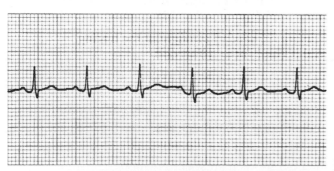

FIGURE 9-10 Sinus tachycardia. From Davis D: *Differential diagnosis of arrhythmias,* ed 2, Philadelphia, 1997, Saunders.

3. **Sinus arrhythmia**
   a. Rate: 60 to 100 beats/min
   b. Rhythm: irregular
   c. Wave pattern abnormalities: R to R cycles vary more than 0.16 s. **In Figure 9-11, note how the distance between the R wave of the QRS complex varies and is inconsistent.**
   d. Cause: none; normal in young, healthy individuals; heart rate may increase during inspiration and decrease during expiration.
   e. Treatment: none necessary

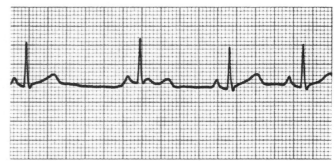

FIGURE 9-11 Sinus arrhythmia. From Davis D: *Differential diagnosis of arrhythmias,* ed 2, Philadelphia, 1997, Saunders.

4. **Premature Atrial Contraction**
   a. Rate: 60 to 100 beats/min. **Less than 6 PACs per minute is considered a minor arrhythmia; more than 6 PACs per minute is considered major arrhythmia.**
   b. Rhythm: regular, except for PAC
   c. Wave pattern abnormalities: the premature P wave looks different than the sinus P wave; the PAC occurs sooner than the next beat would be expected.
   d. Cause: atrial irritability caused by organic heart disease, CNS disturbances, sympathomimetic drugs, tobacco, caffeine
   e. Treatment: if more than 6 PACs per minute, lidocaine may be used

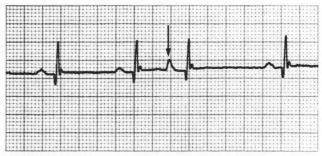

FIGURE 9-12 Premature atrial contraction (PAC). From Davis D: *Differential diagnosis of arrhythmias,* ed 2, Philadelphia, 1997, Saunders.

5. **Premature Ventricular Contraction**
   a. Rate: 60 to 100 beats/min; less than 6 PVCs per minute is considered minor and more than 6 PVCs per minute is considered major.
   b. Rhythm: regular, except for PVCs

> **Exam Note**
>
> When every other beat is a PVC, the arrhythmia is termed **bigeminy**, which is considered a dangerous arrhythmia.

   c. Wave pattern abnormalities: the shape of the QRS complex is abnormal and wider than 0.12 s.
   d. Cause: ventricular irritability caused by hypoxia, acid–base disturbances, electrolyte abnormalities, excessive dose of digitalis, CHF, myocardial inflammation, coronary artery disease
   e. Treatment: lidocaine IV or other antiarrhythmia drugs, such as procainamide or propranolol if more than 6 PVCs per minute

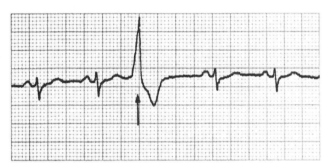

FIGURE 9-13 Premature ventricular contraction (PVC). From Davis D: *Differential diagnosis of arrhythmias,* ed 2, Philadelphia, 1997, Saunders.

6. **Atrial fibrillation**
   a. Rate: variable; atrial rate greater than 350 beats/min
   b. Rhythm: irregular
   c. Wave pattern abnormalities: P waves cannot be distinguished and have an uneven baseline; PR interval is also indistinguishable.

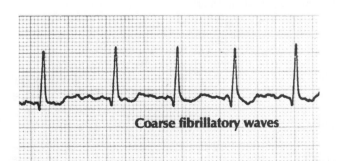

Coarse fibrillatory waves

FIGURE 9-14 Atrial fibrillation. From Davis D: *Differential diagnosis of arrhythmias,* ed 2, Philadelphia, 1997, Saunders.

   d. Cause: hypoxia, arteriosclerotic heart disease, mitral stenosis, valvular heart disease
   e. Treatment: cardioversion, propranolol, digitalis

> **Exam Note**
>
> Atrial fibrillation is considered to be a major arrhythmia, whereby the atria fail to pump blood adequately to the ventricles, which results in a significant decrease in cardiac output.

7. **Atrial flutter**
   a. Rate: atrial, 200 to 400 beats/min; ventricular, 60 to 150 beats/min
   b. Rhythm: regular or irregular
   c. Wave pattern abnormalities: P waves have a characteristic sawtooth pattern and thus are often referred to as "F" waves
   d. Cause: hypoxia, arteriosclerotic heart disease, MI, rheumatic heart disease
   e. Treatment: cardioversion, carotid artery massage, procainamide, digitalis, tranquilizers

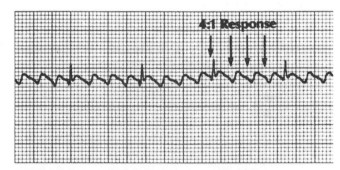

4:1 Response

FIGURE 9-15 Atrial flutter. From Davis D: *Differential diagnosis of arrhythmias,* ed 2, Philadelphia, 1997, Saunders.

> Atrial flutter is an arrhythmia that results in blockade of atrial impulses in what is called a 2:1, 3:1, or 4:1 block. In a 2:1 block, there are two atrial impulses for each ventricular beat, and there are three or four impulses to each ventricular beat in a 3:1 or 4:1 block, respectively.

8. **Ventricular tachycardia (lethal)**
   a. Rate: 140 to 200 beats/min
   b. Rhythm: regular
   c. Wave pattern abnormalities: P waves and PR intervals are absent or hidden in the QRS complex; each QRS is wider than normal and is a run of three or more PVCs.
   d. Cause: arteriosclerotic heart disease, coronary artery disease, myocardial ischemia, mitral valve prolapse, hypertensive heart disease
   e. Treatment: lidocaine, defibrillation, CPR

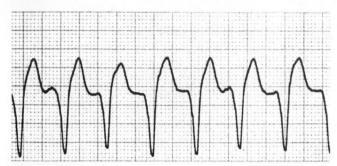

FIGURE 9-16 Ventricular tachycardia (lethal). From Davis D: *Differential diagnosis of arrhythmias,* ed 2, Philadelphia, 1997, Saunders.

9. **Ventricular fibrillation (lethal)**
   a. Rate: cannot be determined
   b. Rhythm: cannot be determined
   c. Wave pattern abnormalities: no distinguishable waves
   d. Cause: coronary artery disease, hypertensive heart disease, acute MI, digitalis overdose
   e. Treatment: defibrillation, CPR. If this arrhythmia is not reversed, death soon results because there is essentially no blood being pumped out of the heart.

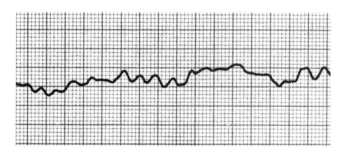

FIGURE 9-17 Ventricular fibrillation (lethal). From Davis D: *Differential diagnosis of arrhythmias,* ed 2, Philadelphia, 1997, Saunders.

10. **First-degree heart block**
    a. Rate: 60 to 100 beats/min
    b. Rhythm: regular
    c. Wave pattern abnormalities: PR interval longer than 0.20 s

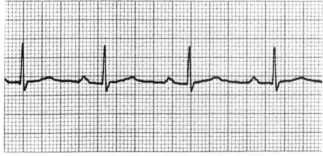

FIGURE 9-18 First-degree heart block. From Davis D: *Differential diagnosis of arrhythmias,* ed 2, Philadelphia, 1997, Saunders.

   d. Cause: complication of digoxin or beta blockers, ischemia of the AV node
   e. Treatment: atropine, isoproterenol

11. **Second-degree heart block**
    a. Rate: 60 to 100 beats/min
    b. Rhythm: regular or irregular
    c. Wave pattern abnormalities: the QRS complex is normal but may be preceded by two to four P waves.
    d. Cause: myocardial ischemia; may be a progression from first-degree block
    e. Treatment: isoproterenol, atropine; pacemaker

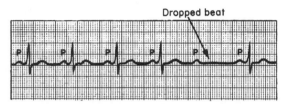

FIGURE 9-19 Second-degree heart block. Electrocardiographic (ECG) tracing showing the widened QRS complex. From Levitsky MG, Cairo JN, Hall SM: *Introduction to respiratory care,* Philadelphia, 1990, Saunders.

12. **Third-degree heart block**
    a. Rate: atrial rate, normal; ventricular rate, less than 40 beat s/min
    b. Rhythm: Atrial and ventricular rhythm are regular but are independent of each other.
    c. Wave pattern abnormalities: PR interval cannot be determined; QRS complex may be normal or widened.
    d. Cause: myocardial ischemia, AV node damage
    e. Treatment: pacemaker

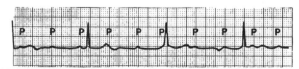

FIGURE 9-20 Third-degree heart block. Electrocardiographic (ECG) tracing showing the widened QRS complex. From Levitsky MG, Cairo JN, Hall SM: *Introduction to respiratory care,* Philadelphia, 1990, Saunders.

13. **Pulseless Electrical Activity (PEA)**
    a. A condition in which there is dissociation between the electrical and mechanical activity of the heart. The ECG pattern that appears on the oscilloscope (or ECG monitor) does not reflect the actual mechanical activity of the heart.
    b. For example, the ECG may show regular QRS complexes, but the patient has no pulse. Certainly, the tracing should be ignored and chest compressions started.

c. Although PEA is not common, it is often associated with cardiac trauma, tension pneumothorax, severe electrolyte disturbances, and severe acid–base imbalances.

K. **Electric Cardiac Pacemakers**

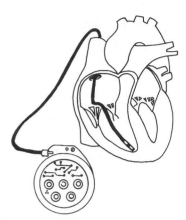

FIGURE 9-21 Electric cardiac pacemaker.

1. Electric pacemakers are devices used to replace the heart's natural pacemaker (SA node); they control the contractions of the heart by a series of rhythmic electrical discharges.
2. External pacemaker: The electrodes that deliver the discharges are placed on the outside of the chest.
3. Internal pacemaker: The electrodes are placed inside the chest wall.
4. The transvenous pacemaker, a **temporary** internal pacer, is introduced into a peripheral vein and, with the use of fluoroscopy and ECG monitoring, is advanced through the superior vena cava and right atrium and positioned in the right ventricle.

    Indications for the temporary transvenous pacemaker are second- and third-degree heart blocks, ventricular asystole, and other arrhythmias resulting in symptomatic bradycardia.
5. A pacer spike is a straight line observed on the ECG strip.
6. To treat permanent arrhythmias, permanent pacemakers are surgically implanted.
7. The electrodes are attached to a battery-operated pace generator, which fires impulses at a specific rate continuously, or to a demand-type pacer, which fires if the patient's heart rate slows to a pre-set rate.
8. The RCP must know whether the patient has a temporary pacemaker before beginning a treatment, such as CPT, because this type of pacemaker can be dislodged with vigorous movement.

L. **Holter Monitoring**
1. A Holter monitor is a portable, battery-powered recording device that records the patient's ECG tracing while the patient conducts daily activities. The monitoring is generally done over 24 h.
2. The patient keeps a diary of activity throughout the day so that it can be compared with the ECG recording. The patient records any symptoms in the diary, which are later correlated to the ECG at that specific time.
3. Because arrhythmias and inadequate blood flow to the heart may occur only briefly or unpredictably, this method of monitoring is useful in patients experiencing irregular heart beats on an inconsistent basis.

II. **HEMODYNAMIC MONITORING**
CRT Exam Content Matrix: IA8b, IB9i, IB10i, IC10, IIIE3e, IIIE4c
RRT Exam Content Matrix: IA8b, IB9i, IB9r, IB10m, IB10s, IC11-12, IIA9a-b, IIIE3d, IIIE4a, IIIJ6

A. **Arterial Catheter (Arterial "Line")**
1. Systemic arterial blood pressure is most accurately measured by placing a catheter directly into a peripheral artery.
2. Peripheral arterial lines should be used in patients with hemodynamic instability. Along with the measurement of blood pressure, these lines provide a direct route for the frequent blood samples drawn from these patients.
3. The most common peripheral artery sites are as follows
    a. Radial: most common because of easy access and good collateral circulation (with ulnar artery). **The Allen test must be performed before puncture to determine whether collateral circulation is present.** (See Chapter 10 on ABG interpretation.)
    b. Brachial
    c. Femoral
4. Sterile technique should be used when the 18- or 20-gauge catheter is placed into the artery by either surgical cutdown or percutaneous puncture. The catheter is connected to a system that delivers a continuous flow of fluid from an IV bag to maintain patency of the system. The IV bag, which should contain normal saline with added heparin, is pressurized by a hand-bulb pressure pump.
5. The system is also equipped with stopcocks to allow for calibration with atmospheric pressure and for arterial sampling.
6. A **strain gauge pressure transducer** (the most commonly used transducer) is connected to the system to provide a display of the pressure waveform and a digital reading of the arterial pressure in millimeters of mercury.

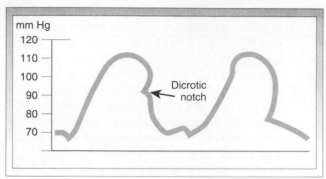

Normal arterial waveform

FIGURE 9-22

7. Pressures measured on the arterial waveform
   a. **Systolic pressure:** equal to the peak of the waveform **(normally 90 to 140 mm Hg).** Systole occurs as the heart contracts, forcing blood through the aorta (to the systemic circulation) and pulmonary arteries (to the lungs).
   b. **Diastolic pressure:** measured at the lowest point of the waveform **(normally 60 to 90 mm Hg).** Diastole occurs in between the contractions of the atria and ventricles (or while the heart is at rest), as these chambers begin refilling with blood.
   c. **Pulse pressure:** the difference between the systolic and diastolic pressures **(normally about 40 mm Hg).**
   d. Mean arterial pressure: represents the average pressure during the cardiac cycle **(normally 80 to 100 mm Hg).**
   e. Note the **dicrotic notch** on the waveform. It represents the closing of the aortic valve. If the dicrotic notch is not visible, the pressure is most likely inaccurate, in that the values are lower than the patient's actual pressure. The dicrotic notch may disappear when the systolic pressure drops below 50 to 60 mm Hg. At this point it is difficult to palpate or hear a cuff pressure.

8. **Complications of arterial catheters**
   a. Infection: risk may be reduced with removal of the catheter within 4 days.

   b. Hemorrhage: make sure all connections in the system are tight.
   c. Ischemia: note the color and temperature of the skin distal to the insertion site to determine distal perfusion.
   d. Thrombosis and embolization: a weak pulse distal to the puncture site may indicate thrombosis. A continuous flush of saline and heparin through the system helps to avoid clot formation.

☑ **Exam Note**

The catheter site and points distal to it should be assessed frequently by the respiratory therapist for signs of the above complications.

9. **Troubleshooting for arterial lines**
   a. "Damped" pressure tracing; causes include
      (1) **Occlusion of the catheter tip by a clot:** correct by aspiration of the clot and flushing with heparinized saline.
      (2) **Catheter tip resting against the wall of the vessel:** correct by repositioning catheter while observing waveform.
      (3) **Clot in transducer or stopcock:** correct by flushing system and, if no improvement is seen in the waveform tracing, change the stopcock and transducer.
      (4) **Air bubbles in the line:** correct by disconnecting transducer and flushing out air bubbles.
   b. Abnormally high or low pressure readings; causes include
      (1) **Improper calibration:** correct by recalibration of monitor and strain gauge.
      (2) **Improper transducer position:** correct by ensuring the transducer is kept at the level of the patient's heart.
   c. No pressure reading; causes include
      (1) **Improper scale selection:** correct by selecting appropriate scale.
      (2) **Transducer not open to catheter:** correct by checking system and making sure the transducer is open to the catheter.

B. **Flow-Directed Pulmonary Artery Catheter (Swan-Ganz Catheter)**

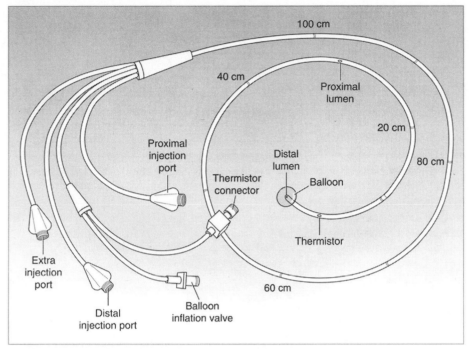

Quadruple (four)-channel Swan-Ganz catheter

FIGURE 9-23

1. The Swan-Ganz catheter is a balloon-tipped catheter made of polyvinyl chloride that is used to measure central venous pressure (CVP), pulmonary artery pressure (PAP), and pulmonary capillary wedge pressure (PCWP), sometimes referred to as pulmonary artery wedge pressure (PAWP).

2. The catheter also allows for the aspiration of blood from the pulmonary artery for **mixed venous blood gas sampling** and injection of fluids to determine cardiac output.

3. The distal channel (lumen) is used for the measurement of PAP and for obtaining mixed venous blood from the pulmonary artery.

4. The proximal channel (lumen) is used for the measurement of CVP or right atrial pressure and for the injection of fluids to determine cardiac output.

5. The balloon inflation channel controls the inflation and deflation of a small balloon, located about 1 cm from the distal tip of the catheter, and is used to measure PCWP.

6. The fourth channel is an extra port for the continuous infusion of fluid, when necessary.

7. This catheter is also equipped with a computer connector to measure cardiac output with the use of the thermodilution technique.

Some catheters are equipped with only two channels, the distal channel and the balloon inflation channel.

8. **Insertion of the Pulmonary Artery Catheter**
   a. The catheter is inserted through the brachial, femoral, subclavian, or internal or external jugular vein.
   b. Continuous monitoring of the catheter pressure and waveform is necessary along with ECG monitoring.
   c. Once the vein is entered, the catheter is advanced into the right atrium, at which time the balloon is inflated and the catheter flows through the right atrium, right ventricle, and into the pulmonary artery, where it "wedges" into a distal branch.
   d. Pressures and pressure waveform tracings are recorded as the catheter passes through the right side of the heart.
   e. Once the catheter "wedges" in a distal branch of the pulmonary artery, the PCWP may be measured, and the balloon should then be deflated, allowing blood flow past the tip of the catheter. Because blood flow is stopped distal to the wedge position when the balloon is inflated, it should not be inflated any longer than **15 to 20 s or pulmonary infarction may occur.**

C. Monitoring of CVP, PAP, and PCWP

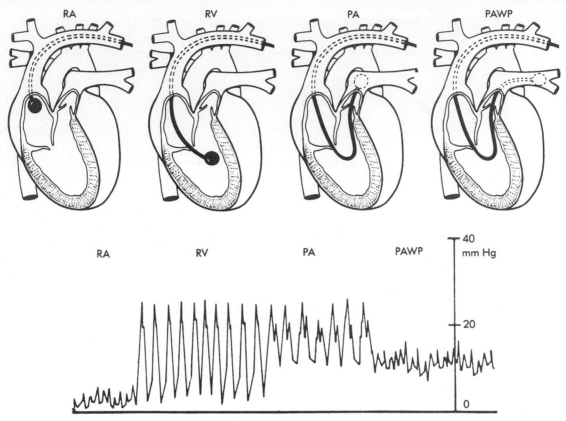

FIGURE 9-24   A normal pressure waveform tracing of the right atrium *(RA)*, right ventricle *(RV)*, pulmonary artery *(PA)*, and pulmonary artery wedge pressure *(PAWP)*. Wilkins RL, Stoller JK, Kacmarek R, *Egan's fundamentals of respiratory care,* ed 9, St Louis, 2009, Mosby.

1. **CVP** may be monitored with a pulmonary artery catheter or from a separate CVP catheter that is inserted through the subclavian, jugular, or brachial vein. The CVP catheter is connected to a water manometer, which reads the pressure in cm H_2O. Measuring the CVP with a pulmonary artery catheter gives the pressure in mm Hg.

> ☑ **Exam Note**
>
> When CVP is monitored with a water manometer, the manometer must be level with the heart while the patient is lying flat. This method of monitoring CVP is not as accurate as using a Swan-Ganz catheter and is not commonly used.

  a. CVP is a measurement of right atrial pressure, which reflects systemic venous return and right ventricular preload. **The normal value is less than 8 cm H_2O or less than 6 mm Hg**.

  b. Conditions that increase CVP
    (1) Hypervolemia (volume overload)
    (2) Pulmonary hypertension
    (3) Right ventricular failure
    (4) Pulmonary valve stenosis
    (5) Tricuspid valve stenosis

    (6) Pulmonary embolism
    (7) Arterial vasodilation, resulting in increased blood volume in the venous system
    (8) Left heart failure
    (9) Improper transducer placement (below the level of the right atrium)
    (10) Positive pressure ventilator breath (measure CVP at end of expiration)
    (11) Severe flail chest or pneumothorax: these conditions may compress the superior and inferior vena cavae, which would decrease venous return and increase CVP as a result of compression of the heart.

> ☑ **Exam Note**
>
> To determine what effect PEEP has on venous return and CVP, measure CVP while the patient continues using PEEP. To determine CVP without the effects of PEEP, discontinue PEEP for the measurement in some patients. However, remember that patients with critical lung conditions using high levels of PEEP cannot tolerate being removed from PEEP; therefore, CVP must be measured while the patient continues using PEEP.

c. Conditions that decrease CVP
   (1) Hypovolemia (inadequate circulating blood volume)
   (2) Vasodilation (from decreased venous tone)
   (3) Leaks or air bubbles in the pressure line
   (4) Improper transducer placement (above the level of the right atrium)
2. **PAP** is an important measurement in the care of critically ill patients with sepsis, ARDS, pulmonary edema, and MI.
   a. It is especially important to monitor PAP and PvO_2 values in patients using at least 10 cm H_2O of PEEP because high levels of PEEP may compromise the cardiac status of the patient by decreasing cardiac output and oxygen delivery to the tissues.
   b. Mixed venous blood sampling (to measure PvO_2) is achieved by obtaining blood from the pulmonary artery. **Normal PvO_2 is 35 to 45 mm Hg.** PvO_2 reflects tissue oxygenation. If this level drops after the initiation of or increase in PEEP, then a decrease in tissue oxygenation has occurred, caused by a drop in cardiac output because of PEEP. PEEP should be decreased to maintain an adequate PvO_2. (See Chapter 11 on ventilator management.)
   c. **Normal systolic PAP is 20 to 30 mm Hg.** Normal diastolic PAP is 5 to 15 mm Hg. Normal mean PAP is 10 to 20 mm Hg.
   d. Conditions that increase PAP
      (1) Pulmonary hypertension (resulting from hypercapnia, acidemia, or hypoxemia, for example)
      (2) Mitral valve stenosis
      (3) Left ventricular failure
   e. Conditions that decrease PAP
      (1) Decreased pulmonary vascular resistance (pulmonary vasodilation); caused by improved oxygenation, for example
      (2) Decreased blood volume
3. **PCWP**
   a. When the balloon at the distal end of the catheter is inflated, it "wedges" in a branch of the pulmonary artery, blocking blood flow from the right side of the heart. The transducer measures the back pressure through the pulmonary circulation, which is equal to pressure in the **left atrium and the left ventricular end-diastolic pressure (LVEDP).**
   b. PCWP, therefore, is a measurement of pressure in the left side of the heart.
   c. As stated, the balloon should not be inflated any longer than 15 to 20 s because blood flow obstructed for any longer may cause pulmonary infarction.

d. **The normal PCWP value is 4 to 12 mm Hg.** A PCWP value of more than 18 mm Hg usually indicates impending pulmonary edema.

> **Exam Note**
>
> PCWP is elevated in patients with cardiogenic pulmonary edema and is normal in patients with noncardiogenic pulmonary edema.

   e. Conditions that increase PCWP
      (1) Left ventricular failure
      (2) Mitral valve stenosis
      (3) Aortic valve stenosis
      (4) Systemic hypertension
   f. Conditions that decrease PCWP
      (1) Hypovolemia
      (2) Pulmonary embolism (PCWP may be normal or decreased)
D. **Complications of Pulmonary Artery Catheter Insertion**
   1. Damage to tricuspid valve
   2. Damage to pulmonary valve
   3. Pulmonary infarction
   4. Pneumothorax
   5. Cardiac arrhythmias
   6. Air embolism
   7. Ruptured pulmonary artery
E. **Measurement of Cardiac Output**
   1. Cardiac output may be measured through the pulmonary artery catheter with the use of the **thermodilution technique.** A cold saline or dextrose solution is injected through the proximal port of the catheter. Heat loss occurs from the injection port to the distal tip of the catheter. The rate of blood flow determines the amount of heat loss and is measured on the cardiac output computer.
   2. Cardiac output may be calculated with the use of the **Fick equation**

$$QT = \frac{VO_2}{[CaO_2 - CVO_2] \times 10}$$

   QT = cardiac output (L/min)
   VO_2 = oxygen consumption (mL/min)
   $[CaO_2 - CVO_2]$ = arterial and mixed venous oxygen content difference (milliliters of oxygen per deciliter of blood), also called vol%

Milliliters per deciliter (mL/dL) must be converted to mL/L to express the cardiac output in L/min. This is accomplished by multiplying the oxygen content difference by 10. Normal cardiac output is 5 L/min.

EXAMPLE:

Calculate a patient's cardiac output given the following information:

$$VO_2 = 250\ mL/min$$

$$CaO_2 - CVO_2 = 5\ vol\%$$

$$QT = \frac{250\ mL/min}{5 \times 10} = \frac{250}{50} = 5\ L/min$$

F. **Measurement of Arterial and Venous O_2 Content**
1. O_2 content refers to the total amount of O_2 dissolved in the plasma and bound to Hb in arterial or mixed venous blood.
2. The difference between arterial and venous O_2 content (arteriovenous O_2 content difference) is used to calculate cardiac output and cardiopulmonary shunting.
3. Total O_2 content of arterial blood (CaO_2) is calculated with the use of the following formula:

$$CaO_2 = 1.34 \times Hb \times SaO_2\ (i.e.,\ mL\ of\ O_2\ bound\ to\ Hb) + PaO_2 \times 0.003\ (mL\ of\ O_2\ dissolved\ in\ plasma)$$

> 1.34 mL of O_2 is capable of binding with 1 g of Hb, and 0.003 mL of O_2 is dissolved in the plasma for each 1 mm Hg of PaO_2.

EXAMPLE:

Calculate the total arterial O_2 content from the following data:

Hb	15 g%
SaO$_2$	98%
PaO$_2$	86 mm Hg

$$1.34 \times 15 \times 0.98 = 19.7\ mL\ of\ O_2\ (bound\ to\ Hb)$$

$$86 \times 0.003 = 0.26\ mL\ of\ O_2\ (dissolved\ in\ the\ plasma)$$

$$CaO_2 = 19.7\ mL + 0.26\ mL = \textbf{19.96 mL/dL (or vol\%)}$$

4. CVO_2 is calculated with the following formula

$$(1.34 \times Hb \times SvO_2) + (PvO_2 \times 0.003)$$

EXAMPLE:

Calculate the total venous O_2 content, given the following data.

Hb	15 g%
SvO$_2$	75%
PvO$_2$	40 mm Hg

$$1.34 \times 15 \times 0.75 = 15\ mL\ of\ O_2\ (bound\ to\ Hb)$$

$$40 \times 0.003 = 0.12\ mL\ of\ O_2\ (dissolved\ in\ plasma)$$

$$CVO_2 = 15\ mL + 0.12\ mL = 15.12\ mL/dL\ (or\ vol\%)$$

☑ **Exam Note**

The normal $C(a-v)O_2$, or arteriovenous O_2 content, difference is 4 to 6 mL/dL (or vol%). In the above calculations, the $C(a-v)O_2$ is

$$19.96 - 15.12 = 4.84\ mL/dL\ (vol\%)$$

An arteriovenous O_2 content difference of less than 4 vol% may be the result of increased cardiac output (less time for tissues to extract O_2; therefore arterial and venous O_2 are closer in value), septic shock, or anemia.

An arteriovenous O_2 content difference of more than 6 vol% may be the result of decreased cardiac output (more time for tissues to extract O_2 because of slower blood flow; therefore a greater difference is seen between arterial and venous O_2 values).

> $C(a-v)O_2$ is useful in determining the effects that PEEP and mechanical ventilation have on the patient's cardiac output and in evaluating the patient's need for more circulatory support.

G. **Intrapulmonary Shunting**
1. Intrapulmonary shunting is defined as the portion of the cardiac output that perfuses through the lungs without coming in contact with ventilated alveoli. This portion of the cardiac output therefore passes through the lungs and into the left side of the heart without being oxygenated.

2. In a healthy person, intrapulmonary shunting occurs. This results from blood flow through the bronchial, pleural, and thebesian veins. These veins return blood to the left atrium, thus bypassing the oxygenation process in the lungs (called an anatomic shunt). **Normally, intrapulmonary shunting is about 2% to 5% of the cardiac output** and is primarily caused by anatomic shunting.

3. Physiologic shunting represents only a small portion of the normal anatomic shunt. Increased physiologic shunting results in a worsening cardiopulmonary status.

4. Conditions that **increase** physiologic shunting
   a. Pneumonia
   b. Pneumothorax
   c. Pulmonary edema
   d. Atelectasis

5. The amount of shunt may be determined with the use of the clinical shunt formula

$$\frac{QS}{QT} = \frac{(PAO_2 - PaO_2)(0.003)}{(CaO_2 - CVO_2) + (PAO_2 - PaO_2)(0.003)}$$

This formula requires a 100% Hb saturation of O_2 in arterial blood.

6. If measurement of PvO_2 is not available (via pulmonary artery catheter), the modified shunt equation may be used:

$$\frac{QS}{QT} = \frac{(PAO_2 - PaO_2)(0.003)}{(4.5 \text{ vol\%}) + (PAO_2 - PaO_2)(0.003)}$$

4.5 vol% represents a normal $CaO_2 - CVO_2$

EXAMPLE:

Calculate a patient's percentage of shunt given the following data

pH	7.37
$PaCO_2$	45 mm Hg
PAO_2	60 mm Hg
FiO_2	0.40
PB	747 mm Hg

$$PAO_2 = (PB - 47)(FiO_2) - (PaCO_2 \times 1.25) *$$

$$(747 - 47)(0.4) - (45 \times 1.25)$$

$$280 - 56 = \textbf{224 torr}$$

$$\frac{QS}{QT} = \frac{(PAO_2 - PaO_2)(0.003)}{(4.5 \text{ vol\%}) + (PAO_2 - PaO_2)(0.003)}$$

$$= \frac{(224 - 60) \times 0.003}{4.5 + (224 - 60)(0.003)} = \frac{0.49}{4.5 + 0.49}$$

$$= \frac{0.49}{5.0} = 0.098$$

$$\frac{QS}{QT} = 0.098 \times 100 = \textbf{9.8\%}$$

*To simplify the math use 7 x O_2% and ($PaCO_2 + 10$) to obtain an answer close enough to get the question correct.

This means that almost 10% of the patient's cardiac output is not being oxygenated in the lungs.

 Exam Note

A simplified method of calculating shunt is as follows: A–a gradient/20 + 4%. Although not as accurate, it should work fine on the NBRC exams.

7. **Interpreting calculated shunt values**
   a. Less than 10% is normal.
   b. Abnormal intrapulmonary status is 10% to 20% and is usually of no significance clinically.
   c. Significant intrapulmonary disease is 20% to 30%, may be life-threatening, and requires cardiopulmonary support.
   d. More than 30% is a serious, life-threatening condition that requires aggressive cardiopulmonary support.

H. **Measuring Cardiac Index**
1. Cardiac output varies according to the patient's body surface area (BSA). The cardiac index (CI) correlates the patient's cardiac output for his or her specific BSA.
2. Formula for calculation

$$CI = \frac{\text{cardiac output (L/min)}}{\text{BSA (m}^2)}$$

3. Normal CI is 2.6 to 4.3 L/min/m^2
4. Factors that **increase** CI
   a. Drugs that increase cardiac contractility (e.g., dopamine, epinephrine, digitalis)
   b. Hypervolemia
   c. Decreased vascular resistance
   d. Septic shock (early stages)
5. Factors that **decrease** CI
   a. Drugs that decrease cardiac contractility (e.g., propranolol and metoprolol)
   b. Hypovolemia
   c. CHF
   d. Increased vascular resistance
   e. MI
   f. Septic shock (late stages)
   g. Positive pressure ventilation
   h. PEEP and CPAP

I. **Measuring Stroke Volume**
1. Stroke volume (SV) is the amount of blood ejected from the ventricle during ventricular contraction.
2. Formula for calculation

$$SV = \frac{\text{cardiac output (mL/min)}}{\text{heart rate (beats/min)}}$$

3. Normal SV is 60 to 120 mL/beat.

J. **Measuring Systemic Vascular Resistance**
1. Systemic vascular resistance (SVR) is a measurement of the resistance that the left ventricle must overcome to eject its volume of blood. This is known as **afterload.**
2. SVR is calculated with the use of the following formula

$$SVR = \frac{\text{MSAP} - \text{CVP (mm Hg)}}{\text{QT (L/min)}}$$

MSAP=mean systemic arterial pressure

This resistance formula may be multiplied by 80 to convert to resistance units of dyne$\times$s$\times$cm^{-5}.

3. Normal SVR is 10 to 18 mm Hg/L/min, or 900 to 1450 dyne$\times$s$\times$cm^{-5}.
4. Factors that **increase** SVR
   a. Vasoconstrictors (dopamine, epinephrine)
   b. Hypovolemia
   c. Hypocapnia
5. Factors that **decrease** SVR
   a. Vasodilators (nitroprusside sodium, morphine, nitroglycerin)
   b. Hypercapnia
   c. Septic shock (early stages)

K. **Measuring Pulmonary Vascular Resistance**
1. Pulmonary vascular resistance (PVR) is a reflection of the afterload of the right ventricle.
2. PVR is calculated with the use of the following formula

$$\frac{\text{MPAP} - \text{PCWP}}{\text{QT}}$$

MPAP=mean pulmonary artery pressure
QT=cardiac output (L/min)
PAWP=pulmonary artery wedge pressure

This resistance formula may be multiplied by 80 to convert to resistance units of dyne$\times$s$\times$cm^{-5}.

3. Normal PVR is 1.5 to 3.0 mm Hg/L/min, or 150 to 250 dyne$\times$s$\times$cm^{-5}.
4. Factors that **increase** PVR
   a. Vasoconstrictors (dopamine, epinephrine)
   b. Hypercapnia
   c. Hypoxemia
   d. Acidemia
   e. Pulmonary embolism
   f. Pneumothorax
   g. Positive pressure ventilation
   h. PEEP and CPAP
5. Factors that **decrease** PVR
   a. Improved oxygenation (pulmonary vasodilator)
   b. Alkalemia (hypocapnia)
   c. Vasodilating agents

L. **Measurement of O$_2$ Consumption (VO$_2$)**
1. VO$_2$ is defined as the amount of O$_2$ (in milliliters) extracted by the peripheral tissues in 1 min. It is also a measurement of the O$_2$ uptake in the lung.
2. VO$_2$ may be calculated with the use of the following formula, which is based on the Fick equation

$$VO_2 = QT[C(a - v)O_2] \times 10$$

10=factor to convert C(a−v)O$_2$ to milliliters of O$_2$ per liter

EXAMPLE:

Given the following data, calculate a patient's O_2 consumption (uptake).

QT	5 L/min
CaO_2	20 vol%
CVO_2	14.5 vol%

$$VO_2 = 5 \times [20 - 14.5] \times 10$$

$$VO_2 = 5 \times 5.5 \times 10$$

$$VO_2 = 275\, mL/min$$

3. Normal O_2 consumption is **150 to 275 mL/min**.
4. Factors that **increase** VO_2
   a. Hyperthermia
   b. Exercise
   c. Seizures
   d. Shivering
5. Factors that **decrease** VO_2
   a. Hypothermia
   b. Cyanide poisoning
   c. Musculoskeletal relaxation

III. **CARDIOPULMONARY STRESS TESTING**
   CRT Exam Content Matrix: IB9r, IB10r, IIIE7e
   RRT Exam Content Matrix: IB9s, IB10t, IIIE7e
   A. **Exercise Stress Testing**
   1. Exercise stress testing is used to evaluate a patient's cardiopulmonary reserve capacity.
   2. The cardiopulmonary stress test is usually conducted with the patient either pedaling a cycle or walking on a treadmill.
   3. Before testing, perform a patient history and physical examination.
      The examination should include
      a. Pulmonary function tests
      b. Carbon monoxide diffusion capacity
      c. Arterial blood gas measurements
      d. Blood pressure
      e. Before and after bronchodilator study (if airflow obstruction exists)
      f. Resting ECG
   4. Some patients are not ideal candidates for cardiopulmonary stress testing. Below is a list of conditions in which stress testing is contraindicated.
      a. CHF
      b. Recent acute MI
      c. Unstable angina
      d. Acute infection
      e. Uncontrolled cardiac arrhythmias
      f. Dissecting aneurysm
      g. Third-degree heart block
      h. Myocarditis
   5. A physician should always be present during the stress test as well as the following emergency equipment

   a. Defibrillator
   b. Oxygen source
   c. Manual resuscitator with mask
   d. Oral airway
   e. Laryngoscope and endotracheal tubes
   f. IV setup with 5% dextrose
   g. Cardiac medications

B. **Cardiac Stress Test**
   1. The patient performs incremental work using either a cycle ergometer or treadmill.
   2. The patient's heart rate, blood pressure, and ECG are monitored before the test.
   3. These same variables are measured at the end of each stage of the test and for at least 15 min after the test or until any cardiopulmonary problems decline.
   4. Most healthy individuals are able to complete all four stages of the exercise without difficulty. Patients with coronary artery disease may not be able to complete all stages because of dyspnea and angina.
   5. This stress test is very useful in diagnosing and treating coronary artery disease but is limited in diagnosing other cardiopulmonary diseases.

C. **Cardiopulmonary Stress Test**
   1. This test requires a cycle ergometer or a treadmill, a system for analyzing exhaled gases, a device for recording ventilation variables, and an oximeter for measuring oxygen saturation or an arterial line for obtaining blood gas measurements.
   2. This test also requires the patient to exercise at certain workload increments.
   3. Values measured during this test include
      a. Blood pressure
      b. Heart rate
      c. ECG
      d. Respiratory rate
      e. Oxygen saturation or blood gases
      f. Oxygen consumption
      g. CO_2 production
      h. Respiratory quotient
      i. Oxygen pulse (volume of oxygen removed from the blood with each heartbeat; calculated by dividing oxygen consumption by the heart rate)
      j. VD/VT ratio
      k. Maximum voluntary ventilation (MVV)
      l. Anaerobic threshold (the point at which the oxygen requirements of the exercising muscles cannot be met and anaerobic metabolism begins providing the cellular energy supply)
      m. The test is discontinued when the patient reaches a predetermined heart rate or if the following signs or symptoms occur
         (1) Physical exhaustion
         (2) Excessive chest pain
         (3) Excessive dyspnea

(4) Excessive fatigue in the legs
(5) PVCs
(6) Ventricular tachycardia
(7) Heart blocks
(8) Hypotension
(9) Patient requests the test to be stopped

POSTCHAPTER STUDY QUESTIONS

1. List four causes of a "damped" arterial pressure waveform.
2. List five conditions that cause an increased CVP.
3. List four conditions that cause a decreased CVP.
4. What are three drugs used to treat PVCs.
5. What is the treatment for ventricular tachycardia?
6. List three conditions that cause an increased PAP.
7. List two conditions that cause a decreased PAP.
8. PAWP is a measurement of what function?
9. List four conditions that cause an increased PCWP.
10. List two conditions that cause a decreased PCWP.
11. List the normal values for CVP, PAP, and PCWP.
12. Calculate the QT of a patient who has a VO_2 of 240 mL/min and a $C(a-v)O_2$ of 6 vol%.
13. In a healthy person, what percentage of the cardiac output makes up the intrapulmonary shunt?
14. Calculate the $C(a-v)O_2$, given the following information

pH	7.43
$PaCO_2$	43 mm Hg
PaO_2	82 mm Hg
SaO_2	95%
PvO_2	37 mm Hg
SvO_2	72%
Hb	14 g/dL

15. List four conditions that increase physiologic shunting.
16. Calculate the percentage of intrapulmonary shunt given the following information

pH	7.39
$PaCO_2$	40 mm Hg
PaO_2	122 mm Hg
FiO_2	0.50
PB	747 mm Hg

17. List four factors that cause an increased SVR.
18. List three factors that cause a decreased SVR.
19. List five factors that cause an increased PVR.
20. List three factors that cause a decreased PVR.
21. Calculate the oxygen consumption given the following information

QT	4.5 L/min
CaO_2	19 vol%
CVO_2	14 vol%

22. List four factors that cause an increased O_2 consumption.
23. List three factors that cause a decreased O_2 consumption.

See answers at the back of the text.

BIBLIOGRAPHY

Davis D, *How to quickly and accurately master ECG interpretation*, Philadelphia, 1985, JB Lippincott.

Davis D: *Differential diagnosis of arrhythmias*, ed 2, Philadelphia, 1997, Saunders.

Des Jardins T, *Cardiopulmonary anatomy and physiology*, ed 5, Albany, NY, 2008, Delmar.

Hess D *and others, Respiratory care principles and practice*, ed 1, Philadelphia, 2002, Saunders.

Levitsky MG, Cairo JN, Hall SM: *Introduction to respiratory care*, Philadelphia, 1990, Saunders.

O'Toole M, editor: *Miller-Keane encyclopedia and dictionary of medicine, nursing, and allied health*, Philadelphia, 2005, Saunders.

Wilkins RL, Stoller JK, Kacmarek R, *Egan's fundamentals of respiratory care*, ed 9, St Louis, 2009, Mosby.

Wilkins R, Krider S, Sheldon R, *Clinical assessment in respiratory care*, ed 6, St Louis, 2010, Mosby.

ABG INTERPRETATION

Answer the pretest questions before studying the chapter. This will help you determine your strong and weak areas in the material covered.

1. Which of the following blood gas measurements determines how well a patient's lungs are being ventilated?

   A. pH
   B. $PaCO_2$
   C. PaO_2
   D. HCO_3^-

2. Which of the following blood gas measurements determines the level of tissue oxygenation?

   A. pH
   B. $PaCO_2$
   C. PaO_2
   D. PvO_2

3. The information below has been obtained from a patient using an aerosol mask at 40% oxygen.

pH	7.42
$PaCO_2$	36 mm Hg
PaO_2	122 mm Hg
HCO_3^-	26 mEq/L

   What is this patient's A−a gradient? PB=747 mm Hg

   A. 45 mm Hg
   B. 77 mm Hg
   C. 113 mm Hg
   D. 235 mm Hg

4. Which of the following conditions shifts the HbO_2 dissociation curve to the right?

   A. Hypercapnia
   B. Hypothermia
   C. Alkalemia
   D. HbCO

5. A patient with a 2 L/min nasal cannula has the following ABG results.

pH	7.51
$PaCO_2$	27 mm Hg
PaO_2	62 mm Hg
HCO_3^-	23 mEq/L

   These results indicate which of the following conditions?

   A. Uncompensated respiratory acidosis
   B. Chronic respiratory alkalosis
   C. Compensated metabolic alkalosis
   D. Acute respiratory alkalosis

6. The respiratory therapist has received an order to obtain ABG levels from a patient, but an Allen test indicates collateral circulation is not present in the right wrist. At this time, the therapist would

   A. Obtain blood from the right radial artery.
   B. Obtain blood from the right brachial artery.
   C. Wait for the physician to evaluate collateral circulation.
   D. Check collateral circulation in the left wrist.

See answers and rationales at the back of the text.

I. **ABG ANALYSIS**
   CRT Exam Content Matrix: IB9f, IB10f, IIIE2a
   RRT Exam Content Matrix: IB9f, IB10f, IIIE2a
   A. Blood gas analysis monitors the following physiologic variables
      1. Arterial oxygenation: PaO_2
      2. Alveolar ventilation: $PaCO_2$
      3. Acid−base status: pH
      4. O_2 delivery to tissues: PvO_2
   B. Arterial samples are used because the values reflect the patient's total cardiopulmonary status.
   C. Mixed venous blood, obtained from the pulmonary artery via a Swan-Ganz catheter, is used to determine O_2 delivery to the tissues (see Chapter 11 on ventilator management).
   D. Blood gases are tested to determine whether to change current therapy or to maintain it.

E. Common sites from which to obtain arterial blood are the radial, femoral, or dorsalis pedis arteries.
1. The radial artery is the most common site because of the presence of good collateral circulation and easy access.
2. A modified Allen test is performed to determine collateral circulation.
   a. Instruct the patient to close his or her hand tightly as you occlude both the radial and ulnar arteries.
   b. Instruct the patient to open his or her hand as you release the pressure on the ulnar artery while watching for the hand to regain normal color.
   c. The hand should "pink up" within 10 to 15 s. This is considered a positive Allen test, and the radial artery may be punctured to obtain arterial blood.
   d. If color is not restored within 10 to 15 s, the test is negative, which means that collateral circulation is not present and blood must not be obtained from this radial artery. Perform an Allen test on the opposite hand to assess collateral circulation.
F. **ABG Sampling** (via radial artery puncture)
1. Explain the procedure to the patient.
2. Perform a modified Allen test.
3. Place a folded towel under the patient's wrist to keep the wrist hyperextended.
4. Clean the puncture site with isopropyl alcohol (70%) or some other appropriate disinfectant.
5. The practitioner must wear gloves for this procedure.
6. A local anesthetic, such as lidocaine (Xylocaine), may be administered subcutaneously around the puncture site, especially in patients who have been punctured several times. Allow 3 to 5 min for the anesthetic to take effect.
7. Aspirate 0.5 mL of a 1:1000 solution of heparin into the syringe using a 22- or 23-gauge needle. Pull the plunger of the syringe back and forth so that the entire portion of the syringe is exposed to the heparin. Then push the plunger all the way in to expel the heparin, making sure there are no air bubbles in the syringe. (Most syringes are previously treated with heparin.)

> The heparin lubricates the syringe, but it is primarily used to prevent the blood from clotting once in the syringe.

8. With the needle/syringe in one hand, palpate the artery with the other hand. The needle should enter the skin at a 45 degree angle with the bevel pointed up. Advance the needle until blood pulsates into the syringe.

9. After obtaining 2 to 4 mL of blood, apply a sterile gauze pad with pressure over the puncture site for 3 to 5 min or until the bleeding has stopped.
10. Air bubbles affect blood gas levels and should be removed from the syringe. Air in the blood causes increased PaO_2 levels and decreased $PaCO_2$ levels.
11. Place a cap or rubber stopper over the needle, or remove the needle and place a cap over the end of the syringe. This prevents air from entering the syringe.
12. Then roll the syringe back and forth in your hands to ensure proper mixing of the blood and heparin to prevent blood clotting. Place the syringe in ice to slow metabolism and keep the ABG levels accurate.
13. Record the following information after the sample is drawn
    a. Patent's name and room number
    b. The patient's FiO_2 level
    c. If the patient is using a ventilator, record
       (1) FiO_2
       (2) VT
       (3) Respiratory rate
       (4) Mode of ventilation (e.g., CMV, SIMV)
       (5) PEEP level
       (6) Mechanical dead space
    d. Patient's temperature: A fever shifts the HbO_2 curve to the right, indicating that Hb more readily releases O_2 to the tissues but does not pick up the O_2 as easily. This may affect the PaO_2 value but not usually to a significant degree.

II. **ARTERIAL OXYGENATION**
   CRT Exam Content Matrix: IB9k, IB10k
   RRT Exam Content Matrix: IB10i
   A. **PaO_2**
   1. The PaO_2 is the portion of O_2 that is dissolved in the plasma of the blood. It is what is left over after the Hb molecules have been saturated.
   2. For every **1 mm Hg of PaO_2,** there is **0.003 mL of dissolved O_2.**
   B. **PAO_2 (alveolar PO_2)**
   1. Is calculated by the following formula (alveolar air equation)

$$PAO_2 = [(PB - 47 \text{ mm Hg})(FiO_2)] - (PaCO_2 \times 1.25)$$

(47 mm Hg is the level of water vapor pressure at body temperature)

$$PAO_2 = [(760 - 47 \text{ mm Hg})(0.21)] - (40 \text{ mm Hg} \times 1.25)$$

$$PAO_2 = (713 \times 0.21) - 50$$

$$PAO_2 = 150 - 50 = \mathbf{100 \text{ mm Hg}}$$

2. This value is often compared with PaO_2 to determine the $P(A-a)O_2$ gradient, which refers to the difference between alveolar O_2 tension and arterial O_2 tension. **The normal gradient on room air is 4 to 12 mm Hg.**

 Exam Note

Because the exam generally uses a barometric pressure of 747 mm Hg, the corrected PB is 700 mm Hg. When multiplying 700 times 0.21, the math can be made simpler by multiplying 7 times 21. Furthermore, instead of multiplying the $PaCO_2$ by 1.25, simply add 10 to the $PaCO_2$. This does not provide an exact answer, but the answer is close enough to get the question correct on the exam. To make the math simpler and faster on the exam, use the equation below.

EXAMPLE:

A patient using a 50% Venturi mask has the following ABG levels

pH	7.36
PaCO₂	45 mm Hg
PaO₂	94 mm Hg

What is this patient's A–a gradient? (PB=747 mm Hg)

$$PAO_2 = (7 \times O_2 \%) - (PaCO_2 + 10)$$
$$= 350 - 55$$
$$= 295 \text{ mm Hg}$$

$$P(A-a)O_2 = PAO_2 - PaCO_2$$
$$= 295 - 94$$
$$= \mathbf{201 \text{ mm Hg}}$$

C. The majority of O_2 carried in the blood is bound to Hb. (See Chapter 1 on oxygen and medical gas therapy.)

D. **HbO_2 Dissociation Curve**

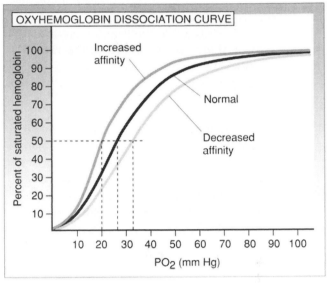

FIGURE 10-1

1. This curve plots the relationship between PaO_2 and SaO_2 and the affinity that Hb has for O_2 at various saturation levels.
2. This S-shaped curve indicates that at PaO_2 levels of less than 60 mm Hg, small increases in PaO_2 result in fairly large increases in SaO_2.

EXAMPLE:

Fifty percent of the Hb molecules would be carrying O_2 at a PaO_2 of only 26 mm Hg. As the PaO_2 increases to 40 mm Hg, the SaO_2 increases substantially, to about 75%. As the PaO_2 continues to increase to 60 mm Hg, the SaO_2 increases to approximately 90%.

3. The flat portion of the curve indicates that at PaO_2 levels above 60 mm Hg, saturation rises slowly: a PaO_2 of 70 mm Hg yields an SaO_2 of 93%, and PaO_2 levels between 80 and 100 mm Hg result in SaO_2 levels of 95% to 100%.

4. Various factors affect the affinity that Hb has for O_2. These factors shift the HbO_2 dissociation curve to the right or the left.

5. If the curve is **shifted to the right,** it indicates that **Hb's affinity for O_2 has decreased,** or Hb will release O_2 to the tissues more readily. **Factors that shift the curve to the right include**
   a. Hypercapnia
   b. Acidosis
   c. Hyperthermia
   d. Increased levels of 2,3-diphosphoglycerate (DPG)

6. If the curve is **shifted to the left,** it indicates that **the affinity of Hb for O_2 has increased,** or Hb will not release O_2 to the tissues as readily. **Factors that shift the curve to the left include**
   a. Hypocapnia
   b. Alkalosis
   c. Hypothermia
   d. Decreased levels of 2,3 DPG
   e. HbCO

7. As O_2 diffuses from the alveoli to the blood (caused by the pressure gradient), it enters an RBC, where it combines with Hb.

8. As O_2 combines with the Hb, the release of CO_2 is enhanced. This is called the **Haldane effect.**

9. As the RBC travels to the tissue, it releases the O_2 because elevated CO_2 levels, which are present around tissues, decrease the affinity of Hb for O_2. This is known as the **Bohr effect.**

10. **Levels of hypoxemia**

60 to 79 mm Hg	Mild hypoxemia
40 to 59 mm Hg	Moderate hypoxemia
<40 mm Hg	Severe hypoxemia

11. **Normal PaO_2 levels:** Subtract 1 mm Hg from 80 mm Hg for each year over age 60 to determine normal PaO_2 by age.

Age (yr)	PaO_2 (mm Hg)
<60	80–100
60	80
65	75
70	70
75	65
80	60

12. **P-50**
   a. The O_2 tension at which 50% of the Hb is saturated when the blood is at 37° C has a PCO_2 level of 40 mm Hg and a pH level of 7.40.
   b. Normal P-50 is 26.6 mm Hg.
   c. Used to describe affinity of Hb for O_2.
      (1) Increased P-50 indicates decreased affinity.
      (2) Decreased P-50 indicates increased affinity.

13. **SaO_2**
   a. Refers to the quantity of O_2 being carried by the Hb compared with the maximum that may be carried.
   b. **Normal SaO_2 level is 95% to 99%.**

III. **CO_2 TRANSPORT AND ALVEOLAR VENTILATION**
A. CO_2 makes up approximately 0.03% of inspired air.
B. CO_2 is the by-product of cellular metabolism, and it is by this mechanism that it enters the blood.
C. After CO_2 enters the blood, it takes one of two routes.
   1. Five percent of the CO_2 dissolves in the plasma.
   2. The remaining 95% enters RBCs.
      a. Approximately 65% of the CO_2 entering the RBC is quickly converted to hydrogen and HCO_3^- ions.
      b. The remaining CO_2 entering the RBC combines with Hb.
      c. Therefore, CO_2 is carried in the blood three ways
         (1) Dissolved in the plasma
         (2) Bound to Hb
         (3) As HCO_3^-
D. **The adequacy of ventilation is determined by the $PaCO_2$ level.**
   1. Normal $PaCO_2$ range is 35 to 45 mm Hg.
   2. $PaCO_2$ levels <35 mm Hg indicate **hypocapnia,** which is excess CO_2 elimination or **hyperventilation.**
   3. $PaCO_2$ levels >45 mm Hg indicate **hypercapnia,** which is inadequate CO_2 elimination or **hypoventilation.**
E. $PaCO_2$ increases when the respiratory rate or VT (minute volume) decreases or dead space increases. $PaCO_2$ decreases when the respiratory rate or VT increases or dead space decreases.

IV. **ACID–BASE BALANCE (pH)**
CRT Exam Content Matrix: IA5, IB9j, IB10j, IC7, IIIE4a
RRT Exam Content Matrix: IA5, IB9j, IB10j, IC8
A. In simple terms, the pH level is determined by the amount of carbonic acid (H_2CO_3) in the blood in relation to the amount of bicarbonate base (HCO_3^-) in the blood. Mathematically, pH is the negative log of the hydrogen ion concentration. Therefore, as hydrogen ions increase, pH decreases.
   1. Henderson-Hasselbalch equation

$$pH = pK + \log \frac{base}{acid}$$

   pK = dissociation constant = 6.1
   2. Clinically, we may state

$$pH = pK + \log \frac{HCO_3^-}{PCO_2}$$

The relationship between pH, HCO_3^-, and CO_2 is vitally important in interpreting blood gas values effectively. HCO_3^- and CO_2 determine the pH level. Understanding the relationship between these three values makes ABG interpretation much easier. To simplify, use the following equation

$$pH = \frac{HCO_3^-}{CO_2}$$

and use simple numbers to see how both HCO_3^- and CO_2 affect pH. If HCO_3^- is 12 and CO_2 is 4, then pH is 3 (12/4). If HCO_3^- increases to 16 and CO_2 does not change, then pH increases to 4 (16/4). Conversely, if HCO_3^- decreases to 8 and CO_2 remains at 4, then pH decreases to 2 (8/4). When HCO_3^- increases, pH increases; when HCO_3^- decreases, pH decreases. Therefore, pH and HCO_3^- have a directly proportional relationship.

Using the same numbers, make changes to the CO_2. If HCO_3^- is 12 and CO_2 is 4, then pH is 3 (12/4). If CO_2 increases to 6, then pH decreases to 2 (12/6). Conversely, if CO_2 decreases to 2, then pH increases to 6 (12/2). When CO_2 increases, pH decreases; when CO_2 decreases, pH increases. Therefore, CO_2 and pH have an indirectly proportional relationship.

Whenever ABG results reveal a *decreased* pH level, either the HCO_3^- is decreased or the CO_2 is increased, or both.

If the ABG result indicates an *increased* pH level, then either the HCO_3^- is increased or the CO_2 is decreased, or both. Practice examples follow in this chapter.

Exam Note

For every 20-mm Hg increase in $PaCO_2$, the pH decreases by 0.10. For every 10-mm Hg decrease in $PaCO_2$, the pH increases by 0.10.

B. The normal plasma pH range is **7.35 to 7.45.**
1. A **pH <7.35** is termed *acidemia* and indicates a higher than normal hydrogen ion concentration. **Acidemia occurs as a result of**
   a. Increased PCO_2 levels
   b. Decreased HCO_3^- levels
2. A **pH >7.45** is termed *alkalemia* and indicates a below-normal hydrogen ion concentration. **Alkalemia occurs as a result of**
   a. Decreased PCO_2 levels
   b. Increased HCO_3^- levels

C. **Respiratory Versus Metabolic Components**
1. When the initial pH change is the result of a PCO_2 change, a respiratory disturbance has occurred.
   a. An **increased** PCO_2 level (>45 mm Hg) decreases the pH (<7.35). This is **respiratory acidemia,** and if the HCO_3^- level is still within normal limits, it is acute or uncompensated. An example of acute (uncompensated) respiratory acidemia is as follows: pH, 7.25; $PaCO_2$, 60 mm Hg; HCO_3^-, 25 mEq/L (normal, 22 to 26 mEq/L).
   b. A **decreased** PCO_2 level (<35 mm Hg) increases the pH (>7.45). This is **respiratory**
   alkalemia, and if the HCO_3^- level is still within normal limits, it is acute or uncompensated. An example of acute (uncompensated) respiratory alkalemia is as follows: pH, 7.53; $PaCO_2$, 29 mm Hg; HCO_3^-, 23 mEq/L.
2. When the initial pH change is the result of a change in HCO_3^-, a metabolic disturbance has occurred.
   a. A **decreased HCO_3^- level** (<22 mEq/L) decreases the pH (<7.35). This is **metabolic acidemia,** and if the $PaCO_2$ level is within normal limits, it is acute or uncompensated. An example of acute (uncompensated) metabolic acidemia is as follows: pH, 7.24; $PaCO_2$, 38 mm Hg; HCO_3^-, 13 mEq/L.
   b. An **increased HCO_3^- level** (> 26 mEq/L) increases the pH (> 7.45). This is **metabolic alkalemia,** and if the $PaCO_2$ level is within normal limits, it is acute or uncompensated. An example of acute (uncompensated) metabolic alkalemia is as follows: pH, 7.54; $PaCO_2$, 41 mm Hg; HCO_3^-, 33 mEq/L.

D. **pH Compensation**
1. The levels of HCO_3^- and CO_2 will change to keep the pH within the normal range. This is called **compensation.** In severe renal disease and end-stage COPD, compensation may be minimal.
2. If the PCO_2 initially changes the pH, then the HCO_3^- changes accordingly to return the pH to normal.

EXAMPLE:

(A)			(B)		
	pH	7.27		pH	7.37
	$PaCO_2$	58 mm Hg		$PaCO_2$	58 mm Hg
	HCO_3^-	31 mEq/L		HCO_3^-	35 mEq/L

The (A) example is a **partially compensated respiratory acidemia.** The elevated $PaCO_2$ level caused the initial drop in pH. The HCO_3^- level is increasing to elevate the pH back to normal. Because the pH is approaching normal but is still low, this makes it **partially compensated.**

As the pH returns to normal (B), resulting from the continued increase in the HCO_3^- level, this is called **chronic** or **compensated respiratory acidemia.**

(A)			(B)		
	pH	7.53		pH	7.43
	$PaCO_2$	26 mm Hg		$PaCO_2$	27 mm Hg
	HCO_3^-	16 mEq/L		HCO_3^-	12 mEq/L

The (A) example is a **partially compensated respiratory alkalemia.** The decreased $PaCO_2$ level caused the initial increase in pH. The HCO_3^- level is decreasing to drop the pH back to normal. Because the pH is approaching normal but is still high, this makes it **partially compensated.**

As the pH returns to normal (B), resulting from the continued decrease in the HCO_3^- level, this is a **chronic or compensated respiratory alkalemia.**

3. If the HCO_3^- level initially changes the pH, then the $PaCO_2$ level changes accordingly to return the pH to normal.

EXAMPLE:

(A)	pH	7.21	(B)	pH	7.36
	$PaCO_2$	22 mm Hg		$PaCO_2$	14 mm Hg
	HCO_3^-	12 mEq/L		HCO_3^-	13 mEq/L

The (A) example is a **partially compensated metabolic acidemia.** The decreased HCO_3^- level caused the initial drop in pH. The patient is hyperventilating (decreasing $PaCO_2$ levels) to elevate the pH back to normal. Because the pH is approaching normal but is still low, this is **partially compensated.** As the pH returns to normal (B), resulting from the continuing drop in $PaCO_2$, this is a **compensated metabolic acidemia.**

(A)	pH	7.50	(B)	pH	7.44
	$PaCO_2$	51 mm Hg		$PaCO_2$	59 mm Hg
	HCO_3^-	31 mEq/L		HCO_3^-	31 mEq/L

The (A) example is a **partially compensated metabolic alkalemia**. The increased HCO_3^- caused the initial increase in pH. The patient is hypoventilating (increasing $PaCO_2$ levels) to drop the pH back to normal. Because the pH is approaching normal but is still high, this is **partially compensated.** As the pH returns to normal (B), resulting from the continuing $PaCO_2$ retention, this is a **compensated metabolic alkalemia.**

☑ Exam Note

When a compensated blood gas measurement is interpreted, if the compensated pH is 7.35 to 7.40, the pH must be assumed to have been acidotic initially. Decide whether the $PaCO_2$ or HCO_3^- caused the initial acidemia. Similarly, if the compensated pH is 7.40 to 7.45, the pH must be assumed to have been alkalotic initially. Decide whether the $PaCO_2$ or HCO_3^- caused the initial alkalemia. Metabolic compensation takes several hours to occur, whereas respiratory compensation may occur in minutes.

E. **Mixed Respiratory and Metabolic Component**
1. When both the $PaCO_2$ and HCO_3^- cause the pH to move in the same direction, this is called a mixed or combined component.
2. An example of a mixed component is

pH	7.21
$PaCO_2$	55 mm Hg
HCO_3^-	18 mEq/L

This is an example of **mixed respiratory and metabolic acidemia.** An elevated $PaCO_2$ level and decreased HCO_3^- level both contribute to acidemia.

V. **ARTERIAL BLOOD GAS INTERPRETATION**
CRT Exam Content Matrix: IA5, IB9j, IB10j, IC7, IIIE4a
RRT Exam Content Matrix: IA5, IB9j, IB10j, IC8

A. **ABG Normal Value Chart Summary**

pH	7.35–7.45
$PaCO_2$	35–45 mm Hg
PaO_2	80–100 mm Hg
HCO_3^-	22–26 mEq/L
Base excess (BE)	−2 to +2
Total base deficit (BD):	−2; total BE: +2

B. **Basic Steps to ABG Interpretation**
1. Determine the acid-base status by observing the pH.
   a. Is the pH acidotic (<7.35)?
   b. Is the pH alkalotic (>7.45)?
2. Determine whether the pH change is the result of a change in $PaCO_2$ or in HCO_3^-.
3. When this is determined, observe for signs of compensation. If the $PaCO_2$ caused the initial pH change, is the HCO_3^- changing to return the pH to normal?
4. Determine oxygenation status by observing PaO_2.

C. **ABG Example Problems**
1. ABG levels are

pH	7.23
$PaCO_2$	57 mm Hg
PaO_2	81 mm Hg
HCO_3^-	24 mEq/L
BE	−1

   a. Acid-base status: **acidemia**
   b. Ventilatory status: **elevated $PaCO_2$; hypoventilation resulting in decreased pH**
   c. Metabolic status: **normal HCO_3^-; no compensation occurring at this time**
   d. Oxygenation status: **normal PaO_2**
   e. Interpretation: **uncompensated (acute) respiratory acidemia**
   f. To correct: **Institute mechanical ventilation** to increase the patient's minute volume, or **increase the ventilator rate or VT if the patient is already receiving mechanical ventilation.**

2. ABG levels are

pH	7.57
$PaCO_2$	25 mm Hg
PaO_2	98 mm Hg
HCO_3^-	25 mEq/L
BE	0

   a. Acid-base status: **alkalemia**
   b. Ventilatory status: **decreased $PaCO_2$; hyperventilation resulting in an increased pH**
   c. Metabolic status: **normal HCO_3^-; no compensation occurring at this time**
   d. Oxygenation: **normal PaO_2**

e. Interpretation: **uncompensated (acute) respiratory alkalemia**

f. To correct: **Decrease the ventilator rate or VT or add mechanical dead space.**

3. ABG levels are

pH	7.45
$PaCO_2$	35 mm Hg
PaO_2	53 mm Hg
HCO_3^-	26 mEq/L
BE	+2

a. Acid-base status: **normal pH**

b. Ventilation status: **normal $PaCO_2$**

c. Metabolic status: **normal HCO_3^-**

d. Oxygenation status: **moderate hypoxemia**

e. Interpretation: **normal acid-base status with moderate hypoxemia**

f. To correct: **If the patient is using 60% or more O_2 mask, initiate CPAP, or add PEEP if ventilator patient is using 60% or more O_2.**

4. ABG levels are

pH	7.38
$PaCO_2$	61 mm Hg
PaO_2	54 mm Hg
HCO_3^-	33 mEq/L
BE	+9

a. Acid-base status: **normal pH**

b. Ventilatory status: **increased $PaCO_2$; hypoventilation resulting in decreased pH**

c. Metabolic status: **elevated HCO_3^-; compensation for initial acidemia**

d. Oxygenation status: **moderate hypoxemia**

e. Interpretation: **compensated (chronic) respiratory acidemia.** Because the compensated pH is between 7.35 and 7.40, assume this was initially an acidemia caused by an elevated $PaCO_2$ level.

f. To correct: **This is a classic example of "normal" ABG levels in a patient with chronic lung disease; therefore, no change in present therapy is needed.**

5. ABG levels are

pH	7.29
$PaCO_2$	43 mm Hg
PaO_2	87 mm Hg
HCO_3^-	16 mEq/L
BE	−7

a. Acid-base status: **acidemia**

b. Ventilatory status: **normal $PaCO_2$**

c. Metabolic status: **decreased HCO_3^- resulting in decreased pH**

d. Oxygenation status: **normal PaO_2**

e. Interpretation: **uncompensated metabolic acidemia.** No compensation is occurring because the $PaCO_2$ is normal.

f. To correct: **Give HCO_3^-.** No ventilator variable changes or oxygenation modifications are necessary at this time.

6. ABG levels are

pH	7.20
$PaCO_2$	22 mm Hg
PaO_2	83 mm Hg
HCO_3^-	15 mEq/L
BE	−10

a. Acid-base status: **acidemia**

b. Ventilatory status: **decreased $PaCO_2$; hyperventilation compensating for initial acidemia**

c. Metabolic status: **decreased HCO_3^- resulting in decreased pH**

d. Oxygenation status: **normal PaO_2**

e. Interpretation: **partially compensated metabolic acidemia.** This was an initial metabolic acidemia followed by hyperventilation. Because more CO_2 is being removed, the pH is returning to normal. It is not fully compensated, in that the pH is not within normal limits at this time. **This is an example of a patient with diabetic acidosis (ketoacidosis).**

f. To correct: **May administer $NaHCO_3^-$.**

VI. **ARTERIAL BLOOD GAS INTERPRETATION CHART**

CRT Exam Content Matrix: IA5, IB9j, IB10j, IC7, IIIE4a

RRT Exam Content Matrix: IA5, IB9j, IB10j, IC8

Key for table: N, normal; I, increased; D, decreased.

	pH	PCO_2	HCO_3^-
Uncompensated (acute)			
Respiratory acidemia	D	I	N
Respiratory alkalemia	I	D	N
Metabolic acidemia	D	N	D
Metabolic alkalemia	I	N	I
Partially compensated			
Respiratory acidemia	D	I	I
Respiratory alkalemia	I	D	D
Metabolic acidemia	D	D	D
Metabolic alkalemia	I	I	I
Fully compensated (chronic)			
Respiratory acidemia	N	I	I
Respiratory alkalemia	N	D	D
Metabolic acidemia	N	D	D
Metabolic alkalemia	N	I	I
Mixed respiratory/metabolic			
Acidemia	D	I	D
Alkalemia	I	D	I

VII. BLOOD GAS ANALYZERS

CRT Exam Content Matrix: IIA10, IIC1, IIC3
RRT Exam Content Matrix: IIA5, IIC1, IIC3

A. Currently, blood gas analyzers have the following capabilities
   1. Accurate measurement of pH, PCO_2, and PO_2
   2. Self-calibration
   3. Accurate measurement of base excess or deficit
   4. Accurate measurement of plasma bicarbonate (HCO_3^-)
   5. Correction for temperature
   6. Self-troubleshooting abilities
   7. Automated blood gas interpretation

B. **Blood Gas Electrodes**
   1. **Sanz electrode: measures pH** by quantifying the acidity and alkalinity of a solution of blood. This is accomplished by the measurement of the potential difference across a pH-sensitive glass membrane.
   2. **Severinghaus electrode: measures PCO_2** by causing the CO_2 gas to produce hydrogen ions by means of a chemical reaction.
   3. **Clark electrode: measures PO_2** as a result of a chemical reaction in which electron flow is measured.

C. **Point of Care (POC) Analyzers**
   1. POC analyzers are portable blood gas analyzers that allow blood gas testing to be done at or near the patient bedside.
   2. POC testing is accurate and results in a quicker response time for the analysis than when the blood is drawn from the patient and then transported to the laboratory.
   3. POC analyzers are often handheld devices and usually require only a few drops of blood for analysis. The blood is placed in a disposable cartridge. Separate cartridges are used depending on the test to be done. Blood gas levels as well as hemoglobin, hematocrit, electrolytes, glucose, blood urea nitrogen, and creatinine may be analyzed.
   4. The sensor on the POC analyzer is automatically calibrated. The POC analyzer calculates, displays, and stores the results. The results can also be placed into the hospital information system or central laboratory for storage and reporting.

D. **Quality Control Procedures**
   1. Blood gas analyzers should undergo one- and two-point calibrations on a routine basis. The process should include high and low values for pH, PCO_2, and PO_2 electrodes.
   2. A one-point calibration should be performed before a blood gas sample is run unless the analyzer automatically performs the calibration at programmed intervals.
   3. A two-point calibration is usually performed every 8 h.

4. Two different buffers are used to perform a two-point calibration on the pH (one buffer for a one-point). The PCO_2 electrode is calibrated with the use of two gas concentrations (5% and 10%). The PO_2 electrode uses a gas mixture of 0% O_2 and another with either 12% or 20% O_2 for the two-point calibration.
5. The criteria for acceptable results are below
   a. pH must be within ±0.04 of the target value.
   b. PCO_2 must be within ±3 mm Hg of the target value.
   c. PO_2 must be within ±3 mm Hg of standard deviations.

POSTCHAPTER STUDY QUESTIONS

1. Interpret the following arterial blood gas values
   A. pH 7.21, $PaCO_2$ 43 mm Hg, PaO_2 81 mm Hg, HCO_3^- 14 mEq/L
   B. pH 7.36, $PaCO_2$ 62 mm Hg, PaO_2 58 mm Hg, HCO_3^- 36 mEq/L
   C. pH 7.57, $PaCO_2$ 27 mm Hg, PaO_2 89 mm Hg, HCO_3^- 24 mEq/L
   D. pH 7.22, $PaCO_2$ 51 mm Hg, PaO_2 71 mm Hg, HCO_3^- 17 mEq/L
   E. pH 7.44, $PaCO_2$ 28 mm Hg, PaO_2 80 mm Hg, HCO_3^- 18 mEq/L
   F. pH 7.32, $PaCO_2$ 52 mm Hg, PaO_2 84 mm Hg, HCO_3^- 31 mEq/L
2. What do the results of an Allen test mean?
3. What conditions shift the HbO_2 dissociation curve to the right?
4. When the HbO_2 curve is shifted to the right, how is the affinity of Hb for O_2 affected?
5. Calculate the $P(A-a)O_2$, given the following data
   PB 747 mm Hg
   ABG levels in a patient using 40% O_2

pH	7.42
$PaCO_2$	45 mm Hg
PaO_2	80 mm Hg
HCO_3^-	25 mEq/L

6. Which ABG value best reflects the patient's ability to ventilate?
7. List a set of ABG levels that are typical of a patient with diabetic ketoacidosis.

See answers at the back of the text.

BIBLIOGRAPHY

Cairo JM, Pilbeam S, *Mosby's respiratory care equipment*, ed 8, St Louis, 2009, Mosby.
Hess D and others: *Respiratory care principles and practice*, ed 1, Philadelphia, 2002, Saunders.
Wilkins RL, Stoller JK, Kacmarek R, *Egan's fundamentals of respiratory care*, ed 9, St Louis, 2009, Mosby.
Wilkins R, Krider S, Sheldon R: *Clinical assessment in respiratory care*, ed 5, St Louis, 2005, Mosby.

VENTILATOR MANAGEMENT

PRETEST QUESTIONS

Answer the pretest questions before studying the chapter. This will help you determine your strong and weak areas in the material covered.

1. The following information has been obtained from a ventilator patient.

Peak inspiratory pressure	48 cm H_2O
Plateau pressure	27 cm H_2O
VT	850 mL
PEEP	4 cm H_2O

On the basis of these data, the patient's static lung compliance is approximately which of the following?

A. 18 mL/cm H_2O
B. 20 mL/cm H_2O
C. 31 mL/cm H_2O
D. 37 mL/cm H_2O

2. A volume-cycled ventilator is in the control mode and the I:E inspiratory/expiratory ratio alarm is sounding. Which control adjustment would correct this problem?

A. Decrease the flow rate.
B. Increase the VT.
C. Increase the respiratory rate.
D. Increase the flow rate.

3. Mechanical ventilation can lead to which of the following complications?

1. **Increased renal output**
2. **Barotrauma**
3. **Increased cardiac output**

A. 1 only
B. 2 only
C. 1 and 2 only
D. 2 and 3 only

4. Static lung compliance will decrease as a result of which of the following?

A. Bronchospasm
B. Mucosal edema
C. Atelectasis
D. Bronchial secretions

5. These data have been collected from a patient whose ventilator was in the control mode.

		ABGs:	
VT	800 mL	pH	7.50
Rate	15/min	$PaCO_2$	30 mm Hg
FiO_2	0.45	PaO_2	98 mm Hg

To increase this patient's $PaCO_2$ to 40 mm Hg, the ventilator rate should be adjusted to what level?

A. 10/min
B. 11/min
C. 12/min
D. 13/min

6. The following data have been collected from a patient using a volume ventilator in the control mode.

		ABGs:	
VT	700 mL	pH	7.44
Rate	10/min	$PaCO_2$	42 mm Hg
FiO_2	0.50	PaO_2	58 mm Hg

Based on this information, the respiratory therapist should recommend which of the following ventilator changes?

A. Increase FiO_2 to 0.60.
B. Increase VT to 800 mL.
C. Add 5 cm H_2O of PEEP.
D. Initiate CPAP with 4 cm H_2O and an FiO_2 of 0.50.

See answers and rationales at the back of the text.

REVIEW

I. **MECHANICAL VENTILATORS**
   CRT Exam Content Matrix: IIA6a-b, IIA11a, d, IIID2c, IIID10, IIIF2i6,9, IIIG3f,i,k, l
   RRT Exam Content Matrix: IIA2a-b, IIID2c, IIID8, IIIF2e6, IIIG3f,h,k

A. **Positive Pressure Ventilation**
  1. Types of positive pressure ventilators
     a. Preset volume ventilators (volume-limited or volume-cycled)
     b. Preset pressure ventilators (pressure-limited or pressure-cycled)
  2. **Volume ventilators**
     a. A preset VT is delivered to the patient in each machine breath, and once it is delivered, inspiration ends.
     b. The volume-limited ventilator can develop an inspiratory pressure that maintains the preset VT when changes in airway resistance and compliance occur (i.e., volume is constant, pressure is variable).
     c. Used for mechanical ventilation of the lungs of adult patients.
  3. **Pressure-cycled ventilators**
     a. A preset inspiratory pressure is delivered to the patient, and once it is reached, inspiration ends.
     b. The delivered VT is unknown but varies with changes in airway resistance and lung compliance (i.e., volume varies, pressure is constant).
     c. When lung compliance decreases, delivered VT decreases. In other words, as the patient's lungs become stiffer and harder to ventilate, the delivered VT decreases.
     d. The pressure control is used like the volume control. When inspiratory pressure is increased, delivered VT is increased and vice versa.
     e. Used to ventilate the lungs of infants and postoperative patients and to administer IPPB treatments. Inspiration ends on most infant ventilators when a preset time is reached. The set inspiratory pressure is reached during that time.
     f. Recently, **pressure control ventilation (PCV)** has been used as a mode of ventilation, especially for adult patients with ARDS in whom conventional volume ventilation with PEEP has not improved ventilation or oxygenation.
     g. Specific indications for PCV vary, but generally the patient should be used to the following ventilator variables before PCV is instituted
        (1) FiO_2, 1.0
        (2) PEEP >15 cm H_2O
        (3) PIP >50 cm H_2O
        (4) Assist/control rate >16/min
     h. Initial settings for PCV should include
        (1) Whatever the FiO_2 was set on prior to PCV

 Exam Note

PIP should be set to obtain a specified exhaled VT. In other words, if the "target" exhaled VT is 600 mL and the actual exhaled VT is 500 mL, then PIP should be increased.

---

        (2) VT, 6 to 10 mL/kg of ideal body weight (IBW)
        (3) PEEP of about 50% of the volume ventilator setting
        (4) I:E, 1:2

 Exam Note

PCV is often combined with inverse I:E ratio ventilation. Because this type of ventilation may be uncomfortable, the patient should be sedated and paralyzed.

---

     i. Studies have shown that PCV improves gas exchange, increases oxygenation, reduces PIP, increases mean airway pressure, reduces required PEEP levels, and decreases minute ventilation, especially when it is combined with an inverse I:E ratio. It has also been shown to reduce cardiovascular side effects and barotrauma compared with volume ventilation with PEEP.
     j. It is important that exhaled VT is monitored during PCV. Because inspiration is pressure-limited, the volume varies with changes in lung compliance and airway resistance.

Exam Note

When a ventilator scenario is given with a patient receiving PCV and the exhaled VT decreases with no change in ventilator settings, either compliance has decreased or airway resistance has increased. Remember, in PCV, inspiratory pressure is limited and cannot increase if compliance decreases or resistance increases. Therefore, delivered tidal volume will decrease.

---

     k. If an inverse I:E ratio of *greater* than 2:1 is used, intrinsic PEEP, also referred to as auto-PEEP, may occur. Auto-PEEP may be detected by monitoring expiratory waveform curves, which reveal the expiratory flow not returning to zero before the next breath. Auto-PEEP may result in barotrauma, decreased venous return and cardiac output, and increased patient effort to initiate a breath if the patient is assisting.

l. Extensive monitoring of the patient's cardiovascular and respiratory variables is vital for patients receiving PCV.

m. The ARDS network has developed guidelines and lung protective strategies to help better ventilate the lungs of patients with ARDS. Below is a summary of those strategies
   (1) Target VT of 6 mL/kg of IBW
   (2) Maintenance of alveolar (plateau) pressure ≤30 cm H_2O
   (3) Use of relatively high PEEP levels (up to 24 cm H_2O)
   (4) Permissive hypercapnia: With the use of lower tidal volumes and therefore lower peak pressures, CO_2 levels may begin to rise, resulting in respiratory acidosis. Studies indicate that a higher percentage of patients recover with minimal side effects from the acidosis if the pH does not drop below 7.20. In fact, acidosis may produce some positive effects. As CO_2 increases, the patient will become sleepy and easier to control while using the ventilator. Also, an acidotic environment shifts the oxyhemoglobin curve to the right, which means that hemoglobin releases oxygen to the tissues more easily and increases the level of tissue oxygenation.
   (5) Oxygenation target: PaO_2, 55 to 80 torr; SpO_2, 88% to 95%; PEEP/FiO_2 adjustments should be assessed at least every 4 h.
   (6) Target pH of 7.30 to 7.45
   (7) Avoidance of excessively high FiO_2 levels (try to maintain below 0.60)

n. Another type of pressure ventilation is **bilevel positive airway pressure, or Bi-PAP.** Bi-PAP may be used on intubated or nonintubated patients. Because patients with COPD have difficulty being weaned from mechanical ventilation, Bi-PAP is used to ventilate the lungs of these patients through a nasal mask, which avoids intubation and conventional volume ventilation. Bi-PAP may buy time for the patient to get past the initial ventilatory crisis and avoid intubation and ventilation. Although it is not always successful, it is becoming a first step in ventilating the lungs of many patients with COPD.

o. Bi-PAP is also used in home ventilation for patients with neuromuscular dysfunction, obstructive sleep apnea, and other conditions that result in hypoventilation.

p. Bi-PAP may be time-triggered or patient-triggered. Once inspiration begins, a preset **inspiratory positive airway pressure** (IPAP) is reached. Expiratory positive airway pressure (EPAP) should be preset to avoid CO_2 buildup in the nasal mask. EPAP is the equivalent of PEEP.

q. The initial IPAP setting is usually 10 to 15 cm H_2O, and the EPAP setting is 4 to 5 cm H_2O. The difference between the IPAP and EPAP settings is the pressure support. In this example, pressure support is 6 cm H_2O. IPAP settings range from 2 to 25 cm H_2O, and EPAP ranges from 2 to 20 cm H_2O.

r. A frequency control determines the timed breath rate and is adjustable from 6 to 30 cycles/min. The % IPAP control is set to determine the time spent in inspiration and functions as the I:E ratio control.

s. Bi-PAP is not a life-support ventilator. The practitioner should use an IPAP that results in an exhaled VT of 8 to 10 mL/kg IBW.

t. Criteria for Bi-PAP mask ventilation include stable hemodynamics, a cooperative patient, minimal airway secretions, and no need for airway protection.

II. **VENTILATOR CONTROLS**
   CRT Exam Content Matrix: IIID2b,d, IIIF2i1-5, 11, IIIG3a-e
   RRT Exam Content Matrix: IIID2b,d, IIIF2e1,2,3,4,5,9, IIIG3a-e
   A. **Ventilator Modes (Volume Ventilators)**
      1. **Control mode**
         a. Patient is not able to trigger a ventilator breath.
         b. Inspiration is strictly time-triggered.

EXAMPLE:

Control rate of 10: The ventilator delivers a breath every 6 s (60 ÷ 10). The minute volume remains constant because the rate cannot be altered.

---

         c. The patient should be heavily sedated or paralyzed.
      2. **Assist-control mode**
         a. In this mode, each breath is either patient-triggered or time-triggered.
         b. This is a commonly used mode of ventilation.
         c. The patient may initiate as many ventilator breaths as required above the set rate; therefore, the patient's minute volume is not consistent.

3. **Synchronized intermittent mandatory ventilation**
   a. Allows for spontaneous breathing along with positive pressure ventilator breaths. It is built into the ventilator and senses when the patient is breathing spontaneously; therefore, no "breath stacking" occurs.
   b. It is used as both a weaning technique and for ventilation before weaning.
   c. The sensitivity is left on because the patient must open a demand valve to obtain gas flow for spontaneous breathing.
4. **Pressure support ventilation**
   a. This mode of ventilation is found on the new generation of ventilators that aid in the weaning process from the ventilator.
   b. It is a patient-assisted, pressure-generated, flow-cycled breath, which may be augmented with SIMV or used by itself.
   c. It was designed to make spontaneous breathing through the ET tube during weaning more comfortable by overcoming the high resistance and increased inspiratory work caused by the ET tube **(5 to 10 cm H$_2$O is all that is required to overcome tubing resistance).**
   d. An inspiratory pressure is set (usually 5 to 10 cm H$_2$O for weaning purposes). As the patient initiates inspiration, the preset pressure is reached and held constant until a specific inspiratory flow is reached. Then the pressure is terminated.
   e. The inspiratory pressure level may be set to achieve a specific VT.
   f. Pressure support ventilation (PSV) may be used for patients who are ventilating well but are intubated to protect their airway or for patients using CPAP but who have oxygenation deficiencies.
5. **Continuous positive airway pressure**
   a. May be achieved with the use of a CPAP mask, nasal prongs, or intubation and a ventilator.
   b. A preset pressure is maintained in the airways as the patient breathes totally on his or her own. No positive pressure breaths are delivered.
   c. Patients whose PaO$_2$ level cannot be maintained within normal limits using a **60% or more O$_2$ mask and who have normal or low PaCO$_2$ levels should begin using CPAP. CPAP is also indicated for patients with obstructive sleep apnea who gain benefit from the positive airway pressure,** which relieves the obstruction in the upper airway.

   d. CPAP setups should always have a **low-pressure alarm** so that leaks in the system are detected.
   e. CPAP separate from the ventilator, such as a CPAP mask, may be accomplished.
      (1) In this type of setup, the patient's exhaled gas flow enters the expiratory limb of the circuit, where it meets an opposing gas flow entering through a Venturi tube.
      (2) This opposing gas flow causes a resistance to exhalation that the patient must overcome.
      (3) The pressure the patient must generate to overcome this resistance results in a positive pressure that is read on a manometer placed in the setup line. This pressure is the CPAP level.
      (4) The CPAP level may be increased or decreased by adjustment of the opposing gas flow that is passing through the Venturi tube in the expiratory limb.
   f. The indications and hazards of CPAP are the same as those listed for PEEP later in this chapter.

B. **VT Control**
   1. Determines the delivered VT to the patient in milliliters or liters.
   2. Should be set at **8 to 12 mL/kg IBW.** May **use as low as 5 to 6 mL/kg IBW for patients with ARDS.** For patients with COPD, 8 to 10 mL/kg is generally adequate.

> ☑ **Exam Note**
>
> Use tidal volumes that do not cause overdistention of alveoli. It is best to maintain alveolar pressure (static pressure) less than 35 cm H$_2$O. Studies indicate that alveolar pressures greater than 35 cm H$_2$O result in lung damage.

   3. For children, use 5 to 7 mL/kg IBW.
      a. **Calculating IBW** (in lb)
         For males

         $$106 + [6 \times (\text{height in inches} - 60 \text{ in})]$$

         For females

         $$105 + [5 \times (\text{height in inches} - 60 \text{ in})]$$

      b. This is very important when you are asked to determine the ventilator VT for an obese patient.

The physician wants your recommendation for the ventilator VT setting for a 5 ft 3 in female patient who weighs 150 kg (330 lb).

$$105 + 5 \times (63 - 60)$$

$$105 + (5 \times 3)$$

$$105 + 15 = 120 \text{ lb (IBW)}$$

$$120 \text{ lb} \div 2.2 \text{ lb/kg} = 55 \text{ kg}$$

$$VT = 10 \text{ mL/kg} \times 55 \text{ kg} = 550 \text{ mL}$$

 Exam Note

To save time, after determining IBW, simply divide the weight by 2 and add a zero to the end of the number. This will represent an adequate initial VT setting that is close to 10 mL/kg. For example, the patient's IBW is 140 lbs. Divide 140 by 2 and you get 70. Adding a zero makes the number 700. Select the choice that is closest to a 700-mL setting.

4. **Increasing the VT increases alveolar ventilation while also increasing the minute volume. This decreases the PaCO$_2$.**

 Exam Note

The most effective way to improve alveolar ventilation and decrease PaCO$_2$ is by increasing the tidal volume, not by increasing the ventilator rate.

Exam Note

A ventilator scenario may be given indicating the patient has a high PaCO$_2$. Increasing the rate and increasing the VT are both given as choices to correct the hypercapnia. Never assume you always select one over the other in a situation like this. You must review the scenario. If the question states the patient has atelectasis, you must increase the VT, not the rate. Atelectasis indicates an inadequate VT; therefore, increasing the rate is not as beneficial.

5. **Decreasing the VT decreases alveolar ventilation while also decreasing the minute volume. This increases the PaCO$_2$.**

EXAMPLE:

A patient breathing 10/min with a VT of 600 mL has a minute volume of 6 L. (Minute volume is calculated as respiratory rate × VT.) If the patient begins breathing at a respiratory rate of 20/min with a VT of 300 mL, the minute ventilation remains 6 L, but the alveolar ventilation has decreased as a result of the decreased VT.

6. On volume ventilators
   a. Increasing the VT increases the inspiratory time.
   b. Decreasing the VT decreases the inspiratory time.
7. The preset machine VT is not the actual volume reaching the patient's lungs.
   a. Volume is "lost" in the ventilator circuit because of airway resistance from gas flow.
   b. Tubing compliance may be calculated to determine how much volume is being lost in the circuit.
   c. With the ventilator set on a specific VT and the high-pressure limit turned up completely, the machine is cycled into inspiration with the ventilator Y adapter occluded. Observe the manometer pressure reading.
   d. Compliance formula

$$\text{Compliance} = \frac{\text{volume}}{\text{pressure}}$$

EXAMPLE:

Set VT at 200 mL (0.2 L). Peak pressure reached is 40 cm H$_2$O.

$$C = \frac{200 \text{ mL}}{40 \text{ cm H}_2\text{O}} = 5 \text{ mL/cm H}_2\text{O}$$

This means that once the patient has started using the ventilator, 5 mL of the set tidal volume will be lost in the tubing for every 1 cm H$_2$O registering on the manometer.

EXAMPLE:

Tubing compliance, 5 mL/cm H$_2$O
VT, 800 mL
Peak inspiratory pressure, 20 cm H$_2$O

Lost volume = tubing compliance × peak inspiratory pressure

$$5 \text{ mL/cm H}_2\text{O} \times 20 \text{ cm H}_2\text{O} = 100 \text{ mL (lost volume)}$$

Set VT is 800 mL

$$800 \text{ mL} - 100 \text{ mL (lost volume)} = 700 \text{ mL}$$

   e. Lost volume is affected by the water level in the humidifier. Lower water levels allow more compressed volume into the walls of the humidifier; hence, more volume is lost or less volume is delivered to the patient.

f. Volume is also lost in the patient's conducting airways (e.g., trachea and bronchi) as a result of resistance to gas flow. This part of the patient's airway is called the **anatomic dead space.** It is the part of the airway where no gas exchange occurs, and it is often called "wasted air."

Exam Note

Anatomic dead space is equal to 1 mL/lb of the patient's IBW, but it is reduced by 50% in the intubated patient. Thus, anatomic dead space is equal to about 1 mL/kg.

EXAMPLE:

An intubated 75-kg (165-lb) patient has an anatomic dead space of approximately 75 mL. This means that 75 mL of the patient's VT does not reach the alveoli to take part in gas exchange. This may also be subtracted from the ventilator VT setting to obtain a corrected VT.

When the formula for selecting ventilator VT as 10 to 12 mL/kg of body weight is used, this lost volume is taken into account, and this is usually an adequate VT. Some ventilators compensate for volume lost in the tubing by delivering a higher VT automatically.

8. Exhaled VT is measured by an exhaled volume digital display. Exhaled VT is most accurately measured with a respirometer placed between the ET tube and ventilator Y adapter or at the exhalation valve. To most accurately measure **the VT delivered by the ventilator, place a respirometer directly on the ventilator outlet.**
9. Volume may be lost from other causes.
   a. Loose humidifier jar or tubing connections cause low exhaled VT readings.
   b. Leakage around the ET tube cuff results in low exhaled VT readings.

C. **Respiratory Rate Control**
1. **Normal initial setup is 8 to 12 breaths/min.**
2. **Adjusting the rate control alters the expiratory time, therefore altering the I:E ratio.**
   a. Increasing the rate decreases expiratory time.
   b. Decreasing the rate increases expiratory time.
3. **Adjusting the rate alters the minute volume.**
   a. Increasing the rate increases minute volume.
   b. Decreasing the rate decreases minute volume.
4. **Adjusting the rate affects the PaCO₂ level.**
   a. Increasing the rate decreases $PaCO_2$.
   b. Decreasing the rate increases $PaCO_2$.

Exam Note

Adjusting the rate to alter the patient's PaCO₂ level is more beneficial for patients receiving controlled ventilation or SIMV. When the ventilator is on assist/control, the patient may obtain as many machine breaths as needed, no matter what rate is set, so the PaCO₂ is most effectively altered by adjustment of the VT control.

D. **Inspiratory Flow Control**
1. Normal setting: 40 to 60 L/min.
2. Adjusting the flow rate alters the inspiratory time, therefore altering the I:E ratio.
   a. Increasing the flow rate decreases inspiratory time.
   b. Decreasing the flow rate increases inspiratory time.
E. **I:E ratio**
1. A comparison of the inspiratory time with the expiratory time
2. **Normal I:E ratio for the adult is 1:2.** This means that expiration is twice as long as inspiration.
3. Normal I:E ratio for the infant is 1:1.
4. The I:E ratio is established by the use of **three** ventilator controls on the volume ventilator.
   a. **VT control**
      (1) Increasing the VT increases inspiratory time (makes inspiratory time longer).
      (2) Decreasing the VT decreases inspiratory time (makes inspiratory time shorter).
   b. **Flow rate control**
      (1) Increasing the flow rate decreases inspiratory time.
      (2) Decreasing the flow rate increases inspiratory time.
   c. **Respiratory rate control**
      (1) Increasing the respiratory rate decreases expiratory time.
      (2) Decreasing the respiratory rate increases expiratory time.
5. Calculate the I:E ratio with the following formula

$$I:E = \frac{\text{inspiratory flow rate (L/min)}}{\text{minute volume (L/min)}} - 1 \text{ (for inspiration)}$$

EXAMPLE:

VT	800 mL (0.8 L)
Rate	12/min
Flow rate	40 L/min

$$I:E \text{ ratio} = \frac{40 \text{ L/min}}{(0.8 \text{ L} \times 12)} = \frac{40 \text{ L/min}}{9.6 \text{ L/min}} = 4.2 - 1 = 1:3.2$$

6. **Calculation of inspiratory time**

$$I\ time = \frac{total\ cycle\ time}{sum\ of\ I{:}E\ ratio\ parts}$$

EXAMPLE:

Calculate the inspiratory time if the I:E ratio is 1:2 and the ventilator rate is 10/min.

$$Total\ cycle\ time = \frac{60}{10\ (rate)} = 6\ s$$

$$I\ time = \frac{6\ s}{3\ (I{:}E\ parts)} = 2\ s$$

---

7. Inspiratory time should not exceed expiratory time, except in specific situations. This is referred to as an **inverse I:E ratio.** Inverse ratio ventilation is sometimes utilized to increase the PaO_2 when FiO_2 and PEEP levels are already high. It may greatly compromise venous blood return to the heart and increase intrathoracic pressure.

 Exam Note

When given a scenario on the exam where a ventilator patient has a normal $PaCO_2$ with hypoxemia and the PEEP and FiO_2 levels are high, increase the inspiratory time to increase the PaO_2. This allows for a longer time for oxygen to diffuse across the alveolar capillary membrane, thereby increasing the PaO_2.

    a. If the I:E ratio alarm is sounding on the ventilator indicating an inverse I:E ratio, three controls may be altered to correct it.
       (1) Rate: decrease to lengthen expiratory time.
       (2) Volume: decrease to shorten inspiratory time.
       (3) Flow: increase to shorten inspiratory time.

Exam Note

Increasing flow is the most common adjustment to correct for an inverse I:E ratio.

F. **O_2 Percentage Control**
   1. Adjustable from 21% to 100% to maintain normal PaO_2 levels
   2. O_2 percentage should be increased to a maximum of 60% to maintain normal PaO_2 levels. Once 60% is reached, PEEP should be added or increased.

3. O_2 percentage should be reduced first to a level of 60% before decreasing PEEP levels in hyperoxygenated patients.
4. The initial setting should be what FiO_2 level the patient was receiving before the initiation of mechanical ventilation.

 Exam Note

The major ventilator controls have been discussed thus far in the chapter, so let's summarize how to set the variables to initiate mechanical ventilation.
Mode: A/C or SIMV
VT: 8 to 12 mL/kg IBW
Ventilator rate: 8 to 12/min
FiO_2: whatever the FiO_2 the patient was receiving before the initiation of ventilation

G. **Sensitivity Control**
   1. This determines the amount of patient effort required to cycle the ventilator into inspiration.
   2. Should be set so that the patient generates **−0.5 to −2.0 cm H_2O pressure.**
   3. If the ventilator self-cycles, the sensitivity is too high. Decrease the sensitivity.
   4. **If it takes more than −2.0 cm H_2O pressure to cycle the ventilator into inspiration, increase the sensitivity.**
   5. In the control mode of ventilation, the sensitivity is turned off and does not allow the patient to trigger a machine breath.
H. **Sigh controls**
   1. The sigh rate should be set at 6 to 12 sighs/h.
   2. The sigh volume should be set 1.5 to 2.0 times the VT.
   3. Sighs aid in preventing atelectasis.
   4. Usually not functional in the SIMV mode

 Exam Note

Although sighs are not commonly used in practice in many areas, the exam may still offer questions on the subject.

I. **Inflation Hold Control**
   1. Adjustable from 0 to 2 s
   2. The mechanism keeps the exhalation valve closed, causing the ventilator VT to be held in the lungs for a preset time.
   3. Used to improve oxygenation by reducing atelectasis and shunting and increasing the diffusion of gases.
   4. Using an inspiratory hold causes an increase in intrathoracic and mean airway pressure, which may result in reduced venous return and cardiac output.

5. Used to obtain a plateau pressure to calculate static lung compliance.

J. **Expiratory Retard (Expiratory Resistance)**
1. Used to prevent premature airway collapse during expiration.
2. Increases the expiratory time, therefore altering the I:E ratio and increasing intrathoracic pressure.
3. Expiratory retard causes an increase in intrathoracic and mean airway pressure, which may result in reduced venous return and cardiac output.

☑ Exam Note

Although expiratory resistance is rarely an option on ventilators, exam questions may appear on the subject.

K. **Positive End-Expiratory Pressure**
1. Used to maintain positive pressure in the airway after a ventilator breath.

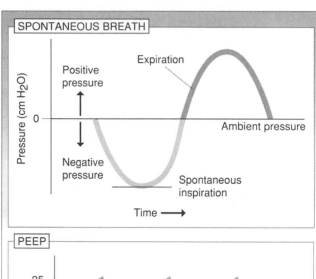

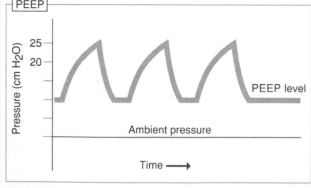

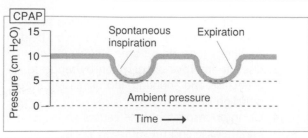

FIGURE 11-1 Positive end-expiratory pressure (PEEP) curves compared with other curves.

2. **Indications for PEEP**
   a. Atelectasis
   b. Hypoxemia with the use of 60% or more O_2
   c. Decreased functional residual capacity (FRC)
   d. Lowering O_2 percentage to safe levels (less than 60%)
   e. Decreased lung compliance
   f. Pulmonary edema
3. Hazards of PEEP
   a. Barotrauma
   b. Decreased venous return
   c. Decreased cardiac output
   d. Decreased urinary output
4. Excessive PEEP levels may lead to decreases in PaO_2 and lung compliance by overdistending already open alveoli and shunting blood to collapsed alveoli.
5. A decreased cardiac output (or cardiac index) caused by PEEP is indicated by a decrease in blood pressure and PvO_2 values.
6. **Optimal PEEP: the level of PEEP that improves lung compliance without decreasing the cardiac output.**
7. A mixed venous PO_2 (PvO_2) level may be obtained from the pulmonary artery by means of a pulmonary artery catheter and reflects changes in the cardiac output.
   a. **Normal PvO_2 is 35 to 45 mm Hg.**
   b. **A PvO_2 of less than 35 mm Hg indicates a possible decrease in cardiac output. If the PvO_2 decreases after initiation of PEEP, it is an indicator of reduced venous return and cardiac output caused by PEEP.**
   c. The PvO_2 value indicates the adequacy of tissue oxygenation.
   d. **Use the PEEP level that provides the best lung compliance and PvO_2 value.**

EXAMPLE:

Determining optimal PEEP
  Which of the following represents optimal PEEP?

PEEP (cm H_2O)	PaO_2 (mm Hg)	PvO_2 (mm Hg)
4	68	34
6	74	37
8	78	33
10	82	32

Notice how the PvO_2 decreased after the increase in PEEP from 6 cm H_2O to 8 cm H_2O. This indicates a drop in cardiac output with this PEEP change. Therefore, return to the PEEP level that maintains the highest

PvO$_2$. In this example, the optimal PEEP level is 6 cm H$_2$O.

Remember that the PaO$_2$ does not determine optimal PEEP level. Even though the PaO$_2$ in this example continued to increase at increasing PEEP levels, it did so at the expense of a decreasing cardiac output. This indicates a worsening oxygenation status.

Another method of determining optimal PEEP levels is the determination of upper and lower inflection points on a pressure/volume curve. The lower inflection point indicates the alveolar critical opening pressure. The upper inflection point indicates the point of alveolar overdistention.

Setting the PEEP level at the lower inflection point ensures that the alveoli remain open at end exhalation. This reduces damage to the alveoli by preventing the opening and closing of the alveoli with each breath, which results in shear force damage. Not allowing the peak inspiratory pressure to exceed the upper inflection point ensures that the lowest airway pressure is being used to ventilate the lungs adequately without overdistending the alveoli and causing alveolar damage and a possible pneumothorax. Lower airway pressure also reduces the potential for cardiac side effects.

Allowing PIP above the upper inflection point results in higher PIP levels with little or no increase in delivered tidal volume.

Figure 11-2 shows the lower inflection point (best PEEP level) to be about 10 cm H$_2$O and the upper inflection point (best PIP level) to be about 28 to 30 cm H$_2$O. Using a PEEP of 10 cm H$_2$O keeps the alveoli from collapsing at end exhalation. Using a PIP of 28 to 30 cm H$_2$O ventilates the lungs effectively while preventing overdistention of the alveoli.

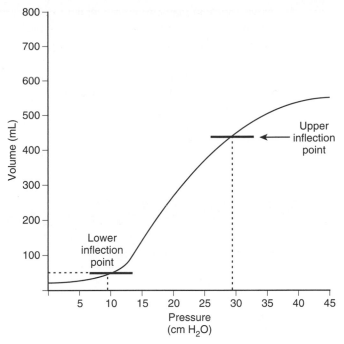

FIGURE 11-2   Best PEEP and PIP levels.

III. **VENTILATOR ALARMS AND MONITORING**
CRT Exam Content Matrix: IA7d-e, IB9c,m, IB10c, IC6, IC9, IIIE4e, IIIE7b, IIIE9, IIIF2i7, IIIG3g
RRT Exam Content Matrix: IA7d-e, IB9c,m, IB10c, IIIE4b, IIIE5, IIIE7b
A. **Low-Pressure Alarm**
   1. Should be set 5 to 10 cm H$_2$O below peak inspiratory pressure.
   2. This alarm is activated by leaks in the ventilator circuit, leaks around the chest tube, a ruptured ET tube cuff, inadequate cuff pressure, or patient disconnection.
B. **High-Pressure Alarm**
   1. Should be set 5 to 10 cm H$_2$O above peak inspiratory pressure.

2. When the high-pressure limit is reached on a volume ventilator, inspiration ends prematurely, decreasing delivered VT.
3. This alarm may be activated by
   a. Decreasing lung compliance
   b. Increasing airway resistance caused by
      (1) Airway secretions
      (2) Bronchospasm
      (3) Water in the ventilator tubing
      (4) Kink in the ventilator tubing
      (5) Patient coughing

 Exam Note

The PIP level should be maintained at less than 35 to 40 cm H_2O to prevent lung tissue damage.

C. **Low PEEP/CPAP Alarm**
   1. Should be set 2 to 4 cm H_2O below the baseline level.
   2. This alarm is activated for the same reasons as stated previously for the low-pressure alarm.
D. **Apnea Alarm**
   1. Set according to the patient's respiratory rate.
   2. This alarm is activated after a preset time passes with no inspiratory flow through the tubing.
   3. Important alarm for patients receiving ventilation in the CPAP mode or with low SIMV rates
E. **Low Tidal Volume Alarm**
   1. Should be set approximately 10% below the set tidal volume.
   2. This alarm is activated for the same reasons as stated previously for the low-pressure alarm.
F. **Mean Airway Pressure ($\bar{P}aw$) Monitoring**
   1. $\bar{P}aw$ is the average pressure applied to the airway over a specific time.
   2. $\bar{P}aw$ is directly affected by
      a. Ventilator rate
      b. Peak inspiratory pressure
      c. Inspiratory time
      d. Inspiratory hold
      e. Expiratory retard
      f. PEEP level
      g. Pressure waveform
      h. I:E ratio
   3. $\bar{P}aw$ is commonly measured by a digital reading on a $\bar{P}aw$ monitor, or it may be calculated with the use of the following equation

$$\bar{P}aw = 0.5 + [PIP - PEEP] \times \frac{\text{(inspiratory time)}}{\text{total respiratory cycle}}$$

   4. Optimal $\bar{P}aw$ is the level that improves oxygenation and ventilation without resulting in cardiovascular side effects and barotrauma.
   5. Studies have shown that $\bar{P}aw$ levels above 12 cm H_2O result in an increased risk of barotrauma.
   6. If there has been no change in dynamic compliance or ventilator variables and if $\bar{P}aw$ decreases, it indicates less pressure required to ventilate the patient's lungs or an increased static lung compliance. An increased $\bar{P}aw$ indicates higher pressure required to ventilate or a decreased static lung compliance.
G. **End-Tidal CO_2 Monitoring (Capnography)**
   1. Capnography is a technique by which exhaled CO_2 is measured. This measurement is obtained by the use of a mass spectrometer. (End-tidal CO_2 is abbreviated $PETCO_2$.)
   2. Normal $PETCO_2$ is approximately the same as alveolar CO_2, which is equal to arterial PCO_2. $PETCO_2$ therefore is a noninvasive technique to obtain the patient's $PaCO_2$ level.
   3. $PETCO_2$ may be expressed as partial pressure or a percentage. Normal $PETCO_2$ is 35 to 45 mm Hg **or 4.5% to 5.5%.**
   4. There is a difference of approximately 2 to 5 mm Hg between normal $PaCO_2$ and $PETCO_2$.
   5. $PETCO_2$ readings may decrease as a result of any of the following. (A low reading results from decreased perfusion to the pulmonary capillaries, rendering an inaccurate $PETCO_2$ reading. $PaCO_2$ may actually be increasing.)
      a. Hyperventilation
      b. Apnea (reading falls to zero)
      c. Total airway obstruction (reading falls to zero)
      d. Conditions in which perfusion is decreased (e.g., hypotension, pulmonary embolism, decreased cardiac output)
   6. $PETCO_2$ readings may increase as a result of the following
      a. Hypoventilation
      b. Hyperthermia (increased CO_2 production)
   7. Continuous $PETCO_2$ monitoring with tracings is becoming an important technique in monitoring critically ill patients. The tracing records CO_2 readings during inspiration (which should be zero because little CO_2 is in inspired air) and during expiration, when CO_2 begins to increase.
   8. A $PETCO_2$ measurement by itself should not be used to predict $PaCO_2$ in patients with left ventricular failure (decreased cardiac output), pulmonary embolism, or COPD because of inaccurate readings under these conditions.

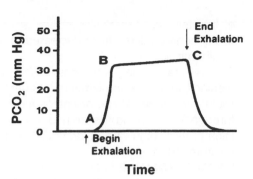

FIGURE 11-3 Capnography. From Wilkins RL, Stoller JK, Kacmarek R: *Egan's fundamentals of respiratory care*, ed 9, St Louis, 2009, Mosby.

IV. **INDICATIONS FOR MECHANICAL VENTILATION**

CRT Exam Content Matrix: IA7c,e, IB9d-e,j, IB10d,f
RRT Exam Content Matrix: IA7c,e, IB9d-e,j, IB10d,f

A. **Apnea**
B. **Acute Ventilatory Failure**
  1. $PaCO_2$ of greater than 50 mm Hg indicates ventilatory failure and a need for mechanical assistance.
  2. To determine ventilatory failure in a patient with COPD who chronically retains CO_2, note whether the pH is below 7.30. If so, there may be a need for ventilator assistance.
C. **Impending Acute Ventilatory Failure**
  1. Sometimes normal ABG levels can be deceiving. A patient may have normal ABG levels, but the respiratory rate may be 30/min to 40/min to achieve this normal PCO_2 level. This indicates pending ventilatory failure. The patient is likely to tire soon, which would result in an increasing $PaCO_2$ level and ventilatory failure.
  2. A patient with a neuromuscular disease, such as Guillain-Barré syndrome, must be monitored closely for lung muscle involvement. **Measurement of the patient's maximal inspiratory pressure (MIP) and vital capacity will help determine the lung status.**
D. **Oxygenation**
  1. The patient's lungs may be ventilating adequately but oxygenating poorly.
  2. Mechanical ventilation is indicated if O_2 deficiency is directly related to an abnormal ventilatory pattern or an increased work of breathing.
  3. A patient using an O_2 mask at **60% or more** whose lungs are being ventilated well (normal or low $PaCO_2$) but are not being oxygenated adequately (low PaO_2) is probably exhibiting a large intrapulmonary shunt. This may be corrected with CPAP. Mechanical ventilation may not be necessary initially.

V. **COMMON CRITERIA FOR INITIATION OF MECHANICAL VENTILATION**

CRT Exam Content Matrix: IA7b,c,e, IB9d-e,j,m, IB10d-f
RRT Exam Content Matrix: IA7b,c,e, IB9d-e,j,m, IB10d-f

A. Vital capacity (VC) of less than 10 to 15 mL/kg; normal is 65 to 75 mL/kg.
B. $P(A-a)O_2$ of greater than 450 mm Hg with the use of 100% O_2; normal is 25 to 65 mm Hg.
  1. When the PaO_2 is low and the $P(A-a)O_2$ is normal for ambient conditions and the patient's age, hypoxemia is most likely the result of hypoventilation.
  2. When the PaO_2 is low and the $P(A-a)O_2$ is high, hypoxemia is most likely the result of either a V/Q mismatch, diffusion defect, or shunting. In this situation, the patient may be hyperventilating to compensate for the hypoxemia.
C. VD/VT ratio of greater than 60%; normal is 25% to 35%.

$$\frac{VD}{VT} = \frac{PaCO_2 - PeCO_2}{PaCO_2}$$

D. Unable to obtain a MIP of at least −20 cm H_2O; normal is −50 to −100 cm H_2O.
E. PEP of less than 40 cm H_2O; normal is 100 cm H_2O.

☑ **Exam Note**

An MIP of greater than −20 cm H_2O or a PEP of less than 40 cm H_2O indicates that the patient cannot generate an adequate cough to maintain secretion clearance.

F. Respiratory rate of greater than 35/min; normal is 10/min to 20/min.

VI. **COMPLICATIONS OF MECHANICAL VENTILATION**

CRT Exam Content Matrix: IA7a, IB2-4, IB7a-b, IIIE6
RRT Exam Content Matrix: IA7a, IB2-4, IIIE6

A. **Barotrauma** (resulting from excessive airway pressure)
  1. Pneumothorax: may be characterized by **subcutaneous emphysema** (air in the subcutaneous tissues)
  2. Pneumomediastinum
  3. Pneumopericardium
B. **Pulmonary Infection**
  1. Debilitated patients have lower resistance.
  2. Contaminated equipment
  3. Improper airway care (e.g., tracheostomy care, suctioning)
  4. Retained secretions as a result of ET tube and poor ability to cough

5. Ciliary dysfunction caused by ET tube
6. Ventilator-associated pneumonia (VAP). (See section XVII of this chapter.)

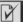 **Exam Note**

The most cost-effective method of preventing cross-contamination of patients and equipment is proper hand washing techniques.

C. **Atelectasis**
1. Using a minimum VT of 8 to 10 mL/kg of body weight prevents this (5 to 6 mL/kg IBW should be used for patients with ARDS).
2. Use of PEEP to prevent alveolar collapse

D. **Pulmonary O$_2$ Toxicity**
1. May result in ARDS.
2. Results from the use of high O$_2$ concentrations for prolonged periods.
3. Characterized by
a. Impaired surfactant production
b. Capillary congestion
c. Edema
d. Fibrosis
e. Thickening of alveolar membranes
f. Decreased lung compliance, resulting in high peak pressures being required to ventilate the patient's lungs. (See Chapter 12 on disorders of the respiratory system.)

E. **Tracheal Damage**
1. Usually at the cuff site

F. **Decreased Venous Blood Return to the Heart**
1. Results from **the positive airway pressures** being transferred onto the large veins returning blood to the heart, which causes decreased pulmonary blood flow, decreased cardiac output, and decreased blood pressure.

G. **Decreased Urinary Output**
1. Results from decreased renal blood flow (caused by decreased cardiac output).
2. Also results from an increased production of antidiuretic hormone **(ADH).**
a. ADH production increases because of baroreceptors in the atria of the heart, which sense the decreased venous return.
b. These receptors send a message to the hypothalamus, which stimulates the pituitary gland to secrete more ADH, thereby reducing urinary output.

H. **Lack of Nutrition**
1. Malnutrition may lead to
a. Difficulty weaning from the ventilator as a result of weakened respiratory muscles.
b. Reduced response to hypoxia and hypercarbia.
c. Impaired wound healing.
d. Decreased surfactant production.

e. Infection.
f. Pulmonary edema from decreased serum albumin levels.
2. Because oral feeding is not possible, nasogastric feedings should be implemented. Other feeding routes include an IV line or enteral feedings through a catheter in the stomach.
3. High-protein, high-carbohydrate diets are recommended.

VII. **DEAD SPACE VOLUME (VD)**
CRT Exam Content Matrix: IB9k, IB10i, IB10k
RRT Exam Content Matrix: IB10i
A. VD is that portion of the VT that does not take part in gas exchange.
B. **Types of VD**
1. **Anatomic VD** (discussed earlier) consists of the conducting airways from the nose and mouth to the terminal bronchioles (i.e., air that does not reach the alveolar epithelium where gas exchange occurs).
a. Anatomic VD=1 mL/lb body weight
b. **A tracheostomy decreases the anatomic VD** by bypassing the upper airway.
2. **Alveolar VD**
a. Air reaches the alveoli but does not take part in gas exchange.
b. Results from lack of perfusion to air-filled alveoli.
c. May result from hyperinflated alveoli where blood is not able to use all the air.
3. **Physiologic VD**
a. The sum of anatomic and alveolar VD.
b. The most accurate measurement of VD.
4. **Mechanical VD**
a. Ventilator circuits have a certain amount of VD, ranging from 75 to 150 mL.
b. Because anatomic VD decreases when a patient has an ET tube or tracheostomy tube, the VD created by the circuit is balanced out.
c. Additional mechanical dead space (VD) may be added to the ventilator circuit **between the ventilator Y adapter and the ET tube adapter to increase PaCO$_2$ levels**. This results from some of the patient's exhaled air (which contains CO$_2$) getting trapped in the excess tubing and being rebreathed with each ventilator breath.
(1) For every 100 mL of dead space added, the PaCO$_2$ increases approximately 5 mm Hg.
(2) Mechanical dead space (VD) may be added to the circuits of patients using control or assist/control modes only. **Never add dead space if the patient is receiving SIMV, PSV, or CPAP, which are modes the patient breathes spontaneously. Dead space**

would increase airway resistance and work of breathing in these modes.

 Exam Note

Although adding dead space to the ventilator circuit is rarely used clinically, questions regarding dead space are occasionally asked on the exams.

Exam Note

If a ventilator patient has an elevated $PaCO_2$ and the question indicates the patient has dead space added to the ventilator circuit, **always remove the dead space first**. Do not increase the VT or rate.

VIII. **LUNG COMPLIANCE (CL)**
   CRT Exam Content Matrix: IA7d, IB9m, IB10m, IC6
   RRT Exam Content Matrix: IA7d, IB9m, IB10n, IC7
   A. Lung compliance is defined as the ease with which the lung expands. It varies inversely with the pressure required to move a specific volume of air.

$$CL = \frac{V}{P}$$

   1. The higher the compliance, the easier it is to ventilate the lung. (The lung requires less pressure to ventilate.)
   2. The lower the compliance, the stiffer the lung is and the harder it is to ventilate. (The lung requires more pressure to ventilate.)
   3. **Normal total lung compliance** (sum of the compliance of lung tissue and thoracic cage) is **0.1 L/cm H_2O (100 mL/cm H_2O).**
   B. **Calculation of Lung Compliance**
   1. **Dynamic compliance**
      a. Formula

$$\text{Dynamic CL} = \frac{VT}{PIP - PEEP}$$

EXAMPLE:

Given the following data, calculate the patient's dynamic lung compliance.

VT	600 mL
PIP	35 cm H_2O
PEEP	5 cm H_2O

$$\text{Dynamic CL} = \frac{600 \text{ mL}}{30 \text{ cm } H_2O} = 20 \text{ mL/cm } H_2O$$

   b. Dynamic compliance is measured as air is flowing through the circuit and airways; therefore, it is actually a measurement of airway resistance, or R_{AW} and lung compliance
   c. Dynamic compliance changes with changes in R_{AW} caused by
      (1) Water in the ventilator tubing
      (2) Bronchospasm
      (3) Airway secretions
      (4) Mucosal edema
   d. **Dynamic compliance is not an accurate measurement of lung compliance**.
   2. **Static compliance**
      a. Is a more accurate measurement of lung compliance because it is measured with no air flowing through the circuit and airways (i.e., under static conditions).
      b. Airflow may be stopped with the volume remaining in the lungs by adjustment to a 1- to 2-s inspiratory hold.
      c. Once the flow has stopped, a **plateau pressure** or static pressure occurs after peak pressure has been reached. The drop from peak to plateau pressure represents the pressure that is being generated as gas is flowing through the tubing, rubbing against the sides of the tubing, ET tube, and airways.
      d. Static compliance is calculated as follows

$$\text{Static CL} = \frac{VI}{\text{plateau pressure} - PEEP}$$

EXAMPLE:

VT	800 mL
Plateau pressure	25 cm H_2O
PEEP	5 cm H_2O
Peak pressure	45 cm H_2O

Calculate the static lung compliance.

$$\text{Static CL} = \frac{800 \text{ mL}}{20 \text{ cm } H_2O} = 40 \text{ mL/cm } H_2O$$

Exam Note

Sometimes on the exams, the data provided to calculate static lung compliance will include not only the ventilator tidal volume but also the actual or exhaled volume. **Always use the actual volume in the equation if it is provided in the question.**

C. Important Points Concerning Lung Compliance

1. Increasing plateau pressures indicate that the lung compliance is decreasing, or the lungs are harder to ventilate.
2. If the peak pressures are increasing but the plateau pressure remains the same, then lung compliance is not decreasing. An increased R_{AW} is occurring from bronchospasm, secretions, coughing, tubing obstructions, and so on.

EXAMPLE:

Time	Peak Pressure	Plateau Pressure
6:00 AM	28 cm H_2O	10 cm H_2O
7:00 AM	34 cm H_2O	10 cm H_2O
8:00 AM	42 cm H_2O	10 cm H_2O

In this example, the peak pressures are increasing while the plateau pressures remain stable. This indicates an increase in R_{AW} and not a decreasing lung compliance.

EXAMPLE:

Time	Peak Pressure	Plateau Pressure
1:00 PM	34 cm H_2O	16 cm H_2O
2:00 PM	40 cm H_2O	22 cm H_2O
3:00 PM	44 cm H_2O	26 cm H_2O

In this example, the plateau pressures are increasing along with the peak pressures. This indicates a decreasing lung compliance.

---

3. Decreasing static lung compliance results from
   a. Pneumonia
   b. Pulmonary edema
   c. Consolidation
   d. Atelectasis
   e. Air-trapping
   f. Pleural effusion
   g. Pneumothorax
   h. ARDS
4. Normal static lung compliance in the patient receiving ventilation is 60 to 70 mL/cm H_2O.

 Exam Note

Calculation of lung compliance is also important in the determination of optimal PEEP level.

EXAMPLE:

Optimal PEEP is represented by which of the following?

PEEP (cm H_2O)	Peak pressure (cm H_2O)	Plateau pressure (cm H_2O)	VT (mL)
4	36	20	500
6	39	22	500
8	42	23	500
10	45	27	500

Remember that optimal PEEP is the level of PEEP that produces the highest static lung compliance. There is no need to calculate the compliance for all four PEEP levels in this problem. Because the VT is the same at all PEEP levels, simply subtract the PEEP level from the plateau pressure. The lowest number you get after doing this is the optimal PEEP level because the lower the number divided into the VT, the higher the lung compliance. In other words, a PEEP of 4 resulted in a plateau pressure of 20, which is a difference of 16. A PEEP of 6 also resulted in a difference of 16; a PEEP of 8, a difference of 15; a PEEP of 10, a difference of 17. The lower the number divided into the VT, the higher the compliance result; therefore, the optimal PEEP level in this example is 8 cm H_2O.

 Exam Note

If compliance data and cardiac output are both given in a question regarding optimal PEEP, select the PEEP level before the drop in cardiac output even if a higher PEEP level resulted in the best lung compliance. For example, the static lung compliance increases when the PEEP is increased from 10 cm H_2O to 12 cm H_2O, but the cardiac out drops. Choose 10 cm H_2O as the optimal PEEP. Remember, optimal PEEP is the level of PEEP that results in the best static lung compliance *without* decreasing the cardiac output.

D. **Calculation of Airway Resistance (R_{AW}).** For an intubated ventilator patient, the amount of pressure being delivered to the airways and how much is going to the alveoli must be known. The difference between these two is the amount of pressure lost as a result of R_{AW}. Determine this loss by subtracting the plateau pressure from the PIP. The closer the plateau pressure is to the peak pressure, the lower the pressure loss caused by R_{AW}, and vice versa. When this pressure difference is divided by the inspiratory flow, R_{AW} can be measured

$$R_{AW} = \frac{(PIP - plateau\ pressure)}{flow\ rate}$$

Normal R_{AW} in nonintubated individuals is 0.6 to 2.4 cm H_2O/L/s, based on a flow rate of 30 L/min or 0.5 L/s. Normal R_{AW} in a ventilator patient is approximately 5 cm H_2O/L/s.

⚠ Because R_{AW} is measured in cm H_2O/L/s, flow rate must be converted from L/min to L/s by dividing flow by 60.

EXAMPLE:

The following data have been collected from a patient using a volume ventilator.

Peak inspiratory pressure	35 cm H_2O
Plateau pressure	20 cm H_2O
Flow rate	60 L/min = 1 L/s

$$R_{AW} = \frac{35 \text{ cm } H_2O - 20 \text{ cm } H_2O}{1 \text{ L/s}}$$

$$= \frac{15 \text{ cm } H_2O}{1 \text{ L/s}} = 15 \text{ cm } H_2O/\text{L/s}$$

Because normal R_{AW} in an intubated patient is around 5 cm H_2O/L/s, this example reflects a high R_{AW}.

IX.　VENTILATION IN THE PATIENT WITH HEAD TRAUMA

Note: Although there is nothing in either the CRT or RRT Exam Content Matrix specific to this topic, the exams have questions regarding it.

A. Higher than normal flow rates should be used to make inspiratory time shorter, which would lessen the time of positive pressure in the airways. The longer the time of positive pressure in the airways, the more impedance of blood flow from the head, which increases ICP.

B. Maintain the $PaCO_2$ between 25 and 30 mm Hg to reduce ICP by vasoconstriction of cerebral vessels. ICP should be maintained below 15 mm Hg; normal ICP is <10 mm Hg.

 Exam Note

Studies indicate that hyperventilation to reduce cerebral blood flow may be detrimental because of inadequate perfusion to healthy brain tissue, but the exams consider it acceptable provided the question indicates the patient has an elevated ICP.

Exam Note

To decrease the $PaCO_2$ level, always increase the ventilator rate. Do not increase the tidal volume or inspiratory pressure because this may cause an increased intrathoracic pressure obstructing venous blood flow from the upper body and head back to the heart. Therefore, ICP may increase as the venous blood returning to the heart decreases.

C. If the ICP begins to increase, the patient should be hyperventilated (preferably with a resuscitation bag) to reduce the cerebral blood flow, thus lowering ICP.

D. Caution must be exercised when suctioning because this tends to increase ICP as a result of hypoxemia.

X.　WEANING FROM MECHANICAL VENTILATION

CRT Exam Content Matrix: IIID7, IIIF2i12, IIIG1g
RRT Exam Content Matrix: IIID6, IIIF2e10, IIIG1g

A. **Criteria for Weaning**
1. VT equal to three times the body weight in kilograms
2. VC >10 to15 mL/kg, or twice the VT
3. Ability to achieve an MIP of at least −20 cm H_2O
4. VD/VT <0.60
5. P(A–a)O_2 <350 mm Hg with the use of 100% O_2
6. Rapid shallow breathing index (RR/VT) <105
7. Respiratory rate <25/min
8. PEEP of 10 cm H_2O or less
9. PaO_2/FiO_2 >200
10. Underlying disease or condition stable or improving
11. Alert patient who is able to follow commands
12. Patient not taking any medications that may hinder spontaneous ventilation
13. No life-threatening situations, such as shock or hypotension
14. No anemia, fever, or electrolyte imbalances

B. **Weaning Techniques**
1. SIMV to decrease the number of mechanical ventilator breaths while allowing for more spontaneous breathing
   a. Patient should be using 40% O_2 or less before extubation.
   b. Patient should be receiving an SIMV rate of 4/min or less before removal from the ventilator.
   c. Postoperative patients may be weaned as they begin waking up. When patients have normal blood gas levels and are beginning to awaken, the SIMV rate can begin to be decreased.
2. **Time On–Time Off Method**
   a. The patient stops using the ventilator periodically, is given T-tube flow-by for a specific length of time, then begins using the ventilator again.
   b. The time without the ventilator is gradually increased until the patient is spending more time without the ventilator than he or she is using it.
   c. The patient is often returned to the ventilator while asleep.
   d. The patient must be monitored closely (e.g., blood pressure, VT, heart rate, respiratory rate, ABG levels, SaO_2) while receiving flow-by.
   e. Often, the O_2 percentage is increased 10% while receiving flow-by.

XI. **HIGH-FREQUENCY VENTILATION**
CRT Exam Content Matrix: IIID4
RRT Exam Content Matrix: IIA2c, IIID4

A. High-frequency ventilation (HFV) refers to breathing rates that are four times the normal rate (60/min in the adult). A smaller than normal VT is used, sometimes less than the anatomic VD. HFV has been shown to improve gas exchange without the barotrauma and cardiovascular problems associated with conventional volume-limited and pressure-limited ventilation in both infants and adults.

> ⚠ The ventilator rate or frequency is measured in Hertz (Hz) which is equal to one breath per second. For example, a rate of 60/min is equal to 1 Hz. A rate of 300/min is equal to 5 Hz, or 5 breaths/s.

B. **Three Classifications of HFV**
   1. **High-frequency positive pressure ventilation**
      a. Gas delivery to the patient occurs with the use of a time-cycled or pressure- or volume-limited device through ventilator tubing that has a low compressible volume. This ensures that little volume is lost in the tubing.
      b. Gas is directed through an insufflation catheter that is placed through the ET tube, and the rapid opening and closing of the exhalation valve determines gas flow into and out of the lungs.
      c. The exhalation valve opens and closes in response to a pneumatic or electric source. Some pneumatic units incorporate fluidic gates to accomplish the opening and closing of the exhalation valve.
      d. **Ventilatory rates with high-frequency positive pressure ventilation (HFPPV) are between 60/min and 100/min (1–1.67 Hz), and the VT is small (between 3 and 5 mL/kg of body weight). I:E ratio of 1 : 3 or less are normally used.**
      e. Delivery of a small VT results in lower peak inspiratory pressure and lower mean airway pressure at a much higher rate than conventional ventilation and an improved distribution of gas.
      f. PEEP may also be used with HFPPV to improve oxygenation and cause fewer cardiovascular side effects than conventional positive pressure ventilation and PEEP.
      g. HFPPV has also been used during thoracic surgery, such as lobectomy or pneumonectomy, in which conventional ventilation may not be effective.
   2. **High-frequency jet ventilation (HFJV)**
      a. A high-pressure gas source injects short, rapid bursts of gas through a jet catheter, usually incorporated into a special ET tube. Air is entrained through a separate channel during inspiration, which increases the flow to the patient.
      b. Frequency rates vary from about 100 to 600 cycles per minute (1.67–10 Hz) at I:E ratio of 1 : 1 to 1 : 4. Peak inspiratory pressures are usually about 8 to 10 cm H_2O above baseline. The VT is usually a little larger than the anatomic VD.
      c. A low-pressure alarm set 2 to 3 cm H_2O below peak inspiratory pressure should be incorporated to indicate power loss or system leaks.
      d. A high-pressure alarm should be set 5 to 10 cm H_2O above peak inspiratory pressure. This alarm may be activated by a plugged ET tube, air-trapping (resulting from short exhalation time at high rates), pneumothorax, or airway secretions requiring suctioning.
      e. The gas is most effectively humidified with the use of a heat exchanger that is designed to withstand high pressure. Water and the jet gas mix then pass through the exchanger. This warms the gas and also humidifies it.
      f. An infusion pump may also be used to humidify the inspired gas. The pump places water in front of the jet nozzle, and as the gas passes through the jet, it combines with the water just outside the jet, humidifying the gas.
      g. Because a low VT is delivered with HFV, resulting in an increased potential for atelectasis, PEEP should be employed so that the incidence of atelectasis is reduced.
   3. **High-frequency oscillation**
      a. High-frequency oscillation (HFO) requires an oscillating device that forces small impulses of gas into and out of the patient's airway.
      b. Three types of oscillating devices are used.
         (1) Piston: As the piston moves inward, a small volume of gas is delivered to the patient. As the piston withdraws, the same amount of gas is drawn away from the patient (exhalation). A sine-type flow wave is usually produced.
         (2) Diaphragm: Audio loudspeakers have been used to accomplish HFO. As the diaphragm vibrates, the rapid movement, both forward and backward, moves a volume of gas into and out of the patient's lungs.
         (3) Flow interrupter: As flow is being delivered to the patient's airways, it passes through a rotating bar with a hole in it. Gas flow periodically passes through the hole and is delivered in small bursts to the patient. Exhalation occurs by normal passive recoil of the lung.
      c. Oscillations occur at a rate of 60 to 3600/min (1–60 Hz) at a VT of less than anatomic VD.

d. HFO may be beneficial in treating patients with large degrees of intrapulmonary shunting. It is being used currently to ventilate the lungs of infants with respiratory distress syndrome.

☑ **Exam Note**

To lower the $PaCO_2$ using high frequency ventilation/oscillation, increase the frequency or the oscillatory amplitude.

C. **Potential Advantages of HFV over Conventional Ventilation**
1. Reduced risk of barotrauma
2. Reduced risk of cardiac side effects
3. Less fluctuation in ICP
4. Improvement of mucociliary clearance

XII. **ESTIMATING DESIRED VENTILATOR VARIABLE CHANGES**
CRT Exam Content Matrix: IIID2b, IIIF2i2-3, IIIG3b-c
RRT Exam Content Matrix: IIID2b, IIIF2e2-3, IIIG3b-c

A. **Making Changes in FiO_2**

$$\text{Desired } FiO_2 = \frac{PaO_2(\text{desired}) \times FiO_2(\text{current})}{PaO_2(\text{current})}$$

EXAMPLE:

The data below are from a patient using a volume ventilator.

Mode	Control	ABGs:	
		pH	7.43
VT	750 mL	$PaCO_2$	42 mm Hg
Rate	12/min	PaO_2	53 mm Hg
FiO_2	0.40		

To increase this patient's PaO_2 to 80 mm Hg, to what level must the FiO_2 be changed?

$$\text{Desired } FiO_2 = \frac{80 \times 0.4}{53} = \frac{32}{53} = 0.60$$

B. **Making Changes in the Ventilator Rate**

$$\text{Desired rate} = \frac{\text{Rate (current)} \times PaCO_2(\text{current})}{PaCO_2(\text{desired})}$$

EXAMPLE:

Data collected from a patient using a volume ventilator in the control mode.

		ABGs:		
VT	800 mL	pH	7.51	
FiO_2	0.35	$PaCO_2$	26 mm Hg	
Rate	16/min	PaO_2	94 mm Hg	

To raise the patient's $PaCO_2$ to 35 mm Hg, the ventilator rate should be adjusted to what level?

$$\text{Desired rate} = \frac{16 \times 26}{35} = \frac{416}{35} = 11.8 \text{ or } 12/\text{min}$$

C. **Making Changes in Minute Volume ($\dot{V}E$)**

Formula: $\dot{V}E$ = respiratory rate × VT

$$\text{Desired } (\dot{V}E) = \frac{\dot{V}E(\text{current}) \times PaCO_2(\text{current})}{PaCO_2(\text{desired})}$$

EXAMPLE:

Below are data collected from a patient using a volume ventilator in the control mode.

		ABGs:	
VT	700 mL (0.7 L)	pH	7.28
Rate	10/min	$PaCO_2$	54 mm Hg
FiO_2	0.45	PaO_2	74 mm Hg

Which of the following ventilator settings would decrease the patient's $PaCO_2$ to 45 mm Hg?

VT	650 mL	Rate	10/min
VT	700 mL	Rate	12/min
VT	700 mL	Rate	14/min
VT	750 mL	Rate	10/min

In this question, we use the equation above to derive the necessary $\dot{V}E$ to decrease the $PaCO_2$ to the desired level. Then choose the answer with the appropriate $\dot{V}E$ that has been calculated.

$$\text{Desired } \dot{V}E = \frac{7 \times 54}{45} = \frac{378}{45} = 8.4 \text{ L}$$

The $\dot{V}E$ required to decrease the $PaCO_2$ to 45 mm Hg is 8.4 L. In the example, the second choice gives a minute volume of 8.4 L (700 mL × 12/min).

D. **Making Changes in Alveolar Ventilation $\dot{V}A$**

Formula: $\dot{V}A = (\dot{V}T - \text{anatomic VD}) \times$ respiratory rate

$$\text{Desired } \dot{V}A = \frac{\dot{V}A(\text{current}) \times PaCO_2(\text{current})}{PaCO_2(\text{desired})}$$

EXAMPLE:

Below are data from a patient who is using a volume ventilator in the control mode.

		ABGs:	
VT	800 mL (0.8 L)	pH	7.30
Rate	12/min	$PaCO_2$	50 mm Hg
FiO_2	0.40	PaO_2	76 mm Hg
Anatomic VD	150 mL		

Which of the following ventilator settings would decrease the patient's $PaCO_2$ to 40 mm Hg?

VT	700 mL	Rate	15/min
VT	800 mL	Rate	18/min
VT	800 mL	Rate	15/min
VT	850 mL	Rate	12/min

In this question, use the equation above to derive the alveolar ventilation necessary to bring the $PaCO_2$ down to 40 mm Hg. It is the same equation used in the previous problem, except that we correct for anatomic VD (in this case, 150 mL), which is subtracted from the VT. This value is then multiplied by the respiratory rate to determine the $\dot{V}A$.

$$800 - 150 = 650 \text{ mL or } 0.65 \text{ L}$$

$$0.65 \times 12 = 7.8 \text{ L}$$

$$\text{Desired } \dot{V}A = \frac{7.8 \times 50}{40} = \frac{390}{40} = 9.75 \text{ L}$$

Therefore, an alveolar volume of 9.75 L is required to decrease the $PaCO_2$ to 40 mm Hg. Now choose the appropriate choice from the table above; in this case, it is the third one.

XIII. **PRACTICE VENTILATOR PROBLEMS**
CRT Exam Content Matrix: IIID2b, IIIF2i2-3, IIIG3b-c
RRT Exam Content Matrix: IIID2b, IIIF2e2-3, IIIG3b-c

A. A 75-kg male patient is using a volume ventilator in the control mode. Appropriate data from his chart are as follows

		ABGs:	
VT	700 mL	pH	7.28
Rate	12/min	PaCO₂	54 mm Hg
FiO₂	0.50	PaO₂	74 mm Hg
PEEP	5 cm H₂O	HCO₃⁻	23 mEq/L

Based on this information, the respiratory therapist should recommend which of the following ventilator changes?
1. Increase PEEP to 10 cm H_2O.
2. Add 100 mL of mechanical VD.
3. Increase the FiO_2 to 0.60.
4. Increase the VT to 800 mL.
   Answer: The fourth choice. The patient is hypoventilating as a result of an inadequate VT. The patient weighs 75 kg; therefore, use 10 to 12 mL/kg IBW to determine an adequate VT. The ventilator should be set on a VT between 750 and 900 mL.

B. A patient is using a volume ventilator in the control mode of ventilation. Pertinent data follow.

		ABGs:	
VT	800 mL	pH	7.41
Rate	12/min	PaCO₂	37 mm Hg
FiO₂	0.60	PaO₂	137 mm Hg
PEEP	8 cm H₂O	HCO₃⁻	26 mEq/L

What is the most appropriate ventilator change to recommend at this time?
1. Decrease the FiO_2 to 0.50.
2. Increase the VT to 900 mL.
3. Decrease the rate to 10/min.
4. Decrease the PEEP to 6 cm H_2O.
   Answer: The fourth choice. The patient's lungs are well ventilated but are hyperoxygenated with the use of 60% O_2. **On the board exams, begin weaning the patient from PEEP if the O_2% is 60% or less.**

C. A 46-year-old, 80-kg (176-lb) man's lungs are being mechanically ventilated with a volume ventilator in the assist/control mode. Data follow.

		ABGs:	
FiO₂	0.30	pH	7.48
Rate	12	PaCO₂	32 mm Hg
VT	800 mL	PaO₂	53 mm Hg

What is the most appropriate recommendation at this time?
1. Decrease the rate to 8/min.
2. Decrease VT to 750 mL.
3. Increase the FiO_2 to 0.50.
4. Begin PEEP at 8 cm H_2O for the patient.
   Answer: The third choice. This patient is slightly hyperventilating as a result of hypoxemia. As the PaO_2 increases, hyperventilation should subside. Increasing the FiO_2 or adding PEEP both will elevate the PaO_2, but because the FiO_2 is 0.30, we can safely increase it to as high as 0.60 before adding PEEP.

D. A patient is using the control mode of ventilation with the following settings

VT	800mL
Rate	10/min
FiO₂	0.35

ABG values

pH	7.50
PaCO₂	29 mmHg
PaO₂	97 mmHg
HCO₃⁻	25 mEq/L

What would be the most appropriate ventilator change to make at this time?
1. Increase the inspiratory flow.
2. Add 5 cm H_2O PEEP.
3. Increase the FiO_2 to 0.50.
4. Decrease VT to 700 mL.
   Answer: The fourth choice. This patient is hyperventilating, which is resulting in a low $PaCO_2$. Because the PaO_2 is normal, hypoxemia is not the cause of the hyperventilation. Minute ventilation is too high and can be reduced by decreasing VT, thereby increasing $PaCO_2$.

E. A 60-kg (132-lb) female patient is using a volume ventilator in the control mode with the following settings:

		ABGs:	
VT	800 mL	pH	7.52
Rate	12/min	$PaCO_2$	28 mm Hg
FiO_2	0.40	PaO_2	92 mm Hg

What is the appropriate ventilator change at this time?

1. Increase the FiO_2 to 0.50.
2. Add PEEP of 5 cm H_2O.
3. Decrease rate to 6/min.
4. Decrease VT to 600 mL.

> **Answer:** The fourth choice. The VT setting is more than 12 mL/kg, which is causing the patient to hyperventilate. Decreasing the VT will increase the $PaCO_2$. Decreasing the rate will also increase the $PaCO_2$, but a rate of 6/min (third choice) in the control mode is too low.

XIV. VENTILATOR FLOW, VOLUME, AND PRESSURE WAVEFORMS

CRT Exam Content Matrix: IIID3, IIIF2i8, IIIG3h,k
RRT Exam Content Matrix: IIID3, IIIF2e7, IIIG3g,j

A. Flow Waveforms

1. **Square wave (constant flow)**
   a. With this flow pattern, the flow remains constant throughout inspiration.
   b. Changes in R_{AW} and compliance do not change the flow pattern under normal circumstances.
   c. This type of flow pattern is beneficial to patients with increased respiratory rates.

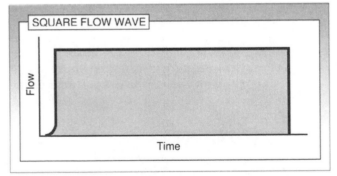

FIGURE 11-4

2. **Sine (sinusoidal) wave**

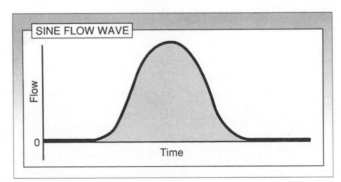

FIGURE 11-5

   a. The flow gradually accelerates from the beginning of inspiration then decelerates toward the end of inspiration.
   b. This flow pattern benefits patients with increased R_{AW} because airway turbulence produced by this flow is decreased.

3. **Decelerating ramp wave**
   a. The initial flow is high and begins decelerating as inspiration continues.
   b. The flow never decreases more than 50% to 55% of initial flow.
   c. The pattern benefits patients with low compliance by allowing ventilation to occur at a decreased pressure.
   d. This flow usually results in optimal distribution of gas, lower PIP, reduced work of breathing, and improved patient comfort.

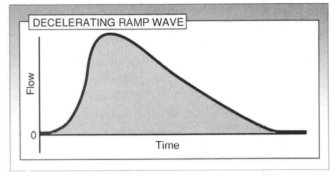

FIGURE 11-6

4. **Accelerating ramp wave**
   a. The flow is initially slow and accelerates to a peak flow by the end of inspiration.
   b. This pattern creates less turbulence of flow in the beginning of inspiration; therefore, more volume may be delivered through narrowed or obstructed airways.

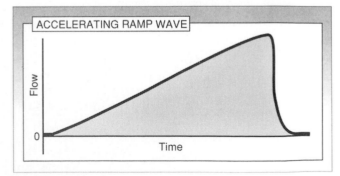

FIGURE 11-7

B. **Volume Waveform**
1. This is a typical volume waveform showing volume in milliliters on the vertical axis and time in seconds on the horizontal axis. Notice how the waveform returns to zero (baseline) during exhalation.

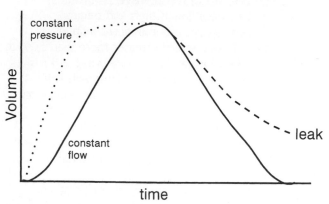

FIGURE 11-8 Typical volume waveform. Modified from Branson R, Hess D, Chatburn R: *Respiratory care equipment,* Philadelphia, 1999, Lippincott, Williams, and Wilkins.

2. If the volume tracing does not return to baseline at the end of exhalation, it is an indication of leaks in the ventilator circuit or around the ET tube cuff or chest tube, or it may result from air-trapping.

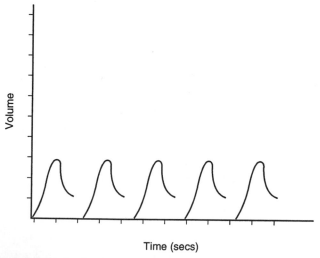

FIGURE 11-9 Atypical volume waveform.

3. If the volume tracing goes below the baseline, this is an indication of auto-PEEP or the patient may be coughing or agitated.

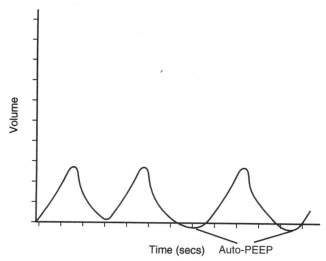

FIGURE 11-10 Typical pressure waveform.

4. Obstructive lung disease causes the tracing to be flat during exhalation as a result of decreased expiratory flows.

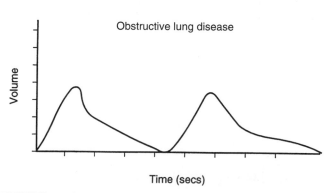

FIGURE 11-11

C. Pressure Waveform

1. This is a typical pressure waveform that is shown during volume ventilation; pressure is shown on the vertical axis, and time is on the horizontal axis. (When pressure ventilation is used, the pressure waveform is almost square.)

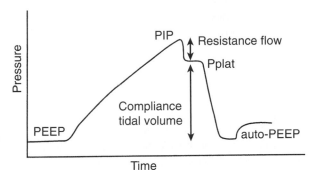

FIGURE 11-12 Lung compliance and auto-PEEP. Modified from Branson R, Hess D, Chatburn R: *Respiratory care equipment,* Philadelphia, 1999, Lippincott, Williams, and Wilkins.

2. Peak pressure rises during inspiration and is determined by VT, R_AW, lung compliance, and inspiratory flow.
3. The difference between peak pressure and plateau pressure is R_AW.
4. If the waveform does not return to baseline during exhalation, the patient is receiving PEEP, or auto-PEEP is occurring.

XV. SUMMARY OF VENTILATOR ADJUSTMENTS ACCORDING TO ABG RESULTS

CRT Exam Content Matrix: IIID2b, IIIF2i2-3, IIIG3b-c
RRT Exam Content Matrix: IIID2b, IIIF2e2-3, IIIG3b-c

ABG Abnormality	Ventilator Adjustment
Decreased pH, increased PaCO₂, decreased or normal PaO₂	Increase VT (Maintain 8 to 12 mL/kg) or increase rate
Increased pH, decreased PaCO₂, normal or increased PaO₂	Decrease VT, decrease rate or add mechanical VD
Normal pH, increased PaCO₂, PaO₂ of 50 to 65 mm Hg, increased HCO₃⁻	No adjustment needed; this is a patient with COPD. May begin weaning if other weaning criteria are met.
Normal or increased pH, normal or decreased PaCO₂, decreased PaO₂	Increase FiO₂ if <0.60. Add or increase PEEP if FiO₂ is 0.60 or more.
Normal pH, normal PaCO₂, increased PaO₂	Decrease FiO₂ if it is higher than 0.60; decrease PEEP if FiO₂ is 0.60 or lower.
Decreased pH, normal PaCO₂, decreased HCO₃⁻	No ventilator changes are necessary; administer HCO₃⁻.

XVI. MAINTENANCE OF THE VENTILATOR CIRCUIT

CRT Exam Content Matrix: IIB3, IIIF2i10, IIIG3j
RRT Exam Content Matrix: IIB2

A. Routine ventilator circuit changes vary from hospital to hospital, but the circuit should be changed no more frequently than once per week. The more frequently the circuit is changed, the higher the risk for VAP. Bacterial culturing of the circuits determines whether more frequent circuit changes are necessary.
B. When the ventilator circuit is changed, the patient should be hyperoxgenated before removal of the circuit. In some cases, when the patient may not tolerate even the shortest time away from the ventilator during the circuit change, the patient's lungs should be manually ventilated by a respiratory therapist or nurse while another therapist changes the circuit.

XVII. VENTILATOR-ASSOCIATED PNEUMONIA

CRT Exam Content Matrix: IIB3
RRT Exam Content Matrix: IIB2

A. Pneumonia which occurs in patients who have been receiving mechanical ventilation for at least 48 hours
B. Even though ET tubes are cuffed to help prevent the aspiration of large volumes of gastric material, oropharyngeal and subglottic secretions can still leak past the cuff and into the lower airway resulting in VAP.
C. VAP will most likely occur within the first 2 wk of mechanical ventilation; the mortality rate ranges from 5% to 40%.
D. Common pathogens responsible for VAP include *Pseudomonas aeruginosa, Klebsiella pneumoniae, Escherichia coli, Serratia marcescens, Staphylococcus aureus,* and *Streptococcus pneumoniae.*
E. Although there is no standard criteria for the diagnosis of VAP, patients generally have three or more of the following presenting symptoms
   1. Fever >38.2° C
   2. Purulent secretions
   3. Increased WBC count (>10,000/mL)
   4. New infiltrates on chest x-ray film
F. Methods to Reduce the Incidence of VAP
   1. Hand washing
   2. Noninvasive ventilation (higher incidence of VAP for intubated patients)
   3. Good oral hygiene procedures
   4. Positioning of patient in the semi-Fowler position: there is a greater incidence of VAP in the supine position
   5. Appropriate ET tube cuff pressure
   6. The use of a closed suction system; this eliminates disconnection from the ventilator for suctioning. The more the patient is disconnected, the higher the risk of contamination.
   7. The use of ET tubes (Hi-Lo Evac tube) that allow for continuous aspiration of subglottic

secretions. Studies indicate a 50% reduction in VAP when continuous aspiration is utilized. (See Chapter 4 on management of the airway.)

8. Less frequent ventilator circuit changes; as mentioned in the previous section, changes should be no more frequent than one per week. Studies indicate that circuits do not need to be changed unless they are visibly soiled or are not functioning properly. Make sure condensate is drained from the tubing so it does not drain into the patient's airway.

9. The use of heat moisture exchangers (HME) rather than heated humidifiers

10. Rotating (kinetic) beds; (proper patient-turning procedures may be just as beneficial in helping reduce the incidence of VAP as these beds)

11. Antibiotic treatment includes vancomycin, tobramycin, cefepime, and gentamicin.

POSTCHAPTER STUDY QUESTIONS

1. Pressure control ventilation is most commonly used for adults with what lung condition?
2. What effect does decreasing lung compliance have on delivered VT in a neonate receiving pressure-limited ventilation?
3. What level of pressure support should be used for weaning so that airway resistance is overcome while breathing is spontaneous?
4. As the oxygenation status of a patient worsens while using an O_2 mask, at what point should CPAP be employed?
5. How is minute ventilation calculated?
6. How is alveolar minute ventilation calculated?
7. Calculate the ventilator tubing compliance when the volume is set at 200 mL (0.2 L) and an inspiratory pressure of 50 cm H_2O is generated.
8. Using the tubing compliance in question number 7, calculate the corrected VT when the patient is receiving a VT of 700 mL with a peak inspiratory pressure of 20 cm H_2O.
9. On the initial ventilator setup, at what range should the ventilator rate be set?
10. How should the appropriate ventilator VT be determined?
11. List six indications for the use of PEEP.
12. List four hazards of PEEP.
13. Define optimal PEEP.
14. After the PEEP level is increased, how can it be determined that cardiac output has been adversely affected?
15. How may the ventilator low-pressure alarm be activated?
16. List ways that the ventilator high-pressure alarm may be activated.

17. How should the high-pressure alarm be set?
18. List some factors that affect airway resistance (R_{AW}).
19. What is normal PETCO$_2$?
20. List four conditions that result in a decreased PETCO$_2$ reading.
21. List two conditions that result in an increased PETCO$_2$ reading.
22. List six criteria that indicate mechanical ventilatory assistance is necessary.
23. List eight complications of mechanical ventilation.
24. Calculate the static lung compliance if the VT is 750 mL, PIP is 46 cm H_2O, PEEP is 8 cm H_2O, and plateau pressure is 28 cm H_2O.
25. List some conditions that result in decreased lung compliance.
26. What is indicated if peak inspiratory pressures are increasing but the plateau pressure is not increasing?
27. List the criteria that patients should meet before they can begin to be weaned from the ventilator.
28. What respiratory rates are used with HFJV?
29. List four advantages of high-frequency ventilation over conventional ventilation.
30. A ventilator patient receiving an FiO$_2$ of 0.30 has a PaO$_2$ of 60 mm Hg. To increase the PaO$_2$ to 80 mm Hg, what change to the FiO$_2$ must be made?
31. A patient using a ventilator in the control mode with a ventilator rate of 8/min has a PaCO$_2$ of 55 mm Hg. To decrease the PaCO$_2$ to 40 mm Hg, what change must be made to the ventilator rate?
32. A 36-year-old woman uses a ventilator in assist/control mode with the following variables: rate, 10/min; VT, 650 mL; and FiO$_2$, 0.40. The ABG results are as follows: pH, 7.27; PaCO$_2$, 54 mm Hg; PaO$_2$, 75 mm Hg; and HCO$_3^-$, 26 mEq/L. What ventilator alteration should be made?
33. A ventilator patient receiving an FiO$_2$ of 0.70 and PEEP of 8 cm H_2O has a PaO$_2$ of 147 mm Hg. What ventilator adjustment should be made to reduce the PaO$_2$?
34. On a volume waveform, if the tracing does not return to baseline, what does this indicate?

See answers at the back of the text.

BIBLIOGRAPHY

Branson R, Hess D, Chatburn R: *Respiratory care equipment*, Philadelphia, 1999, Lippincott, Williams, and Wilkins.

Cairo J, Pilbeam S, *Mosby's respiratory care equipment*, ed 8, St Louis, 2009, Mosby.

Eubanks D, Bone R, *Comprehensive respiratory care*, ed 2, St Louis, 1990, Mosby.

MacIntyre N, Branson R, *Mechanical ventilation*, ed 2, Philadelphia, 2009, Saunders.

Pilbeam SP, *Mechanical ventilation: physiological and clinical applications*, ed 4, St Louis, 2006, Mosby.

Wilkins RL, Stoller JK, Kacmarek R, *Egan's fundamentals of respiratory care*, ed 9, St Louis, 2009, Mosby.

PRETEST QUESTIONS

Answer the pretest questions before studying the chapter. This will help you determine your strong and weak areas in the material covered.

1. Pursed-lip breathing would be most beneficial in which of the following lung disorders?

   A. Emphysema
   B. Pulmonary edema
   C. Pneumonia
   D. Pleural effusion

2. On assessing a patient's laboratory results, you notice a sputum culture that reveals a high eosinophil count. This is characteristic of which of the following pulmonary conditions?

   A. Tuberculosis (TB)
   B. Asthma
   C. Pneumonia
   D. Pulmonary embolism

3. Which lung condition is characterized by consolidation on chest films?

   A. Pulmonary edema
   B. Emphysema
   C. Pneumonia
   D. Pleural effusion

4. A 17-year-old asthmatic girl enters the emergency department in moderate respiratory distress. She states that the attack began about 1 h before she came to the emergency department. You would expect her ABG results to reveal

   A. Acute respiratory acidosis with hypoxemia.
   B. Metabolic acidosis with hypoxemia.
   C. Acute respiratory alkalosis with hypoxemia.
   D. Chronic metabolic alkalosis.

5. Which of the following causative organisms for pneumonia is characteristically seen in patients with acquired immunodeficiency syndrome (AIDS)?

   A. *Pneumocystis carinii*
   B. *Klebsiella* species
   C. *Pseudomonas* species
   D. *Haemophilus influenzae*

6. The drug streptokinase is used to treat which of the following lung disorders?

   A. Pneumonia
   B. Pleural effusion
   C. Pneumothorax
   D. Pulmonary embolism

See answers and rationales at the back of the text.

REVIEW

I. **Chronic Obstructive Pulmonary Disease (COPD)**
   CRT Exam Content Matrix: IA2, IA4, IA5, IA6, IB1a,c, IB4a-c, IB5a-f, IB7e, IB9d-e,i,o,s, IB10e,i,o,s, IC1,5, IIIC1-4, IIID5a-c, IIIE7a-f, IIIG1a, IIIK5
   RRT Exam Content Matrix: IA2, IA4, IA5, IA6, IB1a,c, IB4a-c, IB5a-e, IB9e,i,p, IB10e,i,q, IC2,6, IIIC1-4, IIID5a-c, IIIE1, IIIE7a-f, IIIK5, IIIK8

> COPD is a condition in which there is a chronic obstruction to airflow within the lungs. The following diseases discussed in the outline are classified as **COPD:** emphysema, chronic bronchitis, and asthmatic bronchitis. Typical asthma, cystic fibrosis, and bronchiectasis were considered to be COPD in the past but are no longer classified as such.

   A. **Emphysema**
      1. **Definition:** a permanent abnormal enlargement of the air spaces distal to the terminal bronchioles, associated with destructive changes of the alveolar walls
         a. Panlobular (panacinar) type
            (1) The acinus is the anatomic gas exchange unit of the lung, made up of the respiratory bronchiole, alveolar duct, alveolar sacs, and the alveoli.
            (2) The entire acinus is involved in this emphysema.
            (3) There is significant loss of lung parenchyma.

(4) Alveoli are destroyed.

(5) Bullae are present.

(6) Usually is associated with emphysema resulting from α_1-antitrypsin deficiency.

b. Centrilobular (centriacinar)

(1) Lesion is in the center of the lobules, which results in enlargement and destruction of the respiratory bronchioles.

(2) Usually involves the upper lung fields and is most commonly associated with chronic bronchitis.

c. Bullous emphysema

(1) Emphysematous changes are isolated and accompanied by the development of bullae, which are weak air spaces and susceptible to rupture.

(2) *Bullae* are defined as air spaces in their distended state, more than 1 cm in diameter.

(3) *Blebs* are defined as air spaces adjacent to the pleura, usually less than 1 cm in diameter in their distended state.

2. **Causes**

a. Smoking

b. α_1-Antitrypsin deficiency (hereditary)

3. **Pathophysiology**

a. Elastic recoil of the lung is diminished, which results in premature airway closure.

b. Inspiratory flow rates are normal, while expiratory flow rates are reduced.

c. Air-trapping leads to chronic hyperinflation of the lungs and an **increased FRC.**

d. **Lung compliance is increased** as a result of the destruction of elastic lung tissue.

e. Emphysema diminishes the area over which gas exchange occurs and is accompanied by regional differences in ventilation and perfusion. This accounts for increased physiologic dead space and the abnormal ABG results observed in patients with emphysema.

4. **Clinical signs and symptoms**

a. Dyspnea: initially occurs on exertion, then progressively worsens.

b. Digital clubbing: results from **chronic hypoxemia.**

c. Increased AP chest diameter (barrel chest)

d. The use of accessory muscles during normal breathing

e. Elevated hemoglobin level, hematocrit, and RBC count

f. ABG levels reveal chronic CO_2 retention and hypoxemia (advanced stages of the disease).

g. Reduced breath sounds and hyperresonance to percussion

h. Cyanosis

i. **Right-sided heart failure (cor pulmonale)** in advanced stages

(1) Cor pulmonale results from an increased workload on the right ventricle as it attempts to deliver blood through constricted pulmonary blood vessels.

(2) These vessels are constricted (causing pulmonary hypertension) as a result of arterial hypoxemia and hypercarbia.

(3) Chronic pulmonary hypertension results in right ventricular hypertrophy and, eventually, right-sided heart failure.

(4) **Cor pulmonale results in peripheral edema, such as pedal (ankle) edema, distended neck (jugular) veins, and an enlarged liver.**

(5) **O_2 therapy is essential in the prevention or treatment of cor pulmonale in patients with chronic respiratory failure.** O_2 is a pulmonary vasodilator that decreases pulmonary hypertension.

(6) Diuretic and digitalis therapy is indicated when right ventricular failure supervenes the underlying respiratory problems.

5. **Characteristics on chest x-ray films**

a. Flattened diaphragm

b. Hyperinflation

c. Reduced vascular markings

d. Bullous lesions

6. **Characteristics on pulmonary function studies**

a. Increased residual volume (RV) and FRC

b. Decreased diffusion capacity

c. Decreased VC

d. Decreased forced expiratory volume in 1 s (FEV_1)

e. Decreased FEV_1/forced vital capacity (FVC)

f. Prolonged nitrogen washout

7. **Treatment**

a. Smoking cessation program

(1) Group counseling

(2) Nicotine replacement therapy: nicotine gum, nicotine patch, nicotine inhaler, nicotine lozenge, nicotine nasal spray

(3) Drug therapy: bupropion (Wellbutrin); an antidepressant drug that has proved to be beneficial in smoking cessation

(4) Frequent reminders from health care providers about the need to stop smoking to improve quality of life

(5) Discussions with a respiratory therapist or other health care provider to help the patient understand the effects that smoking has on the cardiopulmonary system

b. Adequate hydration

c. Postural drainage

d. Bronchodilators

e. Prevention of infections by immunizations

f. Exercise (walking)

g. Breathing exercise training

    (1) Diaphragmatic breathing exercises

    (2) **Pursed-lip breathing:** prevents premature airway closure by producing a back pressure into the airways on exhalation.

h. Care must be taken when administering oxygen to patients with emphysema who chronically retain CO_2 and who have chronic hypoxemia. PaO_2 levels should be maintained between 50 and 65 mm Hg to avoid blunting the respiratory drive or increasing V/Q mismatching.

 Exam Note

If the PaO_2 increases above 70 mm Hg and the $PaCO_2$ begins increasing after a patient with severe COPD starts receiving O_2, then the patient's "hypoxic drive" is being knocked out or V/Q mismatching is increasing; decrease the oxygen percentage. Remember to maintain the PaO_2 level at 50 to 65 mm Hg. This is a controversial theory that some disagree with. **The NBRC exams offer questions regarding this theory and recognize it as being valid.**

B. **Chronic Bronchitis**

1. **Definition:** chronic excessive mucus production, resulting from an increase in the number and size of mucus glands and goblet cells. Symptoms are a cough and increased mucus production for at least 3 months of the year for more than 2 consecutive years. Males are most commonly affected.

2. **Cause**

    a. Smoking

3. **Pathophysiology**

    a. Increase in the size of mucus glands

    b. Increase in the number of goblet cells

    c. Inflammation of bronchial walls

    d. Mucus plugs in peripheral airways

    e. Loss of cilia

    f. Emphysematous changes in advanced stages of disease

    g. Narrowing airways, leading to airflow obstruction

4. **Clinical signs and symptoms**

    a. Cough with sputum production

    b. Dyspnea on exertion progressing to dyspnea with less effort

    c. CO_2 retention and hypoxemia in advanced stages

d. Increased pulmonary vascular resistance in advanced stages

e. Increased hemoglobin level, hematocrit, and RBC count in advanced stages

f. Right-sided heart failure (cor pulmonale) in advanced stages

5. **Characteristics on chest x-ray films**

    a. Not significant in early disease

    b. Hyperinflation (in advanced stages)

6. **Characteristics on pulmonary function studies**

    a. None in early disease

    b. Increased RV

    c. Decreased FEV_1

    d. Decreased inspiratory flow rates in obstructive bronchitis

7. **Treatment**

    a. Same as for emphysema

II. **ASTHMA**

CRT Exam Content Matrix: IA2, IA4, IA5, IB1a,c, IB4a-c, IA5a-f, IB7e,IB9d-e,i,o,s, IB10e,i,o,s, IC1,5, IIIC1-4, IIID5a-c, IIIE7a-f, IIIG1a

RRT Exam Content Matrix: IA2, IA4, IA5, IA6, IB1a,c, IB4a-c, IB5a-e, IB9e,i,p IB10e,i,q, IC2,6, IIIC1-4, IIID5a-c, IIIE1, IIIE7a-f

A. **Definition:** a disease characterized by increased reactivity of the trachea and bronchi to various stimuli, resulting in bronchoconstriction (bronchospasm), increased mucus production, and swelling of mucosal tissue

B. **Causes**

1. The exact underlying cause remains unknown.

2. The cause is associated with the following

    a. Allergic response

    b. Heredity

    c. Environmental factors

    d. Infection

    e. Psychosocial factors

    f. Socioeconomic factors

C. **Classifications of Asthma (based on severity)**

1. **Mild intermittent**

    a. This is the least severe of the four classifications.

    b. Symptoms of wheezing or coughing are experienced no more than twice per week.

    c. The patients in this category generally have FEV_1 and peak expiratory flow (PEF) values of at least 80% of predicted.

    d. Routine management generally consists of beta agonists, as needed.

    e. Exacerbation of symptoms rarely results in emergency department treatment or hospitalization.

2. **Mild persistent**

    a. Symptoms of coughing or wheezing are experienced more than twice per week but less than once per day.

b. Symptoms affect the patient's daily activity and sleep during the night; nocturnal coughing, wheezing, or dyspnea is experienced more than twice per month.

c. The patients in this category generally have FEV_1 and PEF values of at least 80% of predicted.

d. Routine management generally consists of a corticosteroid to control symptoms and the use of a beta agonist, as needed.

e. Emergency department treatment for exacerbations occurs periodically and may occasionally result in hospitalization.

3. **Moderate persistent**

a. Symptoms of coughing or wheezing are experienced almost daily in this category.

b. Exacerbation of symptoms are experienced at least twice per week and may persist for several days.

c. Symptoms affect the patient's daily activity and sleep during the night; nocturnal coughing, wheezing, or dyspnea is experienced more than once per week.

d. The patients in this category generally have FEV_1 and PEF values of 60% to 80% of predicted.

e. Daily management generally consists of a long-acting, aerosolized bronchodilator to control nocturnal symptoms, corticosteroids two or three times per day, and a short-acting beta agonist as needed for exacerbations.

f. Patients in this category routinely require emergency department treatment or require hospitalization.

4. **Severe persistent**

a. This is the worst category of the four. Symptoms of coughing or wheezing are experienced almost continually.

b. Exacerbations are frequent and may last for weeks.

c. Symptoms affect the patient's daily activity and sleep during the night; nocturnal coughing, wheezing, or dyspnea is experienced almost every night.

d. The patients in this category generally have FEV_1 and PEF values of 60% or less of predicted.

e. Daily management generally consists of a long-acting, aerosolized bronchodilator to control nocturnal symptoms, corticosteroids, and a short-acting beta agonist two to three times per day.

f. Patients in this category routinely require emergency department treatment or require hospitalization.

D. **Pathophysiology**

1. Mast cells in the bronchial tree are stimulated, which causes the release of
   a. Histamine
   b. Leukotrienes
   c. Slow-reacting substance of anaphylaxis (SRS-A)
   d. Eosinophilic chemotactic factor of anaphylaxis (ECF-A)
   e. Prostaglandins

2. The release of these substances result in
   a. Bronchoconstriction
   b. Mucosal edema
   c. Increased mucus production
   d. Accumulation of eosinophils in the blood and sputum
   e. Vasodilation

E. **Clinical Signs and Symptoms**

1. Mild wheezing and coughing initially, which may progress to severe dyspnea if the attack is not arrested

2. The cough is initially nonproductive, progressing to a productive cough by the end of the episode.

3. Secretions contain high levels of eosinophils.

4. Intercostal and supraclavicular retractions

5. The use of accessory muscles to breathe (in a severe attack)

6. Paradoxical pulse: Systolic blood pressure is 10 mm Hg higher on expiration than on inspiration.

7. Tachycardia and tachypnea

8. ABG levels initially reveal hypoxemia and low $PaCO_2$. $PaCO_2$ increases as the attack worsens and the patient begins to tire.

9. Cyanosis

F. **Characteristics on Chest X-ray Films**

1. Hyperinflation (hyperlucency of lung fields)
2. Atelectasis
3. Infiltrates

G. **Characteristics on Pulmonary Function Studies**

1. Decreased FEV_1
2. Decreased FVC
3. Decreased FEV_1/FVC
4. Increased RV

H. **Treatment (Preventive)**

1. Prevention (avoid known allergens or causative factors)

2. Medications (long-term controllers taken daily to help control or maintain the degree of inflammatory mediator release in the airways)
   a. Long-acting beta agonists (bronchodilators) such as salmeterol (Serevent)
   b. Asthma preventive drugs (not used during an attack)

      (1) Cromolyn sodium (Intal)
      (2) Leukotriene modifier drugs such as zafirlukast (Accolate) or montelukast (Singulair)
    c. Corticosteroids

I. Treatment (During an Attack)

1. Quick-relief, short-acting beta agonists such as albuterol (Ventolin, Proventil) or anticholinergic bronchodilators such as ipratropium bromide (Atrovent)
2. IV fluids
3. O_2 therapy

J. Status Asthmaticus: a severe asthmatic attack that responds poorly to bronchodilator therapy and is associated with signs or symptoms of potential respiratory failure

1. Patient should be hospitalized immediately.
2. Hydration
3. IV corticosteroids
4. Supplemental oxygen
5. Close monitoring of ABG levels and pulse oximetry (SpO_2)
6. Bronchodilating agents
7. CPT (if tolerated) to remove mucus plugs and secretions
8. If the attack is not controlled by previous measures, intubate the patient and institute mechanical ventilation.

K. Nocturnal Asthma

1. Nocturnal (nighttime) symptoms are seen in up to 75% of all patients with asthma and even in those who have mild intermittent or mild persistent asthma.
2. Mechanisms resulting in nocturnal symptoms may be related to changes in vagal tone, body temperature, mediators, epinephrine, inflammation, and $beta_2$–receptor function during sleep.
3. Other causes may include aspiration, sleep apnea, increased mucus production, sinusitis, gastroesophageal reflux, and the normal decrease in lung function when the patient is sleeping.
4. Management generally includes sustained-release theophylline and beta agonists, long-acting beta agonists, and/or inhaled corticosteroids.

L. Occupational Asthma

1. Characterized by increased wheezing or coughing while at work or within several hours after leaving work and improving on days off from work.
2. Diagnosis may be made by measuring peak flows while at work.
3. The most common workplace causes include formaldehyde, grain dust, cigarette smoke, and avian proteins.

M. Exercise-Induced Asthma (EIA)

1. Characterized by symptoms occurring 5 to 15 min after strenuous exercise that spontaneously resolves in about 1 h.
2. The exact cause of EIA is not clear but may be related to
    a. Heat or water loss from the respiratory tract mucosa
    b. Hyperventilation, resulting in the release of bronchoconstricting chemical mediators
    c. Rapid rewarming of the airway, resulting in vascular congestion, increased permeability, and edema causing airway obstruction
3. Beta agonists may be used beneficially before exercise along with asthma preventives such as cromolyn sodium or nedocromil sodium (Tilade) or the leukotriene modifiers such as zafirlukast or montelukast.
4. Other medications that can be beneficial include anticholinergics such as ipratropium bromide, oral beta agonists, theophylline, and antihistamines.
5. Some nonasthma medications such as inhaled furosemide (Lasix) and inhaled heparin have also been used to treat EIA.
6. Nonpharmacologic measures used to reduce the incidence of EIA include
    a. Wear a mask to cover the nose and mouth during exercise in cold weather.
    b. Warm up before exercise.
    c. Exercise in warm, humidified environments.
    d. Allow for a cooling down period after exercise.

III. BRONCHIECTASIS

CRT Exam Content Matrix: IA2, IA4, IA5, IB1a,c, IB4a-c, IA5a-f, IB7e, IB9d-e,i,o,s, IB10e,i,o,s, IC1,5, IIIC1-4, IIID5a-c, IIIE7a-f, IIIG1a

RRT Exam Content Matrix: IA2, IA4, IA5, IA6, IB1a,c, IB4a-c, IB5a-e, IB9e,i,p, IB10e,i,q, IC2,6, IIIC1-4, IIID5a-c, IIIE1, IIIE7a-f

A. Definition: a dilation of the bronchi and bronchioles that is chronic in nature and results in inflammation and damage to the walls of these airways.

B. Causes

1. Chronic respiratory infections
2. TB lesion
3. Secondary to cystic fibrosis
4. Bronchial obstruction

C. Pathophysiology

1. It is not clear whether the chronic dilation is a result of destructive changes in the bronchial walls caused by inflammation and infection or, possibly, a congenital defect of the airways.
2. Bronchial obstruction may render the mucociliary transport system ineffective, which may lead to an accumulation of thick secretions.

3. The bronchial wall is destroyed, which results in atrophy of the mucosal layer.
4. Because of the decreased values in both flows and volumes, this disease may be either obstructive or restrictive in nature (see characteristics on pulmonary function studies).

D. **Clinical Signs and Symptoms**
1. Productive cough with large amounts of thick, purulent secretions that may be foul-smelling. Often, a layering of the sputum occurs.
2. Tachypnea and tachycardia
3. Hemoptysis
4. Recurrent pulmonary infections
5. Digital clubbing
6. Cyanosis
7. Respiratory alkalosis with hypoxemia (in the early stage)
8. Chronic respiratory acidosis with hypoxemia (in the late stage)
9. Barrel chest

E. **Characteristics on Chest X-ray Films**
1. Increased lung markings
2. Flattened diaphragm
3. Segmental atelectasis

F. **Characteristics on Pulmonary Function Studies**
1. Decreased FVC
2. Decreased FRC
3. Decreased FEV_1
4. Decreased $FEF_{25\%-75\%}$

G. **Treatment**
1. CPT
2. Aerosol therapy
3. Bronchodilator therapy
4. Mucolytics (e.g., acetylcysteine [Mucomyst], dornase alfa [Pulmozyme])
5. Antibiotics
6. O_2 therapy
7. Expectorants

IV. **LOWER RESPIRATORY TRACT INFECTIONS**
CRT Exam Content Matrix: IA2, IA4, IA5, IB1a,c, IB4a-c, IA5a-f, IB7e, IB9d-e,i,o,s, IB10e,i,o,s, IC1,4,5, IIIC1-4, IIID5a-c, IIIE7a-f, IIIG1a
RRT Exam Content Matrix: IA2, IA4, IA5, IA6, IB1a,c, IB4a-c, IB5a-e, IB9e,i,p, IB10e,i,q, IC2,5,6, IIIC1-4, IIID5a-c, IIIE1, IIIE7a-f

A. **Pneumonia**
1. **Definition:** acute inflammation of the gas exchange units of the lungs
2. **Cause**
   a. A variety of organisms (discussed later)
   b. Decreased airway defense mechanisms caused by
      (1) Ineffective coughing
      (2) Obtunded airway reflexes
      (3) Impaired mucociliary transport system
      (4) Obstructed airways

c. Various conditions result in a predisposition to pneumonia
   (1) COPD
   (2) Alcoholism
   (3) Malnutrition
   (4) Seizure disorders
   (5) Chronic debilitating illnesses
   (6) Major surgical procedures
   (7) Old age

3. **Pathophysiology**
   a. Pathogenic microorganisms that reach the gas exchange areas of the lung cause an intense tissue reaction, resulting in production of inflammatory exudates and cells.
   b. The WBCs phagocytize the invading organisms, which leads to further inflammation.
   c. As the lungs begin filling with the inflammatory exudates and cells, they become **consolidated.**
   d. If tissue necrosis is not present, the lung heals and returns to normal function.
   e. If tissue necrosis occurs, healing is slow and fibrous scar tissue is produced, which results in pulmonary fibrosis and loss of normal lung function.

4. **Clinical signs and symptoms**
   a. Infection
   b. Malaise
   c. Fever
   d. Chest pain
   e. Dyspnea and tachycardia
   f. Inspiratory crackles and bronchial breath sounds on auscultation

5. **Characteristics on chest x-ray films**
   a. Consolidation
   b. Air bronchogram

6. **Types of pneumonia**
   a. Bacterial
      (1) Causative organism is ***Streptococcus pneumoniae:*** called pneumococcal pneumonia; **most common bacterial pneumonia**
      (2) *Haemophilus influenzae*
      (3) *Klebsiella pneumoniae*
      (4) *Legionella pneumoniae*
      (5) *Pseudomonas aeruginosa*
   b. *Mycoplasma pneumoniae:* smaller than bacteria; disease is more common in children
   c. Viral
      (1) Influenza viruses
      (2) Adenoviruses
      (3) Chickenpox (varicella-zoster virus)
   d. Protozoan
      (1) ***Pneumocystis carinii* pneumonia (PCP)**

(2) This type of pneumonia is seen in 60% of AIDS cases. Definitive diagnosis is made from cultures of lung secretions and tissue.

(3) *P. carinii* pneumonia is commonly treated with the antiprotozoal drug **pentamidine** via aerosolization.

> ⚠ **Bronchoalveolar lavage (BAL)** is a technique whereby sterile saline is instilled through a bronchoscope to a specific lung segment. The saline is then aspirated and collected for culturing. BAL is being used to help diagnose nosocomial pneumonia. Recently, it is being advocated for diagnosing ventilator-associated pneumonia (VAP). VAP is discussed in detail in Chapter 11 on ventilator management.

7. **Treatment** (for pneumonia in general)
   a. Antibiotics
   b. Supplemental O_2
   c. Chest physical therapy
   d. Adequate hydration
   e. Adequate nutrition
   f. Tracheal suctioning (if there has been poor removal of secretions because of ineffective coughing)

B. **Lung Abscess**
1. **Definition:** an infection of the lung that is characterized by a localized accumulation of pus and destruction of the surrounding tissue.
2. **Causes**
   a. The most common causative organisms are anaerobic bacteria.
   b. Aerobic bacteria, including staphylococci, streptococci, and some gram-negative bacteria, may be less common causes.
   c. May occur after aspiration.
   d. Seen in conjunction with lung cancer.
3. **Pathophysiology**
   a. In the acute phase, it looks much like pneumonia.
   b. As progression occurs, necrosis is evident, which may spread to adjacent lung tissue.
4. **Clinical signs and symptoms**
   a. Fever
   b. Cough, initially nonproductive (or minimal production), followed by production of **purulent, foul-smelling secretions.**
   c. Chest pain
   d. Weight loss
   e. Hemoptysis
   f. Digital clubbing
   g. Tachycardia
   h. Tachypnea
5. **Characteristics on chest x-ray films**
   a. Localized area of consolidation
   b. Most common sites are the superior segments of the lower lobes and posterior segments of upper lobes (as a result of position during an aspiration event).
6. **Characteristic laboratory findings**
   a. Increased WBC count
   b. Anemia (decreased RBC count)
   c. Sputum culture reveals purulence and necrosis
7. **Treatment**
   a. Antibiotics
   b. Postural drainage
   c. Adequate nutrition

> ☑ **Exam Note**
>
> If an abscess ruptures into the pleura, pus accumulates in the pleural space. This is called **empyema**, and it should be drained before CPT.

C. **Tuberculosis**
1. **Definition:** a granulomatous bacterial infection, chronic in nature, affecting the lungs and other organs of the body.
2. **Cause:** The inhalation or ingestion of the bacterium, *Mycobacterium tuberculosis*. Infection is usually spread through coughing and sneezing. Diagnosis is based on skin tests, chest films, and sputum culture showing bacilli that are acid-fast, which means not readily decolorized by acid after staining, a specific characteristic of this bacteria.
3. **Pathophysiology**
   a. After the bacillus is inhaled, it enters the alveoli, which results in an inflammatory reaction similar to that seen in pneumonia.
   b. Macrophages enter the infected area and engulf the bacilli without fully killing them.
   c. The lung tissue surrounding this area encapsulates the bacilli, providing a protective covering. This is called a *granuloma,* or tubercle.
   d. The granuloma fills with necrotic material and is referred to as a caseous (cheese-like) granuloma.
   e. If the patient's immunologic system controls this process or if antituberculosis drugs are given, the lung tissue becomes fibrotic and calcifies as healing occurs. This may result in stiffness or decreased lung compliance in the affected area.
   f. In most cases, the patient's own immunologic mechanisms keep the bacilli in check, but the bacillus remains dormant in the lungs for many years, which causes a positive result on TB skin tests. These encapsulated bacilli can escape in later years, causing infection.
   g. Chronic dilation of the bronchi (bronchiectasis) may result during the healing process of TB.

h. In uncontrolled cases, the tubercles increase in size and combine to form larger tubercles, which may rupture and permit air and the infected material to enter the pleural space, bronchi, and bronchioles.

4. **Clinical signs and symptoms**

 Most individuals infected with TB have few, if any, symptoms. The primary TB lesion heals completely, possibly leaving a small scar, which could calcify later in life.

    a. Cough
    b. Sputum production that tests positive for acid-fast bacilli
    c. Tachycardia
    d. Increased cardiac output
    e. Chest pain
    f. Hemoptysis
    g. Dull percussion note
    h. Crackles and rhonchi with chest auscultation
    i. Hyperventilation and hypoxemia (in early stages)
    j. Chronic respiratory acidosis with hypoxemia (in late stages)
    k. Cyanosis (in severe cases)
    l. Night sweats

5. **Characteristics on chest x-ray films**
    a. Enlarged lymph nodes in the hilar region (lymphadenopathy)
    b. Pleural effusion
    c. Cavitation
    d. Ghon complex (lung lesion and lymph node involvement)
    e. Fibrosis
    f. Infiltrates

6. **Characteristics on pulmonary function studies**
    a. Decreased VC
    b. Decreased FRC
    c. Decreased RV
    d. Decreased total lung capacity (TLC)

☑ Exam Note

These findings are characteristic of the restrictive lung processes that occur in TB.

7. **Treatment**
    a. Supplemental O_2
    b. Antituberculosis drugs: These drugs are used in combination for 2 to 4 mo.
      (1) Rifampin
      (2) Isoniazid (INH)
      (3) Ethambutol
      (4) Streptomycin
    c. Placement in respiratory isolation
    d. Routine airway maintenance

V. OTHER LUNG DISORDERS

CRT Exam Content Matrix: IA2, IA4, IA5, IA8a-b, IB1a,c, IB4a-c, IB5a-f, IB7e, IB9d-e,i,o,s, IB10e,i,l,o,s, IC1,5, 10, IIIC1-4, IIID5a-c, IIIE7a-f, IIIG1a, IIII2, IIIJ3

RRT Exam Content Matrix: IA2, IA4, IA5, IA6, IA8a-b, IB1a,c, IB4a-c, IB5a-e, IB9e,i,l,p IB10e,i,m,q,IC2,6, 10, IIIC1-4, IIID5a-c, IIIE1, IIIE7a-f, III I2, IIIJ3,5

A. **Pulmonary Edema (Cardiogenic)**
  1. **Definition:** an excessive amount of fluid in the lung tissues or alveoli, caused by an increase in pulmonary capillary pressure resulting from hydrostatic left-sided abnormal heart function
  2. **Causes**
    a. Left-sided heart failure
    b. Aortic stenosis
    c. Mitral valve stenosis
    d. Systemic hypertension

These four mechanisms cause back up of fluid from the heart into the pulmonary capillaries until they become engorged, which leads to pulmonary edema; PCWP and PAP levels are also increased.

    e. Alveolar capillary membrane leakage caused by injury, such as seen in ARDS (noncardiogenic pulmonary edema). **The PCWP level is normal with an increased PAP in this instance.**
  3. **Pathophysiology**
    a. Fluid balance is maintained within the capillaries by two forces.
      (1) **Plasma oncotic pressure** (pressure trying to keep fluid in the capillaries)
      (2) **Capillary hydrostatic pressure** (pressure trying to push fluid out of the capillaries)
    b. Oncotic pressure is normally much higher than capillary hydrostatic pressure, keeping fluid in the capillaries.
    c. As blood from the heart backs up into the pulmonary circulation, capillary hydrostatic pressure increases above plasma oncotic pressure, and fluid from the blood leaks out into the interstitial spaces.
    d. Excess fluid overwhelms the lymphatic system (which normally drains the interstitial spaces), and the fluid drains into the alveoli, which results in **decreased lung compliance.**
    e. Airway resistance increases because of the excess fluid.
    f. A–a gradient widens as a result of intrapulmonary shunting, and V/Q mismatching results.

4. **Clinical signs and symptoms**
   a. Dyspnea
      (1) **Orthopnea:** dyspnea while lying down (relieved by sitting upright in semi-Fowler or Fowler position)
      (2) **Paroxysmal nocturnal dyspnea:** severe attack of dyspnea that occurs during sleep and awakens the patient (relieved by sitting up in semi-Fowler position)
   b. Productive cough with thin, pink frothy secretions
   c. Crackles may be auscultated in base of lung (or in all lung fields in severe edema).
   d. Tachypnea
   e. Cyanosis
   f. Diaphoresis (sweating)
   g. Distended neck veins
   h. Tachycardia or other arrhythmias
5. **Characteristics on chest x-ray films**
   a. Increased vascular markings
   b. Interstitial edema
   c. Enlarged heart shadow
6. **Treatment**
   a. O_2 administration (percentage based on PaO_2)
   b. CPAP/Bi-PAP
   c. Cardiac glycosides
   d. Ventilatory support with PEEP (if condition is severe)
   e. Adequate airway maintenance
   f. Morphine
   g. IPPB with ethyl alcohol (40% to 50% dilution). Not used commonly in the clinical setting but may appear on the exam.
   h. Diuretics such as furosemide

B. **Pulmonary Embolism (PE)**
   1. **Definition:** obstruction of the pulmonary artery or one of its branches by a blood clot
      Embolus: a clot that travels through the bloodstream from its vessel of origin to lodge in a smaller vessel, obstructing blood flow.
   2. **Causes**
      a. The blood clot usually originates in deep veins of the legs or pelvic area, dislodges, travels back to the heart through the venous system, and lodges in the pulmonary artery.
      b. The clot originally forms because of stagnation or venous stasis from prolonged bed rest, immobility from the pain of trauma or surgery, or paralysis.
      c. Seen in patients with COPD because of venous stasis, resulting from the increased viscosity of their blood.
   3. **Pathophysiology**
      a. Blood flow is obstructed to areas of the involved lung, which contributes to dead space ventilation (ventilation without perfusion).
      b. Lung compliance decreases as atelectasis occurs in the region of the decreased perfusion. This is the lung's response to inadequate perfusion as it attempts to maintain normal V/Q matching.
      c. Widened A–a gradient results from intrapulmonary shunting and V/Q mismatching.
   4. **Clinical signs and symptoms**
      a. Dyspnea
      b. Chest pain
      c. Tachypnea
      d. Cough
      e. Pleuritic pain
      f. Hemoptysis
      g. Tenderness and swelling in lower extremities due to thrombophlebitis
      h. Tachycardia
      i. Cyanosis
      j. Decreased breath sounds over the affected area. Wheezing and crackles may be heard.
   5. **Characteristics on chest x-ray films**
      a. May be normal
      b. Decreased lung volume
      c. Linear densities of atelectasis
      d. Pleural effusion
      e. Elevated hemidiaphragm caused by atelectasis
   6. **Diagnostic procedures. A valuable procedure for the diagnosis of PE is a V/Q lung scan.** Normal results on a perfusion scan should rule out PE. **Pulmonary angiography** is another procedure that is sometimes performed for definitive diagnosis of PE.
      a. **V/Q scan:** The patient inhales a harmless radioactive substance, which is distributed throughout the alveoli. A small amount of radioactive imaging material is injected into a vein, and it too travels to the lung and outlines the blood supply or perfusion to the lung. Areas with inadequate perfusion appear dark on the scan because the radioactive particles are unable to pass to an area of obstruction.
      b. **Pulmonary angiography** is the most accurate method for detecting PE. A dye that is visible on x-ray film is injected into an artery and travels to the pulmonary arteries, where the obstruction is outlined and can be viewed.
      c. MRI and CT are also used to detect PE (see Chapter 3 on assessment of the cardiopulmonary patient); however, pulmonary angiography, although associated

with more risks, is currently the most diagnostic test for PE.

7. **Treatment**
   a. Prevention
      (1) Elastic stockings
      (2) Leg elevation
      (3) Ambulation
      (4) Small doses of heparin (an anticoagulant)
   b. Anticoagulation (antithrombus) therapy
      (1) Heparin
      (2) Warfarin sodium (Coumadin)
      (3) Streptokinase or urokinase in cases of massive embolus
   c. Supplemental O_2
   d. If hypotension is present
      (1) Vasopressors
      (2) Fluids

C. **Acute Respiratory Distress Syndrome (ARDS)**
   1. **Definition:** a group of symptoms causing acute, catastrophic respiratory failure, resulting from pulmonary injury. For the lung condition to be considered ARDS, three criteria must be met
      a. Infiltrates on chest x-ray film confirm that fluid is leaking into the interstitial spaces.
      b. Normal heart function as evidenced by normal PCWP.
      c. PO_2/FiO_2 ratio of less than 200
   2. **Causes**
      a. Diffuse lung injury
         (1) Sepsis
         (2) Aspiration
         (3) Near drowning
         (4) O_2 toxicity
         (5) Shock
         (6) Thoracic trauma
         (7) Extensive burns
         (8) Inhalation of toxic gases (e.g., smoke inhalation)
         (9) Fluid overload
         (10) Fat embolism
         (11) Narcotic overdose
      b. Most patients have no previous pulmonary problems.
   3. **Pathophysiology**
      a. Lung injury occurs and is followed by an inflammatory process.
      b. The alveolar capillary membrane begins to leak, which causes noncardiogenic pulmonary edema.
      c. Fluid builds up in the interstitial spaces, alveoli, and distal airways.
      d. Surfactant production decreases, which results in atelectasis, while excessive fluid fills the alveoli and airways.
      e. Because of inflammatory cells, fibrin, and cellular debris that result from the

inflammatory process, the lungs become stiff and lung compliance decreases.
   f. In severe cases, the lungs may become almost entirely atelectatic, which may lead to massive intrapulmonary shunting.

4. **Clinical signs and symptoms**
   a. Hypoxemia: In severe cases, it is refractory (not responsive) to O_2 therapy.
   b. Cyanosis
   c. Severe dyspnea and coughing
   d. Decreased lung compliance
   e. Suprasternal and intercostal retractions
   f. Widened A–a gradient with the use of 100% O_2 (severe cases)
   g. Tachypnea

5. **Characteristics on chest x-ray films**
   a. Interstitial edema
   b. Alveolar edema (fluffy infiltration)

6. **Treatment**
   a. Patients are usually not managed well on high O_2 concentrations alone because of decreased lung compliance.
   b. Mechanical ventilation with **PEEP** and tidal volumes of 6 mL/kg of ideal body weight.
      (1) Because the lungs are noncompliant, higher peak inspiratory pressures are necessary to maintain normal $PaCO_2$ levels. High peak pressures result in the release of inflammatory chemical mediators, causing more lung damage. **To prevent further lung tissue damage, do not use a peak inspiratory pressure in excess of 35 to 40 cm H_2O and maintain alveolar pressure (static pressure) at less than 30 cm H_2O.** Protecting the lungs by using lower ventilating pressures causes the $PaCO_2$ level to rise. This is referred to as ***permissive hypercapnia***, which results in a decreased pH level. If the pH level does not decrease to less than 7.20, no significant side effects have been noted. (In some studies, pH levels as low as 7.10 have been found to be safe.) The elevated $PaCO_2$ has three advantages
         (a) Causes sedation.
         (b) Shifts the HbO_2 curve to the right, which results in more oxygen delivery to the tissues.
         (c) Decreases production of inflammatory chemical mediators.
      (2) Add PEEP if PaO_2 is below normal when the patient is receiving an FiO_2 of 0.60 or more. The optimal level of PEEP can be determined by observing the lower inflection point on a volume/pressure

curve. (See Chapter 11 on ventilator management.)

   c. Monitoring of heart pressures (PAP, PCWP) with a pulmonary artery catheter (Swan-Ganz)

   d. Diuretics

   e. Routine airway maintenance

D. **Pneumothorax**

1. **Definition:** the presence of air in the pleural space

2. **Causes**

   a. Spontaneous pneumothorax

     (1) Develops without previous trauma.

     (2) Seen most commonly in tall, thin young males as a result of bleb rupture.

     (3) Seen in patients with COPD as a result of bullous disease and bleb rupture.

   b. Traumatic pneumothorax

     (1) Broken ribs

     (2) Puncture wound

     (3) Chest or neck surgery

3. **Pathophysiology**

   a. When air enters the pleural space, the negative pressure in the pleural space becomes atmospheric, which causes the "negative" pull on the lung to be lost. The lung begins to collapse because of its natural recoil properties, diminishing ventilation to the lung.

   b. A **tension pneumothorax** occurs when the opening to the pleural space in the lung acts as a one-way valve, permitting air to enter the space but not allowing the air to exit.

     (1) Ventilation of the affected lung diminishes.

     (2) The trapped air increases pressure on the affected side, pushing the trachea and mediastinum to the unaffected side. Pressure compresses the heart, which results in a decreased cardiac output. This is a life-threatening condition.

     (3) The **immediate action** to take is to relieve the pressure in the pleural space by insertion of a needle in the second or third intercostal space.

   c. The volume of the unaffected lung will increase and more blood will perfuse it, which helps prevent severe hypoxemia.

4. **Clinical signs and symptoms**

   a. Chest pain

   b. Dyspnea

   c. Decreased breath sounds over the affected lung

   d. Hyperresonant percussion note over the affected lung

   e. Asymmetric chest excursion

   f. Crepitus with subcutaneous emphysema (*crepitus* refers to the crackling under the skin that is felt when air enters the subcutaneous tissues)

   g. Tachypnea (in severe cases)

   h. Cyanosis (in severe cases)

5. **Characteristics on chest x-ray films**

   a. Hyperlucency

   b. Deviation of heart, trachea, and mediastinum to the opposite (unaffected) side if tension pneumothorax is present

6. **Diagnostic procedures**

   a. Although chest x-ray films enable a definitive diagnosis of pneumothorax in patients of all ages, transillumination with a fiberoptic probe has been successful in the diagnosis of pneumothorax in infants. The transilluminator has a light on its distal tip, and when it is placed over areas of free air in the pleural space, transillumination is greater than in other areas.

7. **Treatment**

   a. Needle aspiration: **immediately in tension pneumothorax**

   b. Placement of chest tube

   c. Supplemental O_2, as needed (monitor SpO_2 and/or ABG levels)

E. **Pleural Effusion**

1. **Definition:** excessive fluid in the pleural space

   a. Transudate: fluid caused by an imbalance between transcapillary pressure and plasma oncotic pressure

   b. Exudate: fluid caused by increased capillary permeability, as in inflammation

2. **Causes**

   a. Causes of transudative pleural effusion

     (1) CHF (most common cause)

     (2) Cirrhosis of the liver

     (3) Kidney disease

   b. Causes of exudative pleural effusion

     (1) Infections

     (2) Trauma

     (3) Surgery

     (4) Tumors

     (5) PE

3. **Pathophysiology**

   a. Fluid accumulates in the pleural space as a result of an imbalance between the formation of the fluid and how much is absorbed.

   b. Increased fluid formation may cause pleural effusion.

   c. Decreased absorption may cause pleural effusion.

4. **Clinical signs and symptoms**

   a. Chest pain

   b. Dyspnea

   c. Dullness to percussion

   d. Absent breath sounds over the fluid

5. **Characteristics on chest x-ray films**
   a. Blunting of costophrenic angle
   b. Homogeneous density in dependent part of the hemithorax

 Exam Note

A radiograph obtained with the patient in the lateral decubitus position (lying on the side) should confirm the effusion. The fluid moves with gravity as the patient lies on his or her side.

6. **Treatment**
   a. Drain fluid by thoracentesis.
   b. Chest tube drainage may be necessary in chronic cases.
   c. Supplemental O_2, as needed (monitor ABG levels and/or SpO_2)

F. **Atelectasis**
   1. **Definition:** partial or complete collapse of alveoli. It may involve small localized areas of the lung, a lobe, or the entire lung.
   2. **Causes**
      a. Obstructed airways: This may result from secretions, tumors, mucous plugs, or foreign body aspiration. These obstructions to gas flow prevent air from reaching the alveoli for gas exchange. This is referred to as **absorption atelectasis.** Another example of absorption atelectasis occurs when high levels of O_2 are delivered to the lung. This "washes out" the nitrogen in the lung, which results in collapsed alveoli.
      b. Loss of negative pleural pressure: There is subatmospheric pressure present in the pleural space, which creates a pull on the lung that helps to keep it from collapsing. Any condition that results in loss of this subatmospheric (negative) pressure causes the lung to collapse. Pneumothorax and pleural effusion are both causes of the loss of negative intrapleural pressure.
      c. Right mainstem bronchus intubation: If the right mainstem bronchus is inadvertently intubated, no gas flow enters the left lung, which results in atelectasis of the left lung. The same holds true for a left mainstem bronchus intubation, but the incidence is much less common because the angle of the left mainstem bronchus is 45 degrees to 55 degrees; the right mainstem bronchus angles off the trachea at about 25 degrees, which makes right bronchus intubation more likely.
      d. Deficiency or loss of surfactant: Surfactant is present in the fluid that lines the alveolar wall and reduces surface tension so that alveoli do not collapse during exhalation. Conditions

resulting in reduced surfactant include O_2 toxicity, in which high O_2 levels damage the alveolar type II cells that produce surfactant, which leads to ARDS; near-drowning, which results in loss of surfactant from the aspiration of certain substances; and premature birth, in which surfactant is immature, resulting in atelectasis (see Chapter 13 on neonatal and pediatric respiratory care).
      e. Hypoventilation: Decreased VT from any condition eventually results in atelectasis. Examples include chest or abdominal pain, phrenic nerve paralysis, abdominal or thoracic surgery, high-level spinal cord injury, inadequate ventilator VT settings, and unconsciousness.
      f. Decreased pulmonary blood flow: If a PE is blocking blood flow to the alveoli, the lungs compensate by reducing volume to the specific alveoli (resulting in atelectasis) in which there is deficient perfusion; thus, blood will more likely perfuse open alveoli.
   3. **Pathophysiology**
      a. As a result of the conditions resulting in atelectasis mentioned in the previous section, FRC and VC decrease.
      b. Intrapulmonary shunting occurs as capillary blood passes by collapsed alveoli, preventing normal gas exchange from taking place and resulting in hypoxemia.
   4. **Clinical signs and symptoms**
      a. Asymptomatic in mild atelectasis
      b. Hypoxemia
      c. Dyspnea
      d. Cough
      e. Dullness to percussion
      f. Elevated diaphragm
      g. Crackles in lung bases
      h. Diminished or absent breath sounds
      i. Tracheal deviation toward the atelectatic lung
   5. **Characteristics on chest x-ray films**
      a. Increased density (white)
      b. Elevated diaphragm
      c. Displaced interlobar fissures
      d. Mediastinal shift
      e. Altered bronchial and carinal angles
   6. **Treatment**
      a. Prevention of postoperative atelectasis by administration of incentive spirometry or IPPB
      b. Adequate pulmonary hydration to prevent mucus plugs and mobilization of secretions
      c. Treatment of underlying atelectasis with deep-breathing exercises, such as incentive spirometry or IPPB
      d. Initiation of CPAP if patient has hypoxemia with the use of 60% O_2 or more

e. Initiation of PEEP if patient is receiving mechanical ventilation

VI. SLEEP APNEA

CRT Exam Content Matrix: IB9o,t, IB10o,t, IC11
RRT Exam Content Matrix: IA10, IB9p,u, IB10q,v, IC13, IIIK8

A. Sleep apnea is present in patients who have at least 30 episodes of apnea over a 6-h period of sleep.

B. The apneic period may last from 20 s to more than 90 s.

C. **Types of Sleep Apnea**

1. **Obstructive sleep apnea**

   a. Apnea caused by upper airway anatomic obstruction.

   b. During the apneic period, the patient exhibits **strong and often intense respiratory effort. (See waveform pattern below.)**

   c. Although sleep posture (sleeping on the side rather than supine) has some benefits, **the use of CPAP or Bi-PAP while sleeping is the most effective method for treating obstructive sleep apnea.**

   d. Obstructive sleep apnea may be associated with

      (1) Obesity

      (2) Excessive pharyngeal tissue

      (3) Deviated nasal septum

      (4) Laryngeal web

      (5) Laryngeal stenosis

      (6) Enlarged adenoids or tonsils

   e. **Symptoms of obstructive sleep apnea**

      (1) Loud snoring

      (2) Hypersomnolence (excessive sleeping during the day)

      (3) Morning headache

      (4) Nausea

      (5) Personality changes

2. **Central sleep apnea**

   a. Apnea occurs because of the failure of the central respiratory centers (in the medulla) to send signals to the respiratory muscles.

   b. **It is characterized by the absence of inspiratory effort with no diaphragmatic movement (unlike obstructive sleep apnea).**

   c. This type of sleep apnea is associated with CNS disorders.

   d. Central sleep apnea may be associated with

      (1) Hypoventilation syndrome

      (2) Encephalitis

      (3) Spinal surgery

      (4) Brainstem disorders

   e. **Symptoms of central sleep apnea**

      (1) Insomnia

      (2) Mild snoring

      (3) Depression

      (4) Fatigue during the day

> ⚠️ Some patients may have a combination of both obstructive and central sleep apnea, which is defined as **mixed sleep apnea**.

D. **Diagnostic Sleep Studies**

1. Sleep studies are a very effective method for the diagnosis of sleep apnea and other breathing disorders such as sudden infant death syndrome (SIDS).

2. Sleep studies are also valuable in determining the cause, severity, and pathophysiologic effects of the breathing disorder during sleep.

3. *Polysomnography* refers to events that are recorded graphically while the individual is sleeping.

4. Continuous recordings on graph paper **(polysomnogram)** during the sleep study include

   a. Eye movement (electrooculogram)

   b. Brain wave activity (electroencephalogram [EEG])

   c. ECG

   d. Absence of airflow (apnea) is determined with the use of a CO_2 analyzer, thermistor, tracheal sound recorder, or a pneumotachograph

   e. Chest and abdominal movement

   f. O_2 saturation with the use of an ear oximeter

☝ **PES represents esophageal pressure measurements in the diagrams.**

g. Waveform "12-1" is an example of obstructive sleep apnea. Notice there are periods of no airflow with an increase in intensity of chest movement. This indicates that the upper airway is obstructed and the patient struggling to breathe.

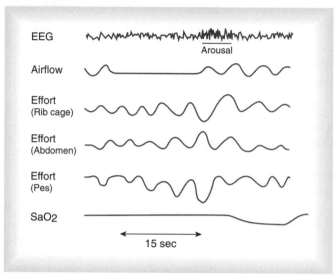

FIGURE 12-1 Obstructive apnea. Spectrum of sleep-related upper airway obstruction. Obstructive apnea. These events are defind as cessation of airflow for 10 s or longer. Paradoxical movement of the rib cage and abdomen in response to the closed airway occurs. Ventilatory effort (*Pes*) usually increases until a threshold is reached that triggers a brief arousal seen on the ECG, and airway opening occurs. Oxyhemoglobin desaturation usually accompanies the event. (From Wilkins RL, Stoller JK, Kacmarek RM: *Egan's fundamentals of respiratory care*, ed 9, St Louis, 2009, Mosby.)

h. Waveform "12-2" indicates central sleep apnea. Note that there is neither airflow nor chest excursion.

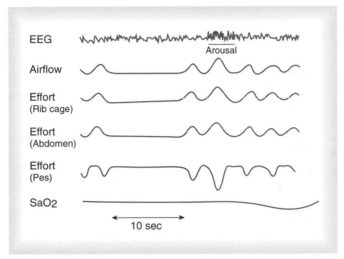

FIGURE 12-2   Central apnea. These events are defined as cessation of airflow for 10 s or longer. Compared to obstructive apnea, no movement of the rib cage or abdomen is present and the airway remains open. During an apneic event, there is a lack of ventilator effort (*Pes*). A brief arousal on the ECG is associated with a maximal ventilator effort that usually follows the episode of apnea. Oxyhemoglobin desaturation may be associated with the event. (From Wilkins RL, Stoller JK, Kacmarek RM: *Egan's fundamentals of respiratory care*, ed 9, St Louis, 2009, Mosby.)

POSTCHAPTER STUDY QUESTIONS

1. List three lung disorders classified as COPD.
2. List the common findings on the chest films of a patient with emphysema.
3. What PaO_2 level should be maintained for a COPD patient with chronic hypoxemia?
4. List the clinical signs and symptoms of cor pulmonale.
5. How does O_2 therapy help prevent or treat cor pulmonale?
6. The count of which type of WBC is characteristically elevated in the sputum and blood of a patient with asthma?
7. What aerosolized medication is used to treat *P. carinii* pneumonia?
8. List four causes of cardiogenic pulmonary edema.
9. List the signs and symptoms of pulmonary edema.
10. List the treatment modalities for pulmonary edema.
11. List the various causes of ARDS.
12. List the signs and symptoms of ARDS.
13. List treatment modalities for ARDS.
14. Define pneumothorax.
15. What is the immediate treatment for a tension pneumothorax?
16. What is the most effective method for treating obstructive sleep apnea?
17. List six variables that are measured during a sleep study.

See answers at the back of the text.

BIBLIOGRAPHY

Farzan S, *A concise handbook of respiratory diseases*, ed 4, Stamford, CT, 1997, Appleton & Lange.

Hess D and others, *Respiratory care principles and practice*, ed 1, Philadelphia, 2002, Saunders.

The Merck manual of medical information, Whitehouse Station, NJ, 1997, Merck.

Wilkins R, Dexter J, *Respiratory disease, a case study approach to patient care*, ed 3, Philadelphia, 2007, FA Davis.

Wilkins RL, Stoller JK, Kacmarek R, *Egan's fundamentals of respiratory care*, ed 9, St Louis, 2009, Mosby.

NEONATAL AND PEDIATRIC RESPIRATORY CARE

PRETEST QUESTIONS

Answer the pretest questions before studying the chapter. This will help you determine your strong and weak areas in the material covered.

1. An APGAR score of 5 is determined 5 min after delivery of a term infant. Which of the following should be done at this time?

   A. Stimulate and deliver low-to-moderate O_2 concentrations.
   B. Intubate and initiate mechanical ventilation.
   C. Intubate and initiate CPAP and 80% O_2.
   D. Initiate nasal CPAP and 100% O_2.

2. The foramen ovale and ductus arteriosus remain patent in infants with persistent fetal circulation as a direct result of which of the following?

   A. Hypocarbia
   B. Pulmonary hypertension
   C. Hyperoxia
   D. Arterial hypotension

3. Which of the following is not an indication for nasal CPAP in an infant?

   A. To increase static lung compliance
   B. To decrease FRC
   C. To decrease PVR
   D. To decrease intrapulmonary shunting

4. Which of the following are complications of an umbilical artery catheter (UAC)?

   1. Pneumothorax
   2. Thromboembolism
   3. Infection

   A. 1 only
   B. 2 only
   C. 1 and 3 only
   D. 2 and 3 only

5. Which of the following may occur as a result of cold stress to an infant?

   1. Hypoxemia
   2. Metabolic acidemia
   3. Hypoglycemia
   4. Decreased O_2 consumption

   A. 1 and 3 only
   B. 2 and 4 only
   C. 1, 2, and 3 only
   D. 1, 2 and 4 only

6. An elevation in the levels of chloride in sweat is diagnostic for which of the following lung conditions?

   A. Bronchiolitis
   B. Cystic fibrosis
   C. Hyaline membrane disease
   D. Epiglottitis

See answers and rationales at the back of the text.

REVIEW

I. **NEONATAL RESPIRATORY CARE**
   CRT Exam Content Matrix: IA7e, IA9, IB1d, IB7c, IB9b,g, IB10b,g, IC7, IIA2, IIA12b, IIA20, IIIE2a-c, IIIE3a, IIIF2d1-2, IIIG2c
   RRT Exam Content Matrix: IA7e, IA9, IB1d, IB7c, IB9b,g, IB10b,g, IC7, IIA1, IIA6, IIA9b, IIIE2a-c, IIIE3a
   A. **The High-Risk Infant**
      1. The term *high-risk infant* describes an infant who is at greater risk of death or who has a higher probability of a permanent disability.
      2. Maternal factors involved with high-risk infants
         a. Maternal age (younger than 16 yr or older than 35 yr)
         b. Diabetes
         c. Drug, alcohol, or tobacco abuse
         d. Maternal infections
         e. Previous cesarean section
         f. High blood pressure
         g. Previous history of an infant with respiratory problems or anomalies
         h. Lack of adequate prenatal care
      3. Other factors that characterize high-risk infants
         a. Premature rupture of membranes (PROM): increases the risk of fetal infection, especially pneumonia

b. Premature delivery (at less than 38 weeks' gestation)

c. Postmature delivery (at more than 42 weeks' gestation)

d. Meconium in amniotic fluid

e. Prolapsed cord

f. Prolonged labor

g. Abnormal fetal presentation (i.e., breech presentation)

B. **Assessment of the Neonate**

1. Assessing gestational age

   a. The **Ballard** scoring system is one of the most accurate means of estimating the baby's gestational age.

   b. The Ballard system scores the infant on neuromuscular criteria and external physical characteristics.

   c. Each specific sign is worth a given number of points, and the infant is given all or part of those points, depending on the assessment of that particular sign or characteristic.

   d. Points from each assessed area are totaled and plotted on a graph, which determines the infant's gestational age.

   e. Areas assessed include skin thickness, color and transparency of skin, amount of vernix present on the infant, plantar creases, posture, and muscle tone.

   f. Normal gestational age is 38 to 42 wk.

   g. The calculated gestational age can then be plotted on a graph, along with the infant's birth weight, to determine whether the infant is appropriate for gestational age (AGA), small for gestational age (SGA), or large for gestational age (LGA).

2. **Apgar scoring system**

   a. This system evaluates the infant's general condition within 5 min after birth.

   b. The five areas of assessment and the 0- to 2-point scoring system for each area are listed in the following table:

	SCORE		
Assessed sign	**0**	**1**	**2**
Heart rate	Absent	<100 beats/min	>100 beats/min
Respiratory effort	Absent	Slow, irregular	Strong cry
Color	Pale, blue	Body pink, extremities blue	Totally pink
Reflex irritability	No response	Grimace	Sneeze or cough
Muscle tone	Limp	Some flexion	Active flexion

   c. The Apgar assessment is done at 1 min after delivery to determine whether immediate intervention is required and again at 5 min after birth.

d. Apgar results at 1 min and the corresponding intervention

   (1) **Score of 7 to 10** is normal; requires routine observation, suction upper airway with bulb syringe, dry the infant, and place under a warmer.

   (2) **Score of 4 to 6** indicates moderate asphyxia; requires stimulation and O_2 administration.

   (3) **Score of 0 to 3** indicates severe asphyxia; requires immediate resuscitation with ventilatory assistance.

e. The 5-min Apgar score is useful in determining the infant's response to intervention; a score of less than 6 is associated with major complications and treatment in an intensive care nursery.

f. The five assessed signs in the Apgar scoring system may be more easily remembered with the use of the following acrostic:

   A for appearance (color)
   P for pulse (heart rate)
   G for grimace (reflex irritability)
   A for activity (muscle tone)
   R for respiration (respiratory effort)

 Exam Note

Acrocyanosis, or cyanosis in the hands and feet, is normal after birth, but cyanosis observed in the mucous membranes or lips indicates that O_2 therapy must be administered immediately.

3. **Silverman scoring system**

   a. This system helps determine the severity of respiratory distress.

   b. The infant is assessed in five areas

      (1) Intercostal retractions

      (2) Xiphoid retractions

      (3) Chest lag or paradoxical breathing

      (4) Nasal flaring: often the first or only sign of respiratory distress

      (5) Grunting: An audible expiratory grunt, caused by the infant partially closing the glottis during exhalation to prevent alveolar collapse, is a common sign of respiratory distress in infants.

   c. Each assessed area is worth from 0 to 2 points; the *lowest* score indicates minimal distress (as opposed to the *highest* score being the best in the Apgar scoring system).

4. **Other clinical assessments**

   a. Respiratory rate: normally 40/min to 60/min

   b. Heart rate: 130 to 150 beats/min

   c. Blood pressure: normal systolic, 60 to 90 mm Hg; normal diastolic, 30 to 60 mm Hg

   d. Temperature: 97.6° F ± 1° F (axillary); 99.6° F ± 1° F (rectally)

Cascade is good

Neonates should be placed in a thermoregulated environment, such as a radiant warmer or incubator immediately after birth to prevent cold stress. Because newborns do not shiver, they warm themselves through brown fat metabolism. This metabolic process uses up oxygen (increased oxygen consumption) and glucose, resulting in hypoxemia and hypoglycemia (decreased glucose level).

e. **Normal ABG levels with room air:**

pH	7.35 to 7.45 (no less than 7.25 at birth)
$PaCO_2$	35 to 45 mm Hg
PaO_2	50 to 70 mm Hg
HCO_3^-	20 to 26 mEq/L
BE	−5 to +5

C. O_2 Delivery Devices for Neonates

1. O_2 hood

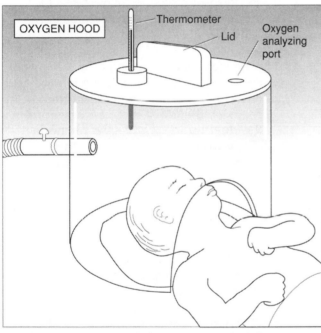

OXYGEN HOOD — Thermometer — Lid — Oxygen analyzing port

FIGURE 13-1 From Scanlan C, Spearman C, Sheldon R: *Egan's fundamentals of respiratory care,* ed 5, St Louis, 1990, Mosby.

a. The O_2 hood is the recommended method for delivering O_2 in the range of 21% to 100% to the infant.

b. A heated nebulizer connected to an O_2 blender is the most common method of O_2 delivery. The aerosol tubing connects into the back of the hood. If a blender is used to regulate the O_2 percentage, the nebulizer must be set on 100% so that no air entrainment occurs, which would alter the blender percentage.

c. A heated humidifier (Cascade or pass-over) is often used rather than a nebulizer to prevent overhydration of the infant.

d. The percentage of O_2 should be analyzed continuously with an O_2 analyzer. A port in the top of the hood makes analyzing possible. **The O_2 percentage should be analyzed as close to the infant's airway as possible because the percentage of O_2 is somewhat higher at the bottom of the hood as opposed to the top.**

e. A heated nebulizer or humidifier should be used because cold gas blowing on the infant's face may induce apnea and colder temperatures in the hood may increase the infant's O_2 consumption.

f. Flows into the hood should be at least 7 L/min to prevent CO_2 buildup in the hood.

g. Temperatures inside the hood should be closely monitored through a port in the top of the hood to avoid overheating or underheating the infant.

h. Noise levels inside the hood have been proven to be a source of hearing loss to the infant. To keep noise levels to a minimum, nebulizers that entrain air should not be used because they produce increased noise levels.

use wick humidify to b noise

2. Nasal catheter or cannula

a. Nasal catheters and cannulas are available in infant sizes and are most commonly used for long-term O_2 therapy in the treatment of bronchopulmonary dysplasia (BPD) and other chronic diseases.

b. The flowmeters used to deliver O_2 through the catheter or cannula should be calibrated so that increments of 0.25 and 0.50 L/min can be used.

3. Incubator

a. An enclosed device used with neonates that has the capability of controlling FiO_2, humidity, and environmental temperature.

b. The temperature and humidity of the gas is servo controlled.

c. The FiO_2 is controlled with an air entrainment device. A metal red flag is attached to a mechanism that blocks the entrainment port, which allows for an FiO_2 of greater than 0.40 when the flag is in the up position. With the flag in the down position, the entrainment port remains open and delivers an FiO_2 of 0.4 or less.

d. The oxygen concentration can be inconsistent and variable when the enclosure is opened to provide care to the infant. Because of this, oxygen is often delivered through an oxygen hood placed over the infant inside the incubator.

e. As with oxygen hoods, it is very important to minimize noise levels within the incubator to prevent hearing impairment in the infant.

4. **Nasal CPAP**
   a. CPAP is most commonly administered to infants with nasal prongs.
   b. CPAP may also be administered with a mask, ET tube, or nasopharyngeal tube.
   c. **Indications for nasal CPAP**
      (1) To improve oxygenation

> ☑ **Exam Note**
>
> To prevent pulmonary tissue damage (such as BPD) from high FiO_2 levels, administer CPAP. The FiO_2 should be no higher than 0.60 to maintain normal PaO_2 levels, if possible. If PaO_2 is less than normal with an FiO_2 of 0.60, institute CPAP; do not increase the FiO_2.

      (2) To increase static lung compliance
      (3) To increase FRC
      (4) To decrease the work of breathing
      (5) To decrease intrapulmonary shunting
      (6) To decrease PVR
   d. **Complications of nasal CPAP**
      (1) Barotrauma (pneumothorax)

> ☑ **Exam Note**
>
> A device known as a **transilluminator** is used on neonates to diagnose a pneumothorax. This device has a small light on its distal end, which is placed over the thin chest wall of the neonate. Normally a small halo of orange light is seen beneath the bulb on the chest. If a pneumothorax is present, a large halo of orange light is seen, indicating air in the thoracic cavity.

> ☑ **Exam Note**
>
> According to the current NBRC exam content matrix, assessing for a pneumothorax with the use of transillumination will appear on the RRT exam only.

      (2) Decreased venous return, resulting in decreased cardiac output

 Decreased venous return is less likely to occur if the infant has decreased static lung compliance caused by respiratory distress syndrome (RDS). Infants with normal lungs would be more susceptible to this complication because the lungs are more compliant and the airway pressure is more easily transferred to the superior and inferior vena cavae.

      (3) Air-trapping
      (4) Pressure necrosis
      (5) Loss of CPAP from crying or displacement
   e. Blood must be drawn frequently to determine ABG levels if CPAP is used to monitor $PaCO_2$ levels. If the $PaCO_2$ begins to rise, mechanical ventilation is necessary.

   f. The use of nasal CPAP for infants is based on the fact that infants are obligate nose breathers. If the baby cries, CPAP is lost.
D. **Hazards of O_2 Therapy in the Neonate**
   1. **Retinopathy of prematurity (ROP)**
      a. This condition is also referred to as *neonatal retinopathy.*
      b. ROP is caused by high levels of O_2 in the blood (**PaO_2 of more than 80 mm Hg**).
      c. ROP occurs primarily in premature infants who have very fragile retinal blood vessels.
      d. Initially, the high arterial O_2 levels cause constriction of the retinal vessels. As the vessels remain constricted, new vessels form in an attempt to oxygenate the retina.
      e. This growth of new vessels leads to hemorrhaging within the retina, retinal detachment, and blindness.
      f. The degree of blindness varies in each situation and infants exposed to supplemental O_2 should have an eye examination before discharge.
      g. ABG samples should be obtained frequently while the infant is receiving O_2 to determine the O_2 level in the blood. **If the infant has a ductal shunt (discussed later in this chapter), the blood must be drawn from the right radial, brachial, or temporal artery to measure the PaO_2 of the blood going to the head.** If no shunt exists, blood may be drawn from the UAC or any peripheral artery.
      h. To reduce the potential of ROP, maintain PaO_2 below 80 mm Hg.
   2. BPD
      a. BPD is caused by long-term supplemental O_2 therapy and mechanical ventilation.
      b. Damage occurs in the alveolar epithelium, causing destruction of pulmonary tissues.
      c. **BPD is discussed in detail later in this chapter.**
E. **Sites for Obtaining Arterial Blood**
   1. **Umbilical artery**
      a. A UAC is normally placed in critically ill infants who require frequent ABG analysis.
      b. Insert the catheter into one of the two umbilical arteries. After insertion, determine the position of the catheter with a radiograph.
      c. Rest the tip of the catheter in the **descending aorta** at either one of the following vertebral levels as seen on a radiographic image
         (1) T6 to T10 (thoracic aorta)
         (2) L3 to L4 (lumbar aorta)
      d. Secure the catheter in place with umbilical tape or sutures attached to the umbilical stump, and then tape the catheter to the abdomen.

e. **Advantages of the UAC**
   (1) Frequent ABG samples are easily obtained.
   (2) Prevents frequent peripheral arterial punctures
   (3) Allows continuous monitoring of blood pressure
   (4) Allows the infusion of drugs and fluids
f. **Complications of the UAC**
   (1) Infection
   (2) Thromboembolism (To help prevent this, flush the line with heparin after a blood sample is drawn.)
   (3) Air embolism
   (4) Hemorrhage
g. Do not leave UACs in place for longer than **7 to 10 days** to help avoid these complications.
h. Generally, no more than 0.5 mL of blood is necessary for ABG analysis.
i. If there is inadequate perfusion to the lower extremities, blanching or cyanosis of the legs or feet will be evident. Withdraw or replace the catheter.

2. **Peripheral artery puncture**
a. Draw arterial blood from one of several arteries in the neonate, including the radial, brachial, temporal, and posterior tibial arteries.
b. The radial artery is the most common site because of its easy accessibility, good collateral circulation, and lack of immediately adjacent nerves or veins.
c. Generally, use a 25- or 26-gauge needle to puncture the artery at a 35 to 45 degree angle to the artery. Face the bevel of the needle up when performing radial puncture.
d. Locate the radial artery by finding a radial pulse or by placing a **transilluminator** under the back of the wrist. This lighted device aids in locating the artery.
e. Because the radial artery in a neonate is very small, it is not uncommon to insert the needle completely through the artery. If, after advancing the needle, you do not obtain blood, withdraw the needle slightly until blood enters the needle.
f. When you obtain an adequate amount of blood, withdraw the needle and apply pressure to the puncture site for approximately 5 min.
g. Remove any air bubbles in the sample before analysis. If this is not done, the blood gas analysis will show erroneous values, indicating a high PaO_2 and low $PaCO_2$.

3. **Arterialized capillary blood sampling**
a. Normally obtain arterialized capillary blood from the heel of the neonate by using a lancet to puncture the capillary.
b. Warm the infant's foot for several minutes (usually by wrapping a warm moist diaper around the foot) to cause peripheral vasodilation, which improves capillary perfusion and arterializes the capillary blood.
c. Then clean the heel with alcohol and puncture the capillary using an appropriate device. Use a heparinized glass capillary tube for the blood.
d. Take care not to squeeze the heel because this may cause damage to the foot and contaminate the sample with venous blood and interstitial fluid.
e. Make sure the capillary tube is as close to the puncture site as possible to avoid contaminating the sample with room air.
f. Once you obtain the sample, apply pressure to the heel until the bleeding stops, and then apply an adhesive bandage.
g. Capillary blood samples offer fairly reliable correlations for arterial pH and PCO_2 but are unreliable for PO_2 values. The capillary PO_2 (PCO_2) may be low, but the PaO_2 may actually be high, which increases the risk of ROP or BPD. It is also possible to have a high PCO_2 when the PaO_2 is low, which risks hypoxic damage. Monitor **arterial** PO_2 levels periodically to prevent this potential hazard. **Normal PCO_2 is 40 to 50 mm Hg.**

F. **Transcutaneous $PaCO_2$ and PaO_2 Monitoring**
1. By applying blood gas electrodes over the skin, you may monitor the neonate's PaO_2 and $PaCO_2$ continuously without having to perform arterial sticks as frequently.
2. Attach the probe to the skin, which warms the skin to 40° to 42° C and results in vasodilation and increased perfusion to the dermal layer of the skin. O_2 and CO_2 diffuse through the skin in concentrations similar to those in arterial blood.
3. **Disadvantages of transcutaneous monitoring**
a. The heated probe may burn the skin. Change the location of the probe every **3 to 4 h** to prevent this. In the more premature infant with very fragile skin, change the probe position every **2 h.**
b. The infant must have adequate perfusion to the area of the skin where the probe is attached to provide accurate readings.
c. Inaccurate readings occur if the probe is inadequately heated, the monitor is not calibrated properly, or the probe becomes loose and air comes between the probe and the skin.
4. The monitor requires calibrating during the initial setup and after probe position changes. This is done with the sensor off the infant and is calculated by (PB: 47 mm Hg) × 0.21. **(Math shortcut for exam: If the corrected PB is 700 mm Hg, then use 7 × 21.)**

5. After calibration, the monitor takes 20 to 30 min to equilibrate before accurate readings are displayed.

G. **Oximetry**

1. Monitoring arterial O_2 saturation with a pulse oximeter (SpO_2) is becoming a popular method of determining the oxygenation status of infants.

2. Oximetry uses photometrics (a light beam shining through the skin or nailbed) to determine SaO_2; therefore, the burning of the skin that is possible with transcutaneous monitoring is not a factor. For more detailed information on oximetry, see chapter 10.

II. **NEONATAL CARDIOPULMONARY DISORDERS**

CRT Exam Content Matrix: IA7e, IA9, IB1d, IB7c, IB9b,g, IB10b,g, IC7, IIA2, IIA12b, IIA20, IIIE2a-c, IIIE3a, IIIF2d1-2, IIIG2c

RRT Exam Content Matrix: IA7e, IA9, IB1d, IB7c, IB9b,g,k, IB10b,g,k, IC7, IIA1, IIA6, IIA9b, IIIE2a-c, IIIE3a

A. **Infant Respiratory Distress Syndrome (IRDS)**

1. **Definition:** a syndrome affecting premature infants that is caused by inadequate amounts of pulmonary surfactant, which leads to massive atelectasis and hypoxemia. (Also known as hyaline membrane disease [HMD].)

2. **Causes**
   a. Immature lungs with surfactant deficiency
   b. **Lecithin–sphingomyelin** (L : S) ratio of less than 2 : 1. These lipid levels may be obtained from amniotic fluid to determine the maturity of the surfactant. A ratio of more than 2 : 1 indicates mature surfactant.
   c. Infants born before 35 weeks' gestation are at risk of IRDS.

3. **Pathophysiology**
   a. Surfactant lines the inner surface of alveoli, decreasing the surface tension and thereby reducing their tendency to collapse.
   b. Immature surfactant or decreased surfactant production, as seen in IRDS, leads to alveolar collapse, decreased lung compliance, hypoxemia, and metabolic acidosis.
   c. Alveolar surface tension increases from the lack of surfactant, which results in fluid being pulled into the alveoli. Because of damage to the capillary endothelial cells by acidosis and hypoxemia, the fluid entering the alveoli contains protein and the blood-clotting component fibrin. This makes the alveoli very stiff (noncompliant) and causes the hyaline membrane formation.

4. **Clinical manifestations**
   a. Nasal flaring
   b. Grunting
   c. Retractions
   d. Tachypnea
   e. Cyanosis
   f. ABG levels reveal hypercapnia and hypoxemia with a mixed respiratory and metabolic acidosis.

5. **Chest x-ray findings**
   a. "Ground glass" appearance
   b. Diffuse atelectasis
   c. Air bronchograms

6. **Treatment**
   a. O_2 therapy to maintain PaO_2 above 50 mm Hg
   b. Nasal CPAP or ET-tube CPAP if the infant's PaO_2 remains below 50 mm Hg with the use of 60% O_2
   c. Positive pressure ventilation with PEEP if $PaCO_2$ is increasing and the pH is less than 7.25
   d. Surfactant replacement
   e. Thermoregulation
   f. Adequate fluids to prevent dehydration
   g. Packed RBCs are given to prevent anemia and blood loss from frequent ABG samples.

B. **Bronchopulmonary dysplasia (BPD)**

1. **Definition:** a form of chronic lung disease seen in infants with severe RDS after prolonged positive pressure ventilation and supplemental O_2. Dysplasia refers to abnormal development, in this case, of the bronchi and lungs.

2. **Causes**
   a. Although the cause of BPD is widely debated, it is thought to occur from prolonged (more than 7 days) exposure to high concentrations of O_2 with positive pressure ventilation.
   b. A major cause of BPD is thought to be high inspiratory pressures associated with mechanical ventilation, which leads to barotrauma.
   c. It occurs more frequently in infants weighing less than 1500 g.

3. **Pathophysiology**
   a. There are four stages of BPD
      (1) **Stage 1** occurs 2 to 4 days after birth and consists of
         (a) Hyaline membrane formation
         (b) Atelectasis
         (c) Necrosis of bronchiolar mucosa
         (d) Bronchiolar metaplasia
      (2) **Stage 2** occurs 4 to 10 days after birth and includes necrosis, repair of alveolar and bronchial epithelium, and emphysematous changes.

(3) **Stage 3** occurs 10 to 20 days after birth and includes
  (a) Interstitial fibrosis
  (b) Atelectasis
  (c) Continuation of bronchiolar metaplasia
  (d) Increased mucus production
  (e) Bullae formation
(4) **Stage 4** occurs 30 days after birth and includes
  (a) Formation of emphysematous alveoli
  (b) Atelectasis
  (c) Continuation of interstitial fibrosis
b. Large amounts of mucus are produced, leading to air-trapping with resultant atelectasis.
4. **Clinical manifestations**
  a. Increased airway resistance
  b. Normal or increased static lung compliance
  c. V/Q mismatching
  d. Hypoxemia when breathing room air
  e. Hypercapnia
  f. Tachypnea
  g. Barrel chest
  h. Retractions
5. **Chest x-ray findings**
  a. "Ground glass" appearance
  b. Opacification
  c. Atelectasis
  d. Hyperlucency
  e. Presence of bullae
6. **Treatment**
  a. O_2 therapy to maintain PaO_2 between 50 and 70 mm Hg (helps prevent pulmonary hypertension resulting from hypoxemia)
  b. A pressure-limited, time-cycled ventilator may be required to maintain normal ABG levels.
  c. Adequate humidification to prevent mucus plugging in the airways or ET tube
  d. Chest physical therapy and suctioning
  e. Adequate nutrition
  f. Maintenance of fluid balance or diuretic administration to minimize the infant's increased risk of cor pulmonale, pulmonary edema, and CHF
  g. Bronchodilator therapy
C. **Meconium aspiration**
  1. **Definition:** Aspiration of meconium is most commonly associated with full-term or postterm infants. Meconium is discharged in the first fetal bowel movement and is composed of mucus, vernix, epithelial cells, and amniotic fluid.
  2. **Causes**
    a. If, while in utero, the infant becomes hypoxic, meconium is passed into the amniotic fluid.
    b. Infants in utero breathe in a shallow manner, moving amniotic fluid into and out of the oropharynx. However, if the infant is stressed or asphyxiated, the breaths are much deeper

and meconium may be aspirated through the vocal cords and into the lungs.
    c. The **postterm** infant is at greater risk of meconium aspiration because less amniotic fluid is present; therefore, there is less dilution of the meconium.
    d. Even if the meconium is present only in the mouth or the glottic area, aspiration may occur with the infant's first few breaths.
  3. **Pathophysiology**
    a. The substances that make up meconium cause it to be very thick; therefore, if aspirated, it plugs airways, which leads to atelectasis and increased airway resistance.
    b. Generally, airflow passes through the obstruction during inspiration but gets trapped during expiration as the airway diameter decreases, which results in hyperinflation.
    c. This air-trapping often leads to pneumothorax.
    d. Infants with this condition often have patent ductus arteriosus (PDA) (discussed later) caused by the intrauterine hypoxia. Hypoxia causes pulmonary vasoconstriction, which prevents the ductus arteriosus and foramen ovale from closing, resulting in a right to left shunt.
  4. **Clinical manifestations**
    a. Long fingernails and peeling skin (signs of postmaturity)
    b. Hypoxemia
    c. Hypercarbia
    d. Tachypnea
    e. Retractions, nasal flaring, grunting
    f. Barrel chest (from air-trapping)
    g. Cyanosis
    h. Crackles and rhonchi on chest auscultation
  5. **Chest x-ray findings**
    a. Patchy infiltrates
    b. Atelectasis
    c. Consolidation
    d. Pneumothorax (commonly observed)
    e. Hyperinflation
  6. **Treatment**
    a. If meconium is observed during delivery, suction the infant's oral and nasal pharynx once the head is delivered and before the first cry, to prevent aspiration of the meconium.
    b. Immediately after delivery, intubate and suction the infant to remove meconium from the lower airway if the infant is not vigorous.
    c. Do not start positive pressure ventilation until all meconium is cleared because this would push it farther into the airways.
    d. Initiate O_2 therapy or mechanical ventilation, depending on the severity of the condition.
    e. Chest physical therapy
    f. Frequent suctioning

D. **Persistent Pulmonary Hypertension of the Newborn (PPHN)**
   1. **Definition:** a condition in which fetal blood circulation through the heart persists after birth because of pulmonary hypertension.
      a. **Normal fetal circulation:** Blood flow through the heart of the infant in utero differs from the pathway the blood takes after birth. Only about 10% of blood returning to the right side of the infant's heart flows on into the pulmonary circulation. The other 90% or so of the blood volume in the right side of the heart shunts over to the left side via two pathways. One is through the foramen ovale, a pathway that allows blood to flow from the right atrium into the left atrium. The second area where shunting occurs is through the ductus arteriosus, which is a communication between the pulmonary artery and the descending aorta.
      b. These two communications between the right and left heart are kept open in utero because of the high pressure in the pulmonary vasculature. After the infant is delivered and begins breathing O_2 from the air, pulmonary vasodilation occurs, reducing the pulmonary hypertension and allowing the foramen ovale and ductus arteriosus to gradually close.
      c. If closure of these two pathways does not occur, blood bypasses the lungs and is shunted directly into the left side of the heart and out to the body without oxygenation. PaO_2 levels do not increase as FiO_2 is increased.
   2. **Causes**
      a. The condition is most common in full-term or postterm infants because the pulmonary vessels are more reactive to hypoxia, leading to pulmonary vasoconstriction
      b. Conditions often accompanied by PPHN
         (1) Perinatal asphyxia
         (2) Meconium aspiration
         (3) Pneumonia
         (4) Sepsis
         (5) Congenital heart defects
         (6) Diaphragmatic hernia
         (7) Hypoplastic lungs
         (8) Hypoglycemia

 Exam Note

Any condition that results in increased pulmonary vascular resistance (PVR) can cause PPHN.

   3. **Pathophysiology**
      a. The foramen ovale and ductus arteriosus remain open as a result of pulmonary hypertension.

      b. This results in right-to-left shunting that causes hypoxemia that is not responsive to O_2 therapy.
   4. **Clinical manifestations**
      a. Tachypnea
      b. Hypoxemia
      c. Cyanosis (not in all cases)
      d. More than a 15-mm Hg difference in the PaO_2 between preductal blood (radial or temporal artery) and postductal blood (umbilical artery) with the use of 100% O_2 (i.e., preductal PaO_2 is higher than postductal PaO_2)

 Exam Note

Even though this is characteristically diagnostic of a right-to-left shunt, PPHN should not be ruled out if this is not observed, because it may still be present. A PDA can be positively identified with the use of ultrasonography. Transcutaneous PO_2 monitors may also be used in place of arterial sticks to determine right-to-left shunting. One $TcPO_2$ probe is placed on the right arm (preductal), one is placed on the abdomen or lower extremities (postductal), and the difference is monitored.

      e. Significant increase in PaO_2 (more than 100 mm Hg) when $PaCO_2$ is maintained at 20 to 25 mm Hg

Exam Note

Maintaining low $PaCO_2$ levels results in pulmonary vasodilation, which should allow less blood flow through the ductus arteriosus and foramen ovale. If shunting is occurring, PaO_2 levels would increase during this test.

   5. **Chest x-ray findings**
      a. May be normal
      b. Decreased pulmonary vasculature
   6. **Treatment**
      a. Mechanical hyperventilation to maintain $PaCO_2$ levels at 20 to 25 mm Hg with an alkaline pH
      b. Maintenance of PaO_2 levels at more than 100 mm Hg

Exam Note

Maintain $PaCO_2$ and PaO_2 levels as mentioned above only for the first few days of therapy to help reverse pulmonary hypertension.

      c. Drug therapy
         (1) Inhaled nitric oxide (see Chapter 1 on oxygen and medical gas therapy for detailed information)
         (2) Tolazoline (Priscoline), a vasodilator
         (3) Nitroprusside sodium (Nipride), a vasodilator
         (4) Sodium bicarbonate to produce alkalemia

(5) Dopamine, which increases systemic vascular resistance and thus reduces the right-to-left pressure gradient, which decreases shunting

d. Weaning from mechanical ventilation should be done slowly because small decreases in ventilator respiratory rates, peak inspiratory pressure, and FiO_2 may result in a return to shunting, which will require even higher ventilator variables (respiratory rate, PIP, FiO_2) than before.

> ☑ **Exam Note**
>
> A PDA may also produce a left-to-right shunt. This occurs in premature infants in whom aortic pressures exceed pulmonary artery pressures, blood flows from the aorta to the pulmonary artery, and the blood is recirculated through the lungs. This may lead to CHF and pulmonary edema. Chest films reveal increased pulmonary vascularity and cardiomegaly. This often results in elevated oxygen levels in the pulmonary artery (PvO_2 and SvO_2).

e. Furosemide (Lasix) is indicated for treatment of the edema, and indomethacin is often used to help constrict the ductus so that blood cannot flow through it.

III. **Extracorporeal Membrane Oxygenation (ECMO)**
ECMO is not specifically mentioned on either exam matrix.

A. Infants who do not respond to conventional mechanical ventilation should begin receiving ECMO.

B. In this procedure, venous blood is removed from the right atrium via an indwelling catheter and pumped through a membrane where the blood is oxygenated. The blood is then returned to the infant via the right jugular vein.

C. Neonatal conditions that may warrant this procedure are
1. Meconium aspiration syndrome
2. RDS
3. PPHN
4. Sepsis
5. Perinatal asphyxia
6. Congenital diaphragmatic hernia

D. To have ECMO initiated, an infant must meet the following criteria
1. Gestational age of more than 35 weeks
2. Reversible lung disease
3. No preexisting head bleeding
4. Significant shunting
5. Reversible anatomic shunting
6. Reversible pulmonary hypertension

IV. **AIRWAY DISORDERS OF THE PEDIATRIC PATIENT**
CRT Exam Content Matrix: IA2, IA6, IB1a, IB1c, IB7d, IB8, IC1, IIA12a, IIID5a, IIIE1, IIIF2c-d
RRT Exam Content Matrix: IA2, IA6, IB1a, IB8, IIIE1

> ☑ **Exam Note**
>
> The matrices are not specific to pediatric and neonatal respiratory care procedures, but questions pertaining to the neonate or pediatric patient with regard to such areas as patient assessment, ventilator management, and airway management will be asked on both exams.

A. **Epiglottitis**
1. **Definition:** a bacterial infection of the epiglottis, most commonly affecting children 3 to 7 years old, resulting in inflammation and edema of the supraglottic area
2. **Causes**
   a. Bacterial infection
   b. Bacterial pathogens responsible for epiglottitis
      (1) *Haemophilus influenzae,* the most common cause
      (2) *Streptococcus* species
      (3) *Staphylococcus aureus*
      (4) *Pneumococcus* species
3. **Pathophysiology**
   a. Bacterial infection leads to inflammation of the epiglottis, glottis, and hypopharynx.
   b. Inflammation leads to swelling of the supraglottic area, resulting in a sudden onset of severe respiratory distress and often precipitating a life-threatening situation.
4. **Clinical manifestations**
   a. High fever
   b. Drooling
   c. Sore throat
   d. Dyspnea
   e. Tachycardia
   f. Inspiratory stridor
   g. Intercostal and sternal retractions
   h. Use of accessory muscles during inspiration
   i. Hoarseness
   j. Sitting up and leaning forward to maintain the airway, as swelling progresses
   k. The epiglottis is swollen and red on direct visualization, which may result in complete upper airway obstruction; thus, if direct visualization is attempted, intubation and tracheostomy equipment must be readily available. Avoid direct visualization if possible.
   l. Initial ABG levels reveal hypoxemia and respiratory alkalosis, progressing to respiratory acidosis if hypoxemia is not reversed.
5. **X-ray findings**
   a. A lateral neck x-ray film will reveal a swollen epiglottis, known as the ***thumb sign*** because it resembles the distal end of a thumb.
6. **Treatment**
   a. Tracheal intubation

(1) Tracheotomy is performed if nasal or oral intubation is impossible.

(2) Usually the patient may be extubated in 36 to 48 h.

b. O$_2$ therapy in uncomplicated cases

c. Antibiotics (for *H. influenzae*)

d. Mechanical ventilation (rarely necessary)

B. **Laryngotracheobronchitis (Croup)**

1. **Definition:** upper airway obstruction resulting from inflammation of the larynx and subglottic area; most commonly seen in children 8 months to 4 years old

2. **Causes**

a. Primarily parainfluenza virus infection

b. May result from adenovirus or respiratory syncytial virus (RSV) infection (discussed later in this chapter)

3. **Pathophysiology**

a. Swelling and edema of the laryngeal and subglottic area results from inflammation that leads to a narrowing airway lumen.

b. The subglottic area is the narrowest portion of the infant's or child's airway, so a small degree of edema causes a significant reduction in the cross-sectional area.

c. The inflammation results in increased mucus production from the mucus glands.

4. **Clinical manifestations**

a. Tachypnea

b. Tachycardia

c. Cyanosis

d. Inspiratory stridor

e. Intercostal and sternal retractions

f. Use of accessory muscles for breathing

g. Barking cough

h. Fever

i. Initial ABG levels reveal hypoxemia and respiratory alkalosis, progressing to respiratory acidosis if hypoxemia is not reversed.

5. **X-ray findings**

a. A lateral neck x-ray film will indicate haziness in the subglottic region.

6. **Treatment**

a. O$_2$ therapy

b. Cool aerosol to reduce swelling (often via croup tent)

c. Aerosolized racemic epinephrine to reduce swelling

d. Adequate hydration

C. **Foreign Body Aspiration**

1. **Definition:** inhalation of a foreign body into the tracheobronchial tree

2. **Causes**

a. Young children often place objects in their mouths and, in some instances, aspirate the object into the respiratory tract.

b. The most commonly aspirated objects are seeds, peanuts, and coins.

3. **Pathophysiology**

a. The aspirated object usually lodges in the right mainstem bronchus because of its angle of bifurcation from the trachea.

b. Certain objects (especially peanuts) may result in a chemical bronchitis that causes mucosal swelling and edema.

c. Commonly, infection distal to the obstruction occurs, resulting in abscess, pneumonia, or bronchiectasis.

4. **Clinical manifestations**

a. Choking or coughing, depending on severity

b. Dyspnea

c. Cyanosis

d. Wheezing (normally unresponsive to bronchodilator therapy)

e. Hemoptysis (uncommon)

5. **Chest x-ray findings**

a. Chest films may indicate hyperinflation of the affected lung.

b. A mediastinal shift away from the side of the aspiration occurs during expiration, as the affected lung becomes hyperinflated.

> Inspiratory and expiratory chest films should be obtained to determine whether a mediastinal shift is present.

6. **Treatment**

a. Abdominal thrusts (severe cases of obstruction)

b. Bronchoscopy to remove foreign object

c. Bronchodilator therapy followed by postural drainage and percussion is often successful in removing the object before bronchoscopy.

D. **Bronchiolitis**

1. **Definition:** an inflammation of the bronchioles that is most commonly seen in children during the first 2 years

2. **Causes**

a. Most commonly results from **RSV** infection

b. Adenovirus and influenza virus infection (less commonly)

3. **Pathophysiology**

a. The viral infection causes inflammation of the bronchioles, mucosal edema, and spasms of the bronchiolar smooth muscle.

b. In severe cases, mucus and fibrin may accumulate in the lumen of the affected bronchioles.

c. Inspiratory and expiratory flows become obstructed, increasing FRC.

d. Atelectasis may result from the inflammation in severe cases.

4. **Clinical manifestations**
   a. Recent upper respiratory tract infection
   b. Fever
   c. Cough
   d. Tachypnea
   e. Dyspnea
   f. Crackles and wheezing on chest auscultation
   g. Apnea (in infants)
   h. Sternal and intercostal retractions
   i. Hypoxemia
5. **Chest x-ray findings**
   a. Marked hyperradiolucency
   b. Infiltrates
6. **Treatment**
   a. Mild cases do not require hospitalization.
   b. **Severe cases**
      (1) O_2 therapy (via hood or tent, depending on the age of the child)
      (2) CPAP to treat severe hypoxemia
      (3) Ribavirin (antiviral drug), administered via a SPAG nebulizer for 12 to 18 h daily through an O_2 hood for 3 to 7 days. This therapy is declining in use and, in fact, is no longer covered on the NBRC exams.
      (4) Mechanical ventilation, if other treatment is unsuccessful
      (5) Adequate hydration
E. **Cystic Fibrosis**
   1. **Definition:** a hereditary disease affecting the exocrine glands of the body that results in the production of thick mucus from these glands. The glands most commonly affected are located in the pancreas, the sweat glands, and the lungs.
   2. **Causes**
      a. Genetic transmission
      b. The mother and father both must be carriers of this recessive gene. Each child of the couple has a one-in-four chance of having the disease.
   3. **Pathophysiology**
      a. Large amounts of thick mucus are produced as a result of the abnormally large numbers of bronchial glands and goblet cells located in the tracheobronchial tree.
      b. Thick mucus stagnates in the airways, leading to airway obstruction and facilitation of bacterial growth.
      c. Mucus plugging results in atelectasis, hyperinflation, and pneumonia.
      d. Abnormalities in the pancreatic ducts and glands result in inadequate absorption and digestion of food, causing malnutrition if not properly treated.
   4. **Clinical manifestations**
      a. Tachypnea
      b. Tachycardia
      c. Cough with thick mucus production

   d. Increased AP chest diameter
   e. Digital clubbing
   f. **Elevated chloride levels in sweat (diagnostic of this disease)**
   g. Use of accessory muscles during normal breathing
   h. Early in the disease process, ABG levels indicate hypoxemia with respiratory alkalosis.
   i. In late stages of disease, ABG levels reveal chronic ventilatory failure with hypoxemia.
   j. Cyanosis
   k. Cor pulmonale, in late stages
   l. Pulmonary function studies reveal decreases in expiratory flow values and increased FRC values
5. **Chest x-ray findings**
   a. Hyperinflation
   b. Flattened diaphragm
   c. Increased lung markings
   d. Cardiomegaly
6. **Treatment**
   a. Aerosolized bronchodilator therapy with a mucolytic, such as acetylcysteine (Mucomyst) or dornase alfa (Pulmozyme), followed by chest physical therapy (flutter valve, PEP therapy, oscillating vest)
   b. O_2 therapy
   c. Expectorants
   d. Continuous aerosol mask
   e. Antibiotics

POSTCHAPTER STUDY QUESTIONS

1. What five conditions are assessed in the Apgar score?
2. Describe the appropriate intervention for the following Apgar scores: 0 to 3; 4 to 6; and 7 to 10.
3. What is often the first sign of respiratory distress in the infant?
4. List the normal ABG levels for an infant.
5. List six indications for nasal CPAP.
6. List five complications of CPAP.
7. List two hazards of O_2 therapy in the neonate.
8. Describe where the tip of the UAC should rest when properly positioned.
9. List four advantages of a UAC.
10. List four complications of a UAC.
11. List six clinical manifestations of IRDS.
12. List the causes of BPD.
13. List eight clinical manifestations of BPD.
14. Describe the chest x-ray findings in infants with BPD.
15. List the treatment modalities for BPD.
16. List the causes of meconium aspiration.
17. List eight clinical manifestations of meconium aspiration.
18. List eight conditions that accompany PPHN.
19. List five clinical manifestations of PPHN.

20. List the treatment modalities for PPHN.
21. List the causes of epiglottitis.
22. List 12 clinical manifestations of epiglottitis.
23. Describe the classic x-ray finding for diagnosis of epiglottitis.
24. List the treatment modalities for epiglottitis.
25. List 12 clinical manifestations of cystic fibrosis.
26. List the treatment modalities for cystic fibrosis.

See answers at the back of the text.

BIBLIOGRAPHY

Hess D and others, *Respiratory care principles and practice*, ed 1, Philadelphia, 2002, Saunders.

Scanlan C, Spearman C, Sheldon R: *Egan's fundamentals of respiratory care*, ed 5, St Louis, 1990, Mosby.

Walsh BK, Czernnske MP, DiBlasi RM: *Perinatal and pediatric respiratory care*, ed 3, St Louis, 2010, Saunders.

Whitaker K, *Comprehensive perinatal and pediatric respiratory care*, ed 3, Albany, NY, 2001, Delmar.

Wilkins RL, Stoller JK, Kacmarek R, *Egan's fundamentals of respiratory care*, ed 9, St Louis, 2009, Mosby.

RESPIRATORY MEDICATIONS

PRETEST QUESTIONS

Answer the pretest questions before studying the chapter. This will help you determine your strong and weak areas in the material covered.

1. With which of the following lung disorders would acetylcysteine (Mucomyst) be indicated?

   1. Emphysema
   2. Bronchiectasis
   3. Cystic fibrosis
   4. Pulmonary edema

   A. 1 and 2 only
   B. 2 and 3 only
   C. 3 and 4 only
   D. 1, 2, and 3 only

2. A patient with glottic edema after extubation is in mild respiratory distress. Which of the following medications would be of benefit in this situation?

   A. Cromolyn sodium
   B. Succinylcholine (Anectine)
   C. Racemic epinephrine
   D. Pentamidine

3. You are having difficulty intubating a combative patient in the emergency department. The respiratory therapist should recommend the delivery of which drug to facilitate intubation?

   A. Succinylcholine (Anectine)
   B. Cromolyn sodium
   C. Atropine sulfate
   D. Epinephrine

4. Which of the following airway disorders may be successfully treated with dexamethasone (Decadron)?

   1. Asthma
   2. Glottic edema
   3. Pulmonary edema

A. 1 only
B. 2 only
C. 1 and 2 only
D. 2 and 3 only

See answers and rationales at the back of the text.

REVIEW

I. **CLASSIFICATION OF RESPIRATORY MEDICATIONS**
   CRT Exam Content Matrix: IIIC3,IIID5a, IIIF2h4, IIIG2b, IIIG4a,b,c,e-k
   RRTExamContentMatrix:IIIC3,IIID5a,IIIG2b,IIIG4b-h
   A. **Diluents**
      1. **Normal saline solution (0.9% NaCl)**
         a. Used to dilute bronchodilating agents
         b. Used to dilute secretions for improved expectoration. Often instilled through ET tubes and tracheostomy tubes, 3 to 5 mL at a time.
      2. **Hypotonic saline solution (0.4% NaCl)**
         a. Used in ultrasonic nebulizers because smaller particles are produced as result of lower concentration.
         b. More stable than sterile water
      3. **Hypertonic saline solution (1.8% NaCl)**
         a. Larger aerosol particles are produced because of the higher concentration of the solution.
         b. Used to stimulate coughing and induce sputum because it is irritating to the airway.
      4. **Sterile distilled water**
         a. Used to dilute other medications
         b. Used to hydrate secretions, thereby decreasing the viscosity for easier expectoration
         c. Used to humidify dry gases
   B. **Mucolytics:** Drugs that break the sputum down chemically for more effective expectoration.
      1. **Acetylcysteine** (Mucomyst)
         a. Available in 10% or 20% solutions
         b. It breaks the **disulfide** bonds in the sputum, thus decreasing the sputum's viscosity.
         c. Often used with bronchodilating agents because a common side effect of acetylcysteine is **bronchospasm.**

179

d. Should be used in treating patients with **thick secretions that are difficult to mobilize**

e. Often used in treating patients with cystic fibrosis or bronchiectasis

f. May be nebulized (1 to 3 mL, three to four times daily) or instilled directly into the trachea

g. If bronchospasm occurs, stop the treatment immediately and administer a bronchodilating agent.

h. Is irritating to mucosal tissues. The patient should rinse mouth after treatment.

2. **Dornase alfa (Pulmozyme, RhDNase)**

a. Used most commonly in patients with cystic fibrosis or other lung conditions in which thick, tenacious sputum is present

b. Must be kept refrigerated and protected from light

c. Do not nebulize in combination with other drugs. Administering a bronchodilator before dornase alfa may help increase the deposition of the drug.

3. **Sodium bicarbonate (2% NaHCO₃)**

a. Increases the pH of the sputum, thereby decreasing its viscosity

b. May be used to improve the mucolytic actions of acetylcysteine

c. Dosage: 2 to 5 mL via aerosol or 2 to 10 mL instilled directly into the trachea every 4 to 8 h

C. **Sympathomimetic Bronchodilators**

 Exam Note

These medications stimulate one or more of the following adrenergic receptors.

Receptor	Location	Response
Alpha	Mucosal blood vessels, bronchial smooth muscle	Vasoconstriction, bronchoconstriction
Beta₁	Heart muscle	Increased heart rate and cardiac output, arrhythmias
Beta₂	Bronchial smooth muscle, peripheral mucosal blood vessels, CNS, and peripheral limb muscles	Bronchodilation, vasodilation, nervousness (CNS), tingling in fingers

---

 Exam Note

The ideal bronchodilator is one that is a pure adrenergic beta₂ receptor stimulator.

---

1. **Epinephrine hydrochloride (Adrenalin Chloride, Sus-Phrine)**

a. Stimulates all three adrenergic receptors

b. Duration of action is 30 min to 2 h

c. Used to stimulate the heart; not commonly used as a bronchodilator

d. Adverse effects
   (1) Increased heart rate
   (2) Hypertension
   (3) Anxiety

e. Dosage: aerosol, 0.1 to 0.5 mL (1 : 100 solution) in 3 to 5 mL of diluent

2. **Racemic epinephrine (microNefrin, Vaponefrin)**

a. Stimulates all three receptors but most strongly the beta₁ receptor

b. Duration of action is 30 min to 2 h

c. Used to decrease mucosal edema and inflammation after extubation or in pediatric patients with croup

d. Has milder effects than epinephrine (half-strength)

e. Dosage: aerosol, 0.2 to 0.5 mL in 3 to 5 mL of diluent every 3 to 4 h

3. **Metaproterenol (Alupent, Metaprel)**

a. Very minor beta₁ and mild beta₂ receptor stimulator

b. Duration of action is 4 to 6 h

c. Used to decrease airway resistance

d. Adverse effects
   (1) Mild cardiac effects
   (2) Mild CNS effects

e. Dosage: 0.1 to 0.3 mL in 3 to 5 mL of diluent every 4 h

4. **Terbutaline sulfate (Brethine, Bricanyl)**

a. **Very minor beta₁ and moderate beta₂ receptor stimulator**

b. Duration of action is 3 to 7 h

c. Used to decrease airway resistance

d. Adverse effects
   (1) Mild cardiac effects
   (2) Mild CNS effects

e. Dosage: 200 mg/puff via MDI every 4 to 6 h

5. **Albuterol (Proventil, Ventolin)**

a. **Mild beta₁ and strong beta₂ receptor stimulator**

b. Duration of action is 4 to 6 h

c. Used to decrease airway resistance

d. Adverse effects
   (1) Mild cardiac effects
   (2) Mild CNS effects
   (3) Nausea
   (4) Tremors

e. Dosage: 2.5 to 5 mg, every 4 to 6 h

6. **Levalbuterol (Xopenex)**

a. Selective beta₂ receptor stimulator

b. Chemically similar to albuterol. The (R)-enantiomer of albuterol, which has the most bronchodilating effects, was isolated and purified for use and called levalbuterol.

c. Lower dosage required than for albuterol: 0.63 mg to 1.25 mg three times per day

d. Action of up to 8 h

e. First line drug for patients with COPD or asthma

f. Mild cardiac side effects, nervousness, and tremors but less than with albuterol

7. **Salmeterol (Serevent)**

a. It is a long-acting beta agonist with stronger $beta_2$ than $beta_1$ effects and is available as a DPI preparation used twice daily.

b. Duration of action: up to 12 h (1 h onset of action)

c. Used to decrease airway resistance

d. Adverse effects

(1) Tachycardia

(2) Hypertension

(3) Nausea

(4) Tremors

8. **Formoterol (Foradil)**

a. It is a long-acting beta agonist with stronger $beta_2$ than $beta_1$ effects and is available as a DPI preparation used twice a day.

b. Indications and adverse effects are the same as for salmeterol.

c. Duration of action is 12 h with a peak effect at 30 to 60 min compared with 3 to 5 h for salmeterol.

9. **Arformoterol (Brovana)**

a. It is a long-acting beta agonist with stronger $beta_2$ than $beta_1$ effects and is available as a liquid aerosolized preparation used twice a day with a small volume nebulizer.

b. The indications, side effects, and onset and duration of action are similar to formoterol.

D. **Parasympatholytic Bronchodilators**

1. **Atropine sulfate**

a. An anticholinergic drug; it blocks the cholinergic constricting influences on the airway and potentiates the adrenergic influences ($beta_2$ stimulation), resulting in bronchodilation.

b. Also inhibits secretion production and increases secretion viscosity.

☑ **Exam Note**

There is more potential for mucus plugging in patients with thick secretions who are given intravenous atropine. Given as an aerosol, atropine has little effect on lung secretions but may dry out the oral mucosa.

---

c. Used to decrease airway resistance, congestion, and cardiac arrhythmias

---

☝ Ipratropium bromide is faster acting, longer lasting, and exhibits fewer side effects than atropine.

---

d. Adverse effects

(1) Increased secretion viscosity

(2) Dry mouth

(3) CNS stimulation

e. Dosage: 1 mg in 3 to 5 mL of diluent, every 4 to 6 h

2. **Ipratropium bromide (Atrovent)**

a. An anticholinergic bronchodilator that acts topically in the lung instead of systemically

b. Peak effect of the drug is 1 to 2 h (compared with 15 min to 1 h with beta agonists with a duration of action of 3 to 4 h).

c. Used to decrease airway resistance, especially in patients with asthma, bronchitis, and emphysema. Some studies have shown ipratropium to be a more potent bronchodilator than beta-adrenergic agents for the treatment of emphysema and bronchitis.

d. Adverse effects

(1) Palpitations

(2) Nervousness

(3) Dizziness

(4) Nausea

(5) Tremors

e. Dosage: 0.5 mg in nebulized solution or two inhalations (36 µg) from a metered-dose inhaler four times daily. Current literature shows that up to 10 puffs four times a day is safe.

3. Tiotropium bromide (Spiriva)

a. An anticholinergic bronchodilator that acts topically in the lung instead of systemically

b. Onset is 30 min with a peak effect at 3 h. The duration of action is 24 h.

c. Same indications as for ipratropium bromide.

d. Adverse effects are similar to those for ipratropium bromide.

e. Dosage: DPI—one capsule, one inhalation daily (18 µg/inhalation)

E. **Phosphodiesterase Inhibitors:** These drugs are called xanthines, and they inhibit the cellular production of phosphodiesterase, an enzyme that readily breaks down cyclic adenosine monophosphate (AMP), another cellular enzyme, which, when produced, results in bronchodilation. It is by the increased production of cyclic AMP that sympathomimetic bronchodilators work.

1. **Theophylline (aminophylline)**

a. Stimulates respiratory rate and depth of breathing and produces pulmonary vasodilation and bronchodilation

b. Used to decrease airway resistance, especially in patients with asthma

c. Duration of action is 4 to 6 h

d. Adverse effects
   (1) Cardiac effects
   (2) CNS effects
   (3) Nausea and vomiting
   (4) Diuresis

e. Dosage: IV loading dose, 6 mg/kg of body weight; maintenance dose, 0.5 mg/kg/h (average dose is 250 mg every 6 h)

f. Theophylline produces effects that provide great benefits for patients with COPD.
   (1) Increased right ventricular output (improves cor pulmonale)
   (2) Improves diaphragmatic function
   (3) Produces pulmonary vasodilation, reducing pulmonary hypertension that results from chronic hypoxemia
   (4) Stimulates breathing by altering the hypoxic response curve when PaO_2 is elevated above 60 mm Hg

 Exam Note

A therapeutic serum level is 10 to 20 mg/L.

F. **Miscellaneous Respiratory Drugs**
   1. **Cromolyn sodium (Intal)**
      a. Stabilizes the mast cell, making it less sensitive to specific antigens and inhibiting the release of histamine
      b. Duration of action is 2 to 6 h
      c. Used as **preventive therapy** for asthma (**not effective during an asthma attack**)
      d. Adverse effects
         (1) Bronchospasm (when delivered in powder form)
         (2) Cough (powder form)
         (3) Local irritation (powder form)

 Exam Note

Cromolyn sodium is most commonly administered in aerosolized form, which is tolerated much better than in the powdered form. The powdered form is delivered through a device called a *Spinhaler*. The capsule is punctured and placed in the device, and the patient inhales deeply, which delivers the powder into the airway. Bronchospasm is a common complication when cromolyn sodium is delivered in this form.

e. Dosage: one 20-mg capsule four times daily (powder form); nebulized form, 20 mg four times daily

 Exam Note

Another mast cell stabilizer similar to cromolyn, but 4 to 10 times stronger, is nedocromil sodium (Tilade), which is available in MDI aerosol only.

2. **Leukotriene modifiers**
   a. During an asthma attack, mast cells in the airway release leukotrienes, which results in an inflammatory response. This response includes bronchoconstriction, mucus production, and vascular permeability. These drugs inhibit the response of the leukotrienes, preventing the inflammatory response from occurring.
   b. These drugs are used to prevent asthma attacks and are for long-term treatment of asthma.
   c. Common drugs of this type are zafirlukast (Accolate), montelukast (Singulair), and zileuton (Zyflo). Zafirlukast and montelukast are referred to as leukotriene receptor antagonists because they block the receptor sites of leukotrienes. Zileuton is referred to as a leukotriene inhibitor because it inhibits the release of leukotrienes.
   d. These drugs are administered as an oral tablet. Zafirlukast is administered twice daily, montelukast once daily, and zileuton four times a day.

3. **Ethanol (ethyl alcohol)**
   a. An antifoaming agent (surfactant) used to decrease the surface tension of frothy, bubbly secretions that are observed with **pulmonary edema**
   b. **Used in the treatment of pulmonary edema** to disperse the edematous bubbles, making the airway more patent. (Not commonly administered clinically but sometimes appears on the NBRC exams.)
   c. Adverse effects
      (1) Mucosal irritation
      (2) Dry mouth
   d. Dosage: 3 to 15 mL of a 40% to 50% solution

G. **Neuromuscular Blocking Agents**
   1. **Succinylcholine (Anectine)**
      a. A depolarizing agent that competes with acetylcholine for cholinergic receptors of the motor end plate of a muscle. If these receptors remain occupied by the depolarizing agent, further stimulation cannot occur and paralysis persists.
      b. Onset of action is 1 min, but the duration of action is only 5 min.
      c. Used as a short-term paralyzing agent to facilitate ET intubation

d. Adverse effects
  (1) Decreased heart rate
  (2) Decreased blood pressure

 Atropine may be administered to counteract these effects.

2. **Tubocurarine chloride**
  a. A nondepolarizing agent (related to curare) that blocks the transmission of acetylcholine at the postjunctional membrane.
  b. Onset of action is 3 to 5 min with a duration of action of 40 to 90 min
  c. Used to paralyze patients who are "fighting" mechanical ventilation
  d. Adverse effects
    (1) Bronchospasm (caused by histamine release)
    (2) Decreased blood pressure
3. **Pancuronium bromide (Pavulon)**
  a. A nondepolarizing agent that is five times stronger than curare and much more commonly used
  b. Onset of action is 4 to 6 min with a duration of 35 to 45 min
  c. Used to paralyze patients who are "fighting" mechanical ventilation
  d. Adverse effects:
    (1) Increased heart rate (mild)
    (2) Increased blood pressure (mild)

 Pancuronium bromide does not cause the release of histamine as curare does; therefore, bronchospasm is not a complication.

Exam Note

The paralyzing effects of the nondepolarizing agents (curare and pancuronium) may be reversed with the administration of edrophonium, neostigmine (Tensilon, Prostigmin).

4. **Vecuronium (Norcuron)**
  a. A nondepolarizing agent similar to pancuronium
  b. The indications, onset of action, and side effects are similar to pancuronium, although vecuronium has a shorter duration time of 60 to 90 min.
5. **Rocuronium (Zemuron)**
  a. A nondepolarizing agent
  b. The indications are the same as the other nondepolarizing drugs, but rocuronium has a

shorter time of onset of only 1 to 2 min. The duration of action is 30 to 60 min.
H. **Antibiotics (Aerosolized)**

Exam Note

A variety of organisms are found in patients with pneumonias, bronchiectasis, cystic fibrosis, and sinusitis; the following medications can be very beneficial in combating these invading organisms.

1. **Gentamicin**
  a. Commonly used in patients with cystic fibrosis
  b. Effective against *Pseudomonas aeruginosa*
  c. May be combined with carbenicillin
  d. May be instilled directly down the ET tube
2. **Amoxicillin**
  a. Used in patients with bronchiectasis
  b. Reduces the purulence of the sputum
3. **Tobramycin (TOBI)**
  a. Commonly used in cystic fibrosis patients
  b. Effective against *Pseudomonas aeruginosa*
  c. Inhaled side effects include alteration of the voice and tinnitus (ringing in the ears)
4. **Amphotericin B**
  a. Used for the treatment of fungal infections
  b. Improvement seen in treatment of pulmonary aspergillosis and the fungus *Candida albicans*
5. **Pentamidine**
  a. An antiprotozoan agent
  b. Used in the treatment of *Pneumocystis carinii* pneumonia (commonly seen in AIDS patients)
  c. Airway side effects of aerosolized pentamidine
    (1) Bronchospasm
    (2) Wheezing
    (3) Bronchial irritation
    (4) Shortness of breath
    (5) Cough

Exam Note

These local airway effects may be prevented or reduced by administering a bronchodilating agent before the delivery of the pentamidine.

  d. The nebulizer used to deliver pentamidine should incorporate a one-way valve that directs the patient's exhaled air through a scavenging filter to prevent contaminating the personnel and surrounding air with this agent.

6. **Ribavirin (Virazole)**
   a. An antiviral agent
   b. Used specifically to treat RSV in neonatal and pediatric patients (declining use in the clinical setting)
   c. Delivered through a SPAG nebulizer (no longer covered on the NBRC exams)
   d. The medication is delivered continuously for 12 to 18 h per day for 3 days to 1 wk, generally through an oxygen hood, oxygen tent, or face tent.
   e. Hazards of ribavirin
      (1) Worsening of respiratory status
      (2) Bacterial pneumonia (from contamination)
      (3) Occlusion of ET tube or ventilator tubing by the hygroscopic particles. Particle filters may decrease the potential of this hazard.

I. **Corticosteroids (Aerosolized):** These antiinflammatory agents are used in respiratory care to prevent or reduce airway inflammation in asthma and upper airway swelling that accompanies glottic edema. Administering these agents via aerosol (usually MDI) reduces systemic side effects, such as cushingoid symptoms (edema, moon face) and adrenal suppression.

Exam Note

The primary indication for inhaled steroids is for antiinflammatory maintenance therapy of mild-to-moderate persistent asthma.

1. Commonly used inhaled steroids
   a. Dexamethasone (Decadron)
   b. Beclomethasone (Beclovent, Vanceril)
   c. Budesonide (Pulmicort)
   d. Flunisolide (AeroBid)
   e. Triamcinolone acetonide (Azmacort)
   f. Fluticasone propionate (Flovent)
2. Side effects (inhaled steroids)
   a. Oropharyngeal fungal infections (candidiasis)
   b. Hoarseness
   c. Cough
   d. Bronchoconstriction

Exam Note

Patients taking MDI-administered corticosteroid therapy must be well educated on the proper use of the MDI and possible side effects of the drugs, such as oral candidiasis (thrush mouth), if overused.

J. **Combination Drugs:** These drugs provide the combined effects of bronchodilation and antiinflammatory responses.
   1. Fluticasone propionate/salmeterol (Advair)
   2. Budesonide/formoterol fumarate (Symbicort)

K. **Analgesics**
   1. **Narcotic analgesics**
      a. This group of drugs reduces pain without the loss of consciousness.
      b. In large doses, these drugs can depress the CNS, producing sleep or sedation.
      c. Morphine, codeine, and meperidine (Demerol) are examples of narcotic analgesics; morphine is the most potent. **Morphine and meperidine are strong respiratory suppressants**. Codeine has a relatively low respiratory suppressant effect.
   2. **Nonnarcotic analgesics**
      a. These drugs are not related chemically to the narcotic analgesics and relieve mild to moderate pain without the loss of consciousness.
      b. Some of these drugs also have antipyretic (fever reducer) and antiinflammatory effects.
      c. The most commonly used nonnarcotic analgesics used are the salicylates, which include aspirin. Aspirin is classified as a nonsteroidal antiinflammatory drug (NSAID). Because it also reduces fever, it may help reduce respiratory distress in critically ill patients with a limited pulmonary reserve.
      d. Aspirin also has anticoagulation properties and is used therapeutically in thromboembolitic diseases.
      e. Other NSAIDs include ibuprofen, which is the most commonly prescribed NSAID for musculoskeletal conditions, because of fewer GI tract side effects, and indomethacin, which is used most commonly to treat pericardial and pleural inflammation. Indomethacin is also used in neonates to help close a patent ductus arteriosus (PDA).
      f. Of the NSAIDs, aspirin seems to have the greatest potential for causing bronchospasm.
      g. Acetaminophen (Tylenol) is a nonsalicylate, nonnarcotic analgesic.

L. **Sedatives**
   1. The most commonly used sedative drugs are those classified as benzodiazepines. These drugs have sedative and antianxiety effects. They have replaced barbiturates because they produce fewer side effects and have fewer drug interactions and less potential for addiction.
   2. These drugs are most commonly used as antianxiety agents and generally do not cause significant respiratory or cardiovascular depression.
   3. One of the most common sedatives used is **midazolam (Versed),** which is often used to provide short-term conscious sedation and relaxation during invasive procedures such as a bronchoscopy. It also has amnesia effects.

4. Another common antianxiety drug that has a longer duration of action than midazolam is diazepam (Valium).

5. Other benzodiazepines include
   a. Alprazolam (Xanax)
   b. Lorazepam (Ativan)
   c. Propofol (Diprivan)

M. **Diuretics**

1. These drugs stimulate urine production and are frequently used in the ICU to promote loss of excess water and salt. Fluid overload can be the result of CHF or large amounts of fluid given IV during resuscitation efforts.

2. The most common type of diuretic is what is classified as a loop diuretic. These drugs block the reabsorption of sodium in the ascending loop of Henle. This results in the excretion of sodium and water. **The most commonly used loop diuretic is furosemide (Lasix).**

3. This type of diuretic is potent and is used over short periods of time. They effectively treat hypertension, pulmonary edema, and peripheral edema.

4. Diuretic use may lead to metabolic alkalosis as evidenced by the elevated bicarbonate level and decreased chloride level. Hypokalemia (decreased potassium) and hypomagnesemia (low magnesium) may also occur, especially with the loop diuretics.

5. Another type of diuretic is the osmotic diuretic, for example, **mannitol (Osmitrol),** which is used to treat oliguria (little urine formation) or anuria (no urine formation) as well as cerebral edema.

II. **DRY POWDER INHALERS**

CRT Exam Content Matrix: IIA22, IIID5b
RRT Exam Content Matrix: IIID5b

A. Two types of DPIs
   1. Single-dose devices: Spinhaler, Rotahaler
   2. Multidose device: used with drugs such as salmeterol and fluticasone

B. DPIs are breath activated and create aerosol by drawing air through a dose of powdered medication. Because DPIs are breath activated, they reduce the problem of the patient having to coordinate inspiration with actuation of the device.

C. High inspiratory flows are required to generate the aerosol; therefore, DPIs are not indicated for acute bronchospasm or in weak, elderly patients or patients younger than 6 years.

D. The powdered medication is in a capsule that is placed in the inhaler. By adjusting the inhaler, the patient punctures the capsule, which allows the powder to be administered as the patient inhales.

III. **VACCINES**

CRT Exam Content Matrix: IIIG4k
RRT Exam Content Matrix: IIIG4h

A. **Influenza vaccine** is recommended annually for the following who are either at high risk of contracting influenza or in close contact with people at higher risk
   1. People older than 50 years
   2. Health care personnel
   3. Nursing home residents
   4. People with chronic lung disease (including asthma) or cardiovascular or renal disorders
   5. Patients with diabetes
   6. People at risk of aspiration (spinal cord injuries, neuromuscular disorders, seizure disorders)
   7. Caregivers of children younger than 5 years and adults older than 50 years of age
   8. Patients with immunocompromised conditions (human immunodeficiency virus [HIV], cancer)
   9. All children 5 to 18 years old
   10. Children 6 months to 4 years of age if at high risk of influenza for reasons given above
   11. Pregnant women during the influenza season

B. Pneumococcal Vaccine (Pneumovax)
   1. This vaccine protects those receiving it from pneumonia caused by *Streptococcus pneumoniae*.
   2. This bacteria is the leading cause of illness in young children and can cause illness and even death among the elderly and people who have underlying medical conditions.
   3. Individuals who are at increased risk of pneumococcal infection and who should be vaccinated include
      a. Children younger than 2 years
      b. Adults 65 years of age or older
      c. People with underlying medical conditions
      d. Immunocompromised people (with HIV, leukemia, lymphoma)
      e. People with chronic cardiac and/or pulmonary disorders
      f. Patients with diabetes
      g. People with sickle cell disease
      h. People who have had a splenectomy

IV. **DRUG CALCULATIONS**

 Exam Note

Drug calculations are not specifically mentioned on either matrix but are occasionally asked about on both exams.

A. **Percentage Strength**
   1. Percentage strength is the number of parts of the solute (ingredient) per 100 parts of solution.
   2. To convert from ratio strength to percentage strength, use the following instructions

a. What is the percentage strength of a 1:2000 solution?

(1) Change 1:2000 to a fraction: 1/2000

(2) Change this to a percentage by dividing 2000 into 1 and multiply by 100.

$$\frac{1}{2000} \times 100 = 0.05\%$$

b. **What is the percentage strength of a 1:500 solution?**

(1) Change 1:500 to a fraction: 1/500

(2) Change this to a percentage by dividing 500 into 1 and multiplying by 100.

$$\frac{1}{500} \times 100 = \mathbf{0.2\%}$$

3. To convert from percentage strength to ratio strength, use the following instructions

a. What is the ratio strength of a 10% solution?

(1) Change 10% to 10/100 or 10:100.

(2) 10:100 is the same as 1:10 (10 goes into 100 ten times).

(3) Therefore, a 10% solution has a 1:10 ratio strength.

B. **Dosage Calculations**

1. **1 mL of a 1% solution (1:100) = 10 mg of solute**

2. **How many milligrams of a 1:100 solution of isoproterenol make up a dose of 0.5 mL of the drug?**

a. A 1:100 solution is a 1% solution (1 divided by 100 × 100).

b. **1 mL of a 1% solution equals 10 mg. (This is a standard rule.)**

c. However, the question is how many milligrams of solution make up **0.5 mL of the drug?**

d. 1 mL of a 1% solution = 10 mg

e. 0.5 mL of a 1% solution = 5 mg (half as much)

3. **How many milligrams in 0.2 mL of a 5% solution of metaproterenol?**

a. Always go back to the **standard rule:** 1 mL of 1% solution = 10 mg

b. 1 mL of a 1% solution = 10 mg

c. 1 mL of a 5% solution = 50 mg (5 times as much)

d. 0.2 mL of 50 mg = 0.2 × 50 mg = 10 mg

POSTCHAPTER STUDY QUESTIONS

1. What is the primary indication for acetylcysteine?

2. What is racemic epinephrine most commonly used for?

3. List four examples of sympathomimetic bronchodilators.

4. List two examples of parasympatholytic bronchodilators.

5. Which neuromuscular blocking agent is used primarily for short-term paralysis during a difficult intubation?

6. How does cromolyn sodium help in the treatment of asthma?

7. List five antibiotics that are aerosolized and the conditions for which they are indicated.

8. List three corticosteroids that are commonly aerosolized.

9. List the side effects of corticosteroid therapy.

10. List three leukotriene modifiers.

11. Leukotriene modifiers are administered for what purpose?

See answers at the back of the text.

BIBLIOGRAPHY

Bills G, Soderberg R, *Principles of pharmacology for respiratory care*, ed 2, Albany, NY, 1998, Delmar.

Oakes D, *Clinical practitioner's pocket guide to respiratory care*, ed 5, Rockville, MD, 1996, Health Educator.

Rau J, *Respiratory care pharmacology*, ed 7, St Louis, 2008, Mosby.

Wilkins RL, Stoller JK, Kacmarek R, *Egan's fundamentals of respiratory care*, ed 9, St Louis, 2009, Mosby.

RESPIRATORY HOME CARE

Answer the pretest questions before studying the chapter. This will help you determine your strong and weak areas in the material covered.

1. Which of the following O_2 systems would be indicated for a very active home care patient?

   A. O_2 concentrator
   B. Liquid O_2
   C. "H" cylinder
   D. "E" cylinder

2. Which of the following is the *LEAST* important area for the respiratory therapist to discuss with the home care patient?

   A. Pathology of the disease process
   B. Cleaning of equipment
   C. Side effects of prescribed therapy
   D. Importance of proper therapy techniques

3. Which of the following IPPB machines is most convenient for use in the home?

   A. Bird Mark 7
   B. Bird Mark 8
   C. Bennett PR-2
   D. Bennett AP-5

4. Diaphragmatic breathing exercises should result in which of the following?

   1. Increased VT
   2. Less dependence on the diaphragm during quiet breathing
   3. Increased FRC
   4. Decreased respiratory rate

   A. 1 and 2 only
   B. 1 and 4 only
   C. 2, 3, and 4 only
   D. 1, 2, and 4 only

See answers and rationales at the back of the text.

I. **HOME REHABILITATION**
   CRT Exam Content Matrix: IIIH1-8
   RRT Exam Content Matrix: IIIH1-8
   A. Goals of Rehabilitation
      1. Help the patient become independent.
      2. Help the patient improve the ability to cope with the disease.
      3. Help the patient gain an understanding of the disease and the limitations that result from it.
      4. Help the patient to set realistic goals for life and then help him or her attain those goals.
   B. **Conditions Requiring Pulmonary Rehabilitation**
      1. Chronic lung diseases
         a. Emphysema
         b. Asthma
         c. Chronic bronchitis
         d. Cystic fibrosis
         e. Bronchiectasis
         f. Pulmonary fibrosis
      2. Neuromuscular diseases
         a. Myasthenia gravis
         b. Guillain-Barré syndrome
         c. Poliomyelitis
         d. Muscular dystrophy
      3. Central respiratory center disorders
         a. CNS injury
         b. Hypoventilation syndrome (nonobese or pickwickian syndrome, sleep apnea)
         c. Ondine curse (primary alveolar hypoventilation)

II. **CARE OF THE REHABILITATION PATIENT**
   CRT Exam Content Matrix: IIA9b-c, IIB1, IIIF2d3, IIIK1,2,5,7
   RRT Exam Content Matrix: IIA4a-c, IIIK2,5,7
   A. **Patient Care Plan**
      1. Humidity therapy
      2. Aerosol therapy
      3. O_2 therapy: **the use of reservoir cannulas and pulse dose O_2 delivery systems aid in conserving O_2.**
      4. Bronchodilator therapy
      5. ABG sampling and analysis or pulse oximeter (SpO_2) monitoring
      6. Oropharyngeal and tracheal suctioning

7. Determination of breath sounds by chest auscultation
8. Chest physical therapy
9. Breathing exercises
10. Sputum induction
11. IPPB therapy: **The Bennett AP-5 unit is commonly used because it operates on electricity rather than compressed gas.**

B. **Periodic Evaluations**
1. Pulmonary function testing
2. Sputum collection and analysis
3. ABG collection and analysis
4. Exercise tolerance testing (6 to 12 min walk)
5. Chest x-ray films

C. **Breathing Exercises**
1. **Pursed-lip breathing**
   a. Teach to patients who experience premature airway closure.
   b. Instruct the patient to inhale through the nose and exhale through pursed lips.
   c. Aids in the patient gaining control of dyspnea.
   d. Provides improved ventilation before a cough effort.
   e. Teaches the patient how to better control the rate and depth of breathing.
   f. Prevents premature airway collapse by generating a back pressure into the airways.
   g. Has psychological benefits.
2. **Diaphragmatic breathing**
   a. Teaches the COPD patient to use the diaphragm during breathing rather than accessory muscles.
   b. The patient or respiratory therapist places a hand over the abdomen as the patient, while lying on his or her back, concentrates on moving the hand upward on inspiration. (A book or weight may be used rather than a hand.)
   c. Increasing the use of the diaphragm results in a decreased respiratory rate, increased tidal volume, decreased FRC, and increased alveolar ventilation.
3. **Segmental breathing**
   a. This is similar to diaphragmatic breathing exercises, except a hand is placed over a specific lung area in which there is atelectasis, secretions, or decreased airflow.

b. The patient should concentrate on moving the hand outward on inspiration.

D. **Cough Instruction**
1. **A VC of less than 10 to 15 mL/kg of ideal body weight indicates inadequate volume for an effective cough.**
2. **Proper cough instruction:** tell the patient to
   a. Inhale slowly and deeply through the nose and hold breath for 3 to 5 s (in a sitting position).
   b. Clasp arms across his or her abdomen and give three sharp coughs without taking a breath while pressing arms into the abdomen.
   c. Use a pillow to "splint" incision sites (e.g., thorax, abdomen)

E. **Home O_2 Administration**
1. **O_2 cylinders**
   a. Probably the least expensive O_2 setup in the home at the present time depending on usage.
   b. Disadvantages of O_2 cylinders in the home
      (1) Heavy and difficult to move
      (2) High pressure hazard
      (3) Difficult for older or debilitated patients to change cylinder or attach a regulator
      (4) Small cylinders are difficult to walk with
      (5) The respiratory therapist should discuss the safety measures and handling of the cylinders with the patient and family members. After instruction, the RT should document the caregivers' ability to operate and handle the equipment safely
      (6) Cylinders are a good supply system for patients using a small volume of oxygen
2. **Liquid O_2 system**
   a. More O_2 in liquid form may be stored than in gaseous form (860 times more).
   b. Liquid is safer than gas stored in high-pressure cylinders.
   c. Portable liquid walkers are more convenient and easier for the patient to handle.
   d. **Calculating the duration of flow for a liquid O_2 system.** (See Chapter 1 on oxygen and medical gas therapy.)
   e. A good supply system for the patients who use high volumes of oxygen.

3. O₂ concentrator

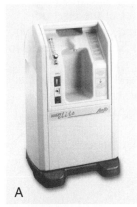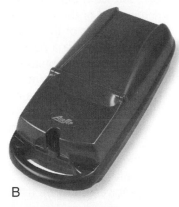

FIGURE 15-1 O₂ concentrator. *A.,* Stationary oxygen concentrator for home care patients *B.,* Light weight portable oxygen concentrator Courtney Airsep, Buffalo, NY.

a. Uses O_2 in the surrounding room air by drawing it into the concentrator and filtering out most of the gases except O_2

b. Two types of concentrators
   (1) Membrane: produces only about 40% O_2 from the unit
   (2) Molecular sieve: much more commonly used and produces 90% to 95% O_2 from the unit. The nitrogen, carbon dioxide, and water vapor is removed as the air passes through sieves containing sodium-aluminum silicate pellets.

c. The concentrator should be placed in the home where air can freely be drawn into it.

d. The concentrator should not be placed near heat vents.

e. The respiratory therapist, on a routine visit, should analyze the delivered O_2 from the concentrator and check all alarms, the flow rate, filters, and batteries. Air inlet filters should be cleaned weekly by the patient or caregiver. If the oxygen concentrator analyzes less than the manufacturer's specifications, the pellets need to be replaced.

f. A backup O_2 system with 1 to 3 days' supply should be available in case of a power outage because concentrators are powered by electricity. Cylinders should be used for the back-up system, not liquid, which evaporates over time.

g. The higher the flow rate used on a concentrator, the less the delivered O_2 percentage. With most concentrators, 1 to 2 L/min will provide 92% to 95% oxygen. Flows of 3 to 5 L/min provide approximately 85% to 92%.

h. **Portable concentrators** are now available that allow for more patient activity. Most models weigh less than 10 lbs and have a battery life of 2 to 5 h. The flow range is generally 1 to 5 L/min and provides oxygen percentages of up to 93%. The flow can be set on a continuous or pulse setting (inspiration only). Some concentrators have been approved for air transportation.

> ⚠ The patient and family should be instructed in all aspects of the proper care and safety of equipment used in the home.

F. **Cleaning Equipment in the Home**
1. All equipment designated "single use only" should be considered disposable and discarded after one use.
2. Nondisposable equipment, such as nebulizers and humidifiers, may be cleaned as follows
   a. Clean first with mild soap.
   b. Rinse.
   c. Disinfect with a solution recommended by the manufacturer.
   d. Rinse again.
   e. Dry the equipment.
   f. Repeat the process every 1 to 3 days.

☑ **Exam Note**

Nebulizing 10 mL of 0.25% acetic acid (vinegar) through nebulizers and room humidifiers is an appropriate cleaning technique. Allowing the equipment to soak in a vinegar solution overnight is also an acceptable method of disinfecting equipment.

---

3. Cannulas should be cleaned with mild soap that does not leave a soap film and then rinsed before a disinfectant is used. They should be replaced every 2 to 4 wk.

4. Humidifiers and nebulizers should be filled with sterile water, and safety relief devices should be incorporated.

5. If heated moisture is delivered, a thermometer should be placed in the line, close to the patient, to monitor inspired gas temperature.

6. Medication nebulizers should be rinsed with water and dried after each treatment. They should be cleaned every day in a mild soap solution, rinsed, disinfected, rinsed again, dried on a paper towel, and placed in a plastic bag until used again.

7. IPPB circuits (nondisposable) may be cleaned in mild soap, rinsed, disinfected, rinsed again, and dried every 1 to 2 days.

8. IPPB machines may be wiped down with a liquid disinfectant every few days.

G. **Respiratory Therapist Responsibilities in Home Care of Pulmonary Patients**
   1. Help set up and maintain equipment.
   2. Instruct the patient and family on the use, care, and safety of all equipment used in the home setting.
   3. Instruct the patient and family in all therapy to be done in the home, including the indications, contraindications, side effects, and hazards of the specific therapy.
   4. Assist in the delivery of therapy to the patient.
   5. Perform simple spirometry tests.
   6. Assess the patient's present cardiopulmonary status and general well-being.
   7. Report to the physician to discuss the present therapy and possible changes needed in current therapy.

III. **HOME APNEA MONITORING**
   CRT Exam Content Matrix: IB9n, IB10n,
   RRT Exam Content Matrix: IB9o, IB10p, IIIK1
   A. Apnea monitoring is most commonly used for infants or pediatric patients who have conditions that cause apnea or bradycardia. Also, infants experiencing apnea from unknown causes and siblings of infants who have died of SIDS should be monitored for apnea.

B. Other patients who may require apnea monitoring are those with BPD, neuromuscular diseases, and tracheostomies and those receiving mechanical ventilation.

C. A soft foam belt with electrodes is fastened around the chest of the infant. The wires of the electrodes send signals of the heartbeat and breathing back to the monitor via a patient cable. These are referred to as impedance monitors.

D. Apnea monitors have audible and visual alarms that detect not only apnea and bradycardia but also malfunctions that occur with the patient cable, electrodes, wires, and battery.

E. Caregivers in the home must be trained thoroughly in the use of and troubleshooting for the monitor.

F. Caregivers must be trained in CPR.

POSTCHAPTER STUDY QUESTIONS

1. List four goals of rehabilitation.
2. List five periodic evaluations of the home care patient that should be conducted by the respiratory therapist.
3. How does pursed-lip breathing benefit patients with emphysema?
4. List two types of O_2 concentrators and the O_2 percentage available with each.
5. What type of evaluations should be made by the respiratory therapist regarding the O_2 concentrators during routine visits?
6. Calculate how long 3 lb of liquid oxygen running through a 2 L/min nasal cannula will last.

See answers at the back of the text.

BIBLIOGRAPHY

Hess D and others, *Respiratory care principles and practice*, ed 1, Philadelphia, 2002, Saunders.
Wilkins RL, Stoller JK, Kacmarek R, *Egan's fundamentals of respiratory care*, ed 9, St Louis, 2009, Mosby.

PULMONARY FUNCTION TESTING

Answer the pretest questions before studying the chapter. This will help you determine your strong and weak areas in the material covered.

1. What is the minimum percent increase in inspiratory flow following a before-and-after bronchodilator study that indicates significant improvement?

   A. 5%
   B. 10%
   C. 15%
   D. 25%

2. In which of the following lung conditions would the FRC be increased?

   1. **Emphysema**
   2. **Cystic fibrosis**
   3. **Pneumonia**

   A. 1 only
   B. 1 and 2 only
   C. 1 and 3 only
   D. 2 and 3 only

3. Which of the following pulmonary function tests would best determine the patient's ability to cough?

   A. VT
   B. Alveolar minute ventilation
   C. FRC
   D. MIP

4. To evaluate the distribution of ventilation to perfusion with a V/Q scan, instruct the patient to inhale which of the following substances?

   A. Helium
   B. CO
   C. Xenon
   D. Argon

5. Following are the results of a patient's spirometry test before and after bronchodilator therapy.

	Before	**After**
FEV_1	32% of predicted	53% of predicted
FVC	38% of predicted	66% of predicted
FEV_1/FVC	50%	64%

Which of the following is the correct interpretation of these results?

A. Mild restrictive disease with significant bronchodilator response
B. Severe obstructive disease with significant bronchodilator response
C. Severe restrictive disease with no significant bronchodilator response
D. Severe obstructive disease with no significant bronchodilator response

See answers and rationales at the back of the text.

I. **LUNG VOLUMES AND CAPACITIES**
   CRT Exam Content Matrix: IA4, IA7b-c, IB9d-e,m,s, IB10d-e,s, IC5, IIC4, IIIE7a-f
   RRT Exam Content Matrix: IA4, IA7b-c, IB9d-e,m,t, IB10d-e,u, IC6, IIC4, IIIE7a-f

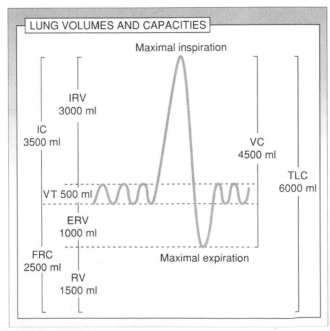

FIGURE 16-1

A. **Lung Volumes**
  1. **Tidal volume (VT)**
     a. The volume of air (usually in milliliters) that is inhaled or exhaled during a normal breath
     b. The exhaled VT is usually measured with a respirometer at the bedside or by spirometry.

> ☑ **Exam Note**
>
> When VT is measured at the bedside, it is most accurately achieved by the patient being instructed to breathe normally through a mouthpiece connected to a respirometer for 1 full min. The volume reading is then divided by the patient's respiratory rate over that 1 min to obtain the VT. Nose clips may be used to ensure mouth breathing only.

     c. VT is decreased or normal in restrictive disease and increased or normal in obstructive disease.
     d. A normal value is 500 mL (or 3 mL/lb of body weight)
  2. **Inspiratory reserve volume (IRV)**
     a. Is the maximum volume of air that can be inspired after a normal inspiration.
     b. Is normally not measured during simple spirometry, but if it is, it should be measured from a slow vital capacity.
     c. IRV could be normal in both obstructive and restrictive disease; therefore its measurement is not clinically significant.
     d. A normal value is 3000 mL.
  3. **Expiratory reserve volume (ERV)**
     a. Is the volume of air exhaled after a normal expiration.
     b. ERV is measured directly by spirometry from a slow VC (i.e., VC − inspiratory capacity).
     c. ERV may be normal or decreased in obstructive or restrictive disease.
     d. A normal value is 1000 mL and 20% to 25% of the VC.
  4. **Residual volume (RV)**
     a. Is the volume of air left in the lungs after a maximal expiration.
     b. It is derived after FRC is calculated, with the use of either the nitrogen washout test or helium dilution test (see FRC section in this chapter).
     c. Once FRC is calculated, subtract the ERV from FRC; this equals the residual volume (i.e., **RV = FRC − ERV**)
     d. RV is increased in obstructive disease and decreased in restrictive disease.
     e. A normal value is 1500 mL.
B. **Lung Capacities**
  1. **Functional residual capacity (FRC)**
     a. Is the amount of air left in the lungs after a normal expiration (i.e., ERV + RV).

  b. Is measured by the helium dilution or nitrogen washout test or by body plethysmography.
  c. **Measurement of FRC by helium dilution test**
     (1) Also called the closed-circuit method
     (2) A spirometer is normally filled with about 600 mL of gas with about 10% helium added to the volume. The volume of the gas and the concentration of helium is measured and recorded before the test.
     (3) The patient is instructed to breathe normally and, at the end of a normal exhalation, is connected to the system.
     (4) The patient rebreathes the gas in the spirometer while carbon dioxide is removed by a CO_2 absorbent.
     (5) Helium is then diluted until equilibrium is reached. This normally takes about 7 min, but in patients with severe lung disease, it may take as long as 30 min for equilibrium to occur. Equilibrium occurs as the helium analyzer falls to a stable level.
     (6) The final concentration of helium is then recorded.
  d. Calculations for FRC

$$\text{System volume} = \frac{\text{helium added (mL)}}{\% \text{ He (first reading)}}$$

$$\textbf{FRC} = \frac{(\%He_1 - \%He_2)}{He_2} \times \text{system vol} \times \begin{array}{c}\text{BTPS correction}\\\text{factor}\end{array}$$

     He_1 = helium concentration before patient is connected to the system

     He_2 = final helium concentration when equilibrium has occurred

     BTPS correction factor = constant to convert volume to body temperature and pressure saturated

> ☑ **Exam Note**
>
> A helium analyzer reads zero when calibrated to room air.

  e. **Measurement of FRC with the use of the nitrogen washout test**
     (1) Also called the open-circuit method
     (2) During this test, the patient breathes in 100% oxygen to wash out the nitrogen in the lungs. The nitrogen concentration in the lungs is approximately 79%.
     (3) The patient is instructed to breathe normally, and at the end of a normal exhalation, the patient is connected to the 100% oxygen breathing system.

(4) During the procedure, the exhaled volume is monitored and recorded and nitrogen percentages are measured.

(5) Complete nitrogen washout occurs in about 7 min.

f. FRC may now be calculated with the use of the following formula:

$$FRC = \frac{expired\ volume \times N_2}{N_1}$$

N_1 = nitrogen percentage in lungs at start of test

N_2 = nitrogen percentage in spirometer at end of test

g. **Measurement of FRC with the use of body plethysmography**

(1) The plethysmograph ("body box") is an airtight chamber in which the patient sits during the procedure.

(2) While being tested, the patient is instructed to seal his or her lips tightly around the mouthpiece and to breathe normally. (The patient may also be tested while being instructed to breathe in shallow, panting breaths.)

(3) As the patient breathes, a pressure transducer measures pressure at the airway as well as inside the chamber.

(4) An electrical shutter is used to periodically close the airway, causing the patient to breathe against a closed airway, at which time volume and pressure values are measured.

(5) The technique of plethysmography is based on Boyle's law, which states that the volume of gas is inversely proportional to the pressure to which it is subjected.

h. FRC can then be calculated with the use of the following formula

$$FRC = \frac{atmospheric\ pressure \times volume\ change}{pressure\ change}$$

i. Body plethysmography also measures thoracic gas volume (VTG), total lung capacity (TLC), and residual volume (RV).

Because body plethysmography actually measures the total amount of gas in the thorax, FRC measurements may be higher than those measured by the helium dilution or nitrogen washout method.

j. FRC is increased in obstructive disease and decreased in restrictive disease.

k. A normal value is 2500 mL.

2. **Inspiratory capacity (IC)**

a. Is the maximum amount of air that can be inspired after a normal expiration (i.e., VT+IRV).

b. Is measured by simple spirometry from a VC.

c. Usually is decreased or normal in obstructive or restrictive disease.

d. A normal value is 3500 mL (75% to 85% of the VC).

3. **Vital capacity (VC)**

a. Is the maximum amount of air that can be exhaled after a maximum inspiration (i.e., VT+IRV+ERV).

b. Is measured by simple spirometry or at the bedside with the use of a respirometer.

 Exam Note

At the bedside, use a mouthpiece connected to a respirometer. Instruct the patient to inhale as deeply as possible and then, slowly, completely exhale through the mouthpiece.

c. VC is decreased in restrictive disease and is normal or decreased in obstructive disease.

d. A normal value is 4800 mL.

 Exam Note

A decreased VC may be the result of pneumonia, atelectasis, pulmonary edema, pulmonary fibrosis, kyphoscoliosis or lung cancer.

4. **Forced vital capacity (FVC)**

a. Is the maximum amount of air that can be exhaled as **fast and forcefully** as possible after a maximum inspiration.

b. Is measured by simple spirometry.

c. Is used to measure FEVs and flows.

d. FVC is decreased in both obstructive and restrictive disease.

5. **Total lung capacity (TLC)**

a. Is the amount of air remaining in the lungs at the end of a maximal inspiration.

b. Is calculated by a combination of other measured volumes (i.e., FRC+IC or VC+RV).

c. TLC is decreased in restrictive disease and increased in obstructive disease.

d. A normal value is 6000 mL.

 Exam Note

TLC decreases as a result of atelectasis, pulmonary edema, and consolidation; TLC increases as a result of emphysema.

6. **RV/TLC (ratio)**
   a. Is the percentage of the TLC that remains in the lungs after a maximal expiration.
   b. Is measured by dividing the RV by TLC and multiplying by 100 to get a percentage.
   c. RV/TLC is normal in restrictive disease and increased in obstructive disease.
   d. A normal value is 20% to 35%.

II. **LUNG STUDIES**
   CRT Exam Content Matrix: IA4, IA7b-c, IB9d-e,m,s, IB10d-e,s, IC5, IIC4, IIIE7a-f
   RRT Exam Content Matrix: IA4, IA7b-c, IB9d-e,m,t, IB10d-e,u, IC6, IIC4, IIIE7a-f
   A. **Ventilation Studies**
      1. **VT** (discussed previously in the chapter)
      2. **Respiratory rate**
         a. Is the number of breaths in 1 min.
         b. Is measured by counting chest excursion for 1 min.
         c. Is increased in hypoxia and hypercarbia and is decreased with central respiratory center depression or depressing hypoxic drive in a COPD patient.
         d. A normal value is 10/min to 20/min.
      3. **Minute volume** (MV, $\dot{V}E$)
         a. Is the total volume of air (in liters) inhaled or exhaled in 1 min. It is calculated by multiplying the respiratory rate times the VT.
         b. Is measured by simple spirometry or at bedside with a respirometer.

 Exam Note

When measuring $\dot{V}E$ at the bedside, use a respirometer with a mouthpiece. Instruct the patient to breathe normally through the mouthpiece as you time the breathing for 1 min. The reading on the respirometer after 1 min is the $\dot{V}E$.

         c. Is increased by hypoxia, hypercarbia, acidosis, or decreased lung compliance and decreased by hypocarbia, alkalosis, and increased lung compliance.
         d. A normal value is 5 to 10 L/min.
   B. **Flow Studies**
      1. **Forced expiratory volume (FEV$_{0.5}$, FEV$_1$, FEV$_3$)**
         a. Is the volume of air that is exhaled over a specific time interval during the FVC maneuver.
         b. Is measured over 0.5, 1, or 3 s (shown as subscript to FEV). The FEV$_1$ is the most common measurement.

   c. The severity of airway obstruction may be determined because it is a measurement at specified time intervals. **FEV is usually decreased in both obstructive and restrictive disease.**

Exam Note

FEV may be decreased in restrictive disease because the FVC is below normal and the measurement of FEV is from the patient's *predicted* FVC, not his or her actual FVC. A better indicator of an obstructive or restrictive disorder is determined from the FEV/FVC ratio, which compares the FEV to the patient's actual FVC (discussed next).

   2. **FEV/FVC (ratio)**
      a. Is a ratio (percentage) of the relationship of FEV to FVC.
      b. Normal values are:
         • 50% to 60% of the FVC is exhaled in 0.5 s
         • 75% to 85% of the FVC is exhaled in 1 s
         • 94% of the FVC is exhaled in 2 s
         • 97% of the FVC is exhaled in 3 s
      c. Obstructive disease is indicated by below normal values of FEV/FVC. Patients with restrictive disease have normal or above normal values.
      d. Because the FEV$_1$ is most commonly measured, look for an **FEV$_1$/FVC of less than 75%** to indicate an obstructive disease.
   3. **FEF$_{200-1200}$**
      a. Is the average flow rate of the exhaled air after the first 200 mL and 1200 mL during an FVC maneuver.
      b. Is measured on the spirograph tracing between the 200-mL mark and the 1200-mL mark to determine the average flow rate from the FVC.
      c. Is decreased in obstructive disease.
      d. A normal value is 6 to 7 L/s (400 L/min).
   4. **FEF$_{25\%-75\%}$**
      a. Is the average flow rate during the middle portion of the FEV.
      b. The 25% and 75% points are marked on the spirographic curve from the FVC.
      c. Values are decreased in obstructive disease.
      d. A normal value is 4 to 5 L/s.
   5. **Peak flow**
      a. Is the maximum flow rate achieved during an FVC.
      b. Is measured from an FVC or by a peak flowmeter.

    c. Is decreased in obstructive diseases

    d. A normal value is 400 to 600 L/min (6.5 to 10 L/s).

6. **Maximum voluntary ventilation (MVV)**

    a. Is the maximum volume of air moved into and out of the lungs voluntarily in 12 to 15 s.

    b. This measurement tests for overall lung function, ventilatory reserve capacity, and air-trapping.

    c. Is decreased in obstructive disease and decreased or normal in restrictive disease.

    d. Normal value is 170 L/min.

7. **Flow volume loop (curve)**

    a. A flow volume loop is displayed on a graph and represents the flow generated during an FEV maneuver followed by a forced inspiratory volume maneuver; both are plotted against volume change.

    b. With the use of a flow volume loop, the following values may be measured

        (1) Peak inspiratory flow (PIF)

        (2) Peak expiratory flow (PEF)

        (3) FVC

        (4) $FEV_{0.5}$, FEV_1, FEV_3

        (5) $FEF_{25\%-75\%}$

    c. The three diagrams (Figure 16-2) show a comparison of flow volume loops representing normal, obstructive, and restrictive disorders.

        (1) The restriction pattern shows a decreased VC and normal expiratory flow rates.

        (2) The obstructive pattern shows a decreased peak expiratory flow rate and a normal exhaled volume.

8. **Diffusion capacity of the lung (DL)**

    a. Represents the gas exchange capabilities of the lungs.

    b. This measurement evaluates how well gas diffuses across the alveolar–capillary membrane into the pulmonary capillaries.

    c. The most common method for measuring DL is the single-breath method.

    d. The patient is connected to a system in which the inspired gas contains a mixture of 10% helium and 0.3% CO. CO is used because of its increased affinity for Hb, which keeps the partial pressure of CO in the capillaries low,

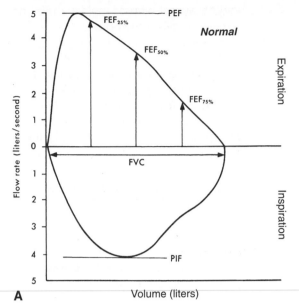

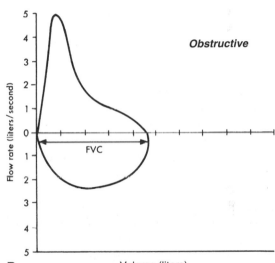

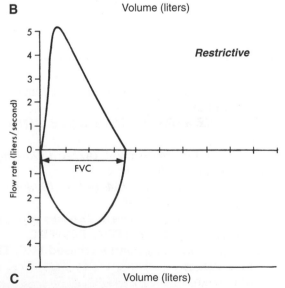

FIGURE 16-2 Comparison of flow volume loops. From Scanlan C, Spearman C, Sheldon R, *Egan's fundamentals of respiratory care*, ed 5, St Louis, 1990, Mosby, and Wilkins RL, Stoller JK, Kacmarek R, *Egan's fundamentals of respiratory care*, ed 9, St Louis, 2009, Mosby.

and because it diffuses rapidly across the alveolar–capillary membrane.

e. The patient is instructed to exhale completely to the RV level, place the mouthpiece in the mouth, inhale as deeply as possible, hold the breath for 10 s, and then exhale.

f. The DLCO (carbon monoxide diffusion capacity), or the measurement of the amount of CO diffusing from the alveoli to the pulmonary blood flow, is calculated with the use of the following formula

$$DLCO = \frac{mL \text{ of CO diffused per min}}{A - a \text{ gradient of CO (mm Hg)}}$$

g. **Normal diffusion capacity is approximately 25 to 30 mL/min/mm Hg.**

h. Diffusion capacity is typically decreased because of either a decreased surface area available for diffusion or thickening of the membrane itself.

i. DLCO is **decreased** as a result of
   (1) O_2 toxicity
   (2) Emphysema
   (3) Sarcoidosis
   (4) Edema
   (5) Asbestosis

9. **V/Q scanning**

a. This radiograph evaluates the relationship of the distribution of ventilation to pulmonary perfusion in the lungs.

b. For the determination of gas distribution, the patient inhales the radioactive isotope **xenon** and holds the breath for 10 to 20 s. Radiographs (photoscintigrams) are obtained to observe how the xenon was distributed in the lung.

c. For the determination of pulmonary perfusion, the patient is injected with a radioactive iodine preparation and photoscintigrams are taken as the blood perfuses the lungs.

III. **OBSTRUCTIVE VERSUS RESTRICTIVE LUNG DISEASES**

CRT Exam Content Matrix: IA4, IA7b-c, IB9d-e,m,s, IB10d-e,s, IC5, IIC4, IIIE7a-f

RRT Exam Content Matrix: IA4, IA7b-c, IB9d-e,m,t, IB10d-e,u, IC6, IIC4, IIIE7a-f

A. **Obstructive Diseases: These diseases result in decreased flow studies (FEV$_1$, FEV/FVC, FEF$_{25\%-75\%}$, FEF$_{200-1200}$) and increased FRC, TLC, and RV values.**
   1. Emphysema
   2. Asthma
   3. Bronchitis
   4. Cystic fibrosis
   5. Bronchiectasis

B. **Restrictive Diseases or Disorders: These diseases result in decreased volumes (FRC, FVC, IC, IRV) and a normal FEV/FVC value.**
   1. Pulmonary fibrosis
   2. Chest wall disease
   3. Pneumonia
   4. Neuromuscular disease
   5. Pleural disease
   6. Postsurgical situations

C. **Severity of disease (by interpretation of pulmonary function tests)**
   1. Normal pulmonary function test results: 80% to 100% of predicted value
   2. Mild disorder: 60% to 79% of predicted value
   3. Moderate disorder: 40% to 59% of predicted value
   4. Severe disorder: less than 40% of predicted value

D. **Predicted values are determined from**
   1. Age
   2. Gender
   3. Height
   4. Ideal body weight
   5. Race

IV. **MISCELLANEOUS PULMONARY FUNCTION STUDIES**

CRT Exam Content Matrix: IA4, IB9d-e,m,s, IB10d-e,m,s, IC5, IIIE7a,f

RRT Exam Content Matrix: IA4, IB9d-e,m,t, IB10d-e,m,u, IC6, IIIE7a-f

A. **Before-and-After Bronchodilator Studies**
   1. Used to determine the reversibility of lung dysfunction and the effectiveness of the bronchodilator.
   2. Patients, most commonly those with asthma, are instructed to perform a peak flow test before administration of a bronchodilating agent. The value is recorded. The administration of the agent is followed by another peak flow study.
   3. Reversibility of obstructed airways and improved flow rates are considered significant if **increases in flow studies are at least 12%.**

$$\text{Percentage of improvement} = \frac{\text{posttreatment value} - \text{pretreatment value}}{\text{pretreatment value}} \times 100$$

B. **Methacholine Challenge Test**
   1. Determines the degree of airway reactivity to methacholine, a drug that stimulates bronchoconstriction.
   2. May be performed in a before-and-after bronchodilator study or before exercise-induced asthma studies.
   3. The objective of the test is to determine the minimum level of methacholine that elicits **a 20% decrease in FEV$_1$.**

4. A physician should be present during testing, and bronchodilators and resuscitation equipment should be readily available.

C. Measurement of Maximal Inspiratory Pressure (MIP)

1. This measurement is also referred to as negative inspiratory force (NIF).
2. This value represents the maximum amount of negative pressure a patient can generate during inspiration.
3. This is measured with an aneroid manometer, which connects to an ET tube via an adapter. The patient is then instructed to inhale as deeply as possible. The manometer records the negative pressure.
4. An adapter attached to the manometer, with a one-way valve that allows for exhalation but not for inspiration, is also an effective method for obtaining an MIP value.

> ⚠ These two methods for determining MIP may cause agitation and anxiety in alert patients. The respiratory therapist should always explain the procedure to the patient before beginning it.

5. Obtain an MIP value in patients who are not intubated by connecting the manometer to a mouthpiece and placing nose clips on the patient.
6. A normal MIP is approximately −50 to −100 cm H_2O.
7. A patient who cannot generate at least −20 cm H_2O of pressure has inadequate respiratory muscle strength. The patient is not capable of generating the necessary negative inspiratory pressures required to cough and maintain a patent airway or to maintain spontaneous ventilation; therefore, mechanical ventilation is most likely indicated.

D. Maximal expiratory pressure (MEP)

1. An aneroid manometer is attached to the patient's ET tube, and the patient is instructed to inhale as deeply as possible and exhale forcefully and completely.
2. The maximum pressure is observed and recorded.
3. Obtain an MEP value in patients who are not intubated by attaching the manometer to a mouthpiece and placing nose clips on the patient.
4. A normal MEP is 90 to 100 cm H_2O.
5. Patients unable to generate an MEP of at least **40 cm H_2O** of pressure are not able to maintain adequate spontaneous ventilation or secretion clearance, which makes mechanical ventilation necessary.

V. INTERPRETATION OF CHART SUMMARY

CRT Exam Content Matrix: IA4, IB9s, IB10s, IIIE7a-c
RRT Exam Content Matrix: IA4, IB9t, IB10u, IIIE7a-c

	Disease	
Function	**Obstructive**	**Restrictive**
FVC	Decreased	Decreased
IC	Decreased or normal	Decreased
ERV	Decreased or normal	Decreased
VT	Increased	Decreased or normal
FRC	Increased	Decreased
RV	Increased	Decreased
RV/TLC	Increased	Normal
FEV₁	Decreased	Normal or decreased
FEF₂₀₀₋₁₂₀₀	Decreased	Normal
FEF₂₅%₋₇₅%	Decreased	Normal
FEV/FVC	Decreased	Normal
MVV	Decreased	Decreased

VI. FLOW-SENSING DEVICES

CRT Exam Content Matrix: IIA16,23
RRT Exam Content Matrix: None

> ☑ **Exam Note**
>
> According to the current NBRC exam content matrix, questions regarding respirometers and other flow-sensing devices (pneumotachometers) will appear on the CRT exam only.

A. Wright Respirometer

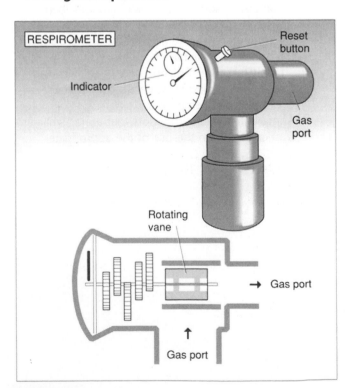

FIGURE 16-3

1. This respirometer is a handheld device that is frequently used at the patient's bedside to measure VC, VT, and V̇E.
2. As the patient's exhaled gas flows through the respirometer, it rotates vanes within the device. Through a gearworks mechanism, the movement of the vane is indicated on a dial calibrated in liters.
3. This device may also be placed in-line to ventilator circuits to measure the patient's exhaled volume. When used for this purpose, it should be placed on the expiratory side of the circuit as close to the patient as possible.

B. **Pneumotachometers**

1. This type of flow-sensing device integrates flow signals to obtain volume measurements.
2. There are three kinds of pneumotachometers; each uses different physical principles to measure flow.
   a. Pressure-drop pneumotachometer: air flows through the tube and meets a resistance, which decreases pressure. The pressure drop is measured by a transducer that converts it into an electronic signal.
   b. Temperature-drop pneumotachometer: uses King's law, which states that the velocity of gas flow over a heated element is proportional to the convective heat loss from the element. It can measure both flow and volume.
   c. Ultrasonic-flow pneumotachometer: this tube has struts inside to cause a turbulence in gas flow. The turbulent flow waves hit the ultrasonic sound waves and changes them. The changes in the ultrasonic sound waves are proportional to the flow of gas and are shown as liters per minute or second.

C. **Bedside (Portable) Spirometers**

1. These flow-sensing spirometers can interface with either a laptop computer or a personal computer. Some utilize microprocessors that are as small as a calculator. With the use of the appropriate software, spirometry can be performed at the bedside.
2. Most portable spirometers use disposable flow sensors that are quite accurate.
3. Most handheld spirometers work on the ultrasonic flow sensor principle. These devices measure FVC, FEV_1, FEV_6, and FEV/FVC ratio.

POSTCHAPTER STUDY QUESTIONS

1. Name a condition that results in an increased RV.
2. What type of lung condition may result in a decreased IC?
3. What device may be used at the patient's bedside to measure VC?
4. What pulmonary function test is the best indicator for distinguishing an obstructive lung disorder from a restrictive one?
5. List three tests that aid in determining the severity of obstructive airway disease.
6. An FEV_1/FVC of less than 75% indicates which type of lung disease?
7. What five values may be measured on a flow volume loop?
8. List five conditions in which DL is decreased.
9. What does a before-and-after bronchodilator test determine?
10. What does MIP, also referred to as NIF, represent?

See answers at the back of the text.

BIBLIOGRAPHY

Hess D and others, *Respiratory care principles and practice*, Philadelphia, 2002, Saunders.

Scanlan C, Spearman C, Sheldon R, *Egan's fundamentals of respiratory care*, ed 5, St Louis, 1990, Mosby.

Ruppell G, *Manual of pulmonary function testing*, ed 9, St Louis, 2009, Mosby.

Wilkins RL, Stoller JK, Kacmarek R, *Egan's fundamentals of respiratory care*, ed 9, St Louis, 2009, Mosby.

EQUIPMENT DECONTAMINATION AND INFECTION CONTROL

PRETEST QUESTIONS

Answer the pretest questions before studying the chapter. This will help you determine your strong and weak areas in the material covered.

1. Which of the following procedures is most often used to decontaminate a bacterial filter used on a mechanical ventilator?

   A. Ethylene oxide sterilization
   B. Autoclaving
   C. Pasteurization
   D. Glutaraldehyde immersion

2. Diseases that may be transmitted via airborne particles include which of the following?

   1. Tuberculosis
   2. Legionellosis
   3. Histoplasmosis

   A. 1 only
   B. 2 only
   C. 1 and 3 only
   D. 1, 2, and 3

3. Which of the following procedures are capable of sterilizing equipment?

   1. Pasteurization
   2. Glutaraldehyde immersion
   3. Acetic acid immersion
   4. Ethylene oxide

   A. 1 and 2 only
   B. 2 and 3 only
   C. 2 and 4 only
   D. 1, 2, and 4 only

4. Which of the following should be worn as a precautionary measure when changing a patient's ventilator circuit?

   1. Gloves
   2. Eye goggles
   3. Gown

   A. 1 only
   B. 1 and 2 only
   C. 1 and 3 only
   D. 1, 2, and 3

5. A high-efficiency particulate air (HEPA) filter should be used in the room of a patient with which type of condition?

   A. Tuberculosis
   B. Adenovirus infection
   C. Epiglottitis
   D. Streptococcal pneumonia

6. Biologic indicators are used in decontamination procedures for which of the following reasons?

   A. They speed up the decontamination process.
   B. They increase the concentration of liquid sterilants.
   C. They indicate what organisms have contaminated the equipment.
   D. They determine whether the decontamination process was effective.

See answers and rationales at the back of the text.

REVIEW

I. **BASIC TERMINOLOGY**
   CRT Exam Content Matrix: IIB1
   RRT Exam Content Matrix: IIB1
   A. Vegetative Organisms: organisms in active growth. **These organisms pose the greatest hazard for infection via respiratory therapy equipment because the most common equipment contaminants are not spore-forming bacteria.**
   B. Spores: organisms in a resting, resistant stage. They are very difficult to kill but pose little threat for infection via respiratory therapy equipment.
   C. Disinfection: killing of all vegetative forms of organisms but not spores. Agents that disinfect equipment are called disinfectants.
   D. Sterilization: killing of all organisms, both vegetative and spores. An agent that sterilizes equipment is called a sterilant.
   E. The suffix *-cidal* means to kill, as in **bactericidal**, which is said of something that kills bacteria.

F. The suffix *-static* means to prevent growth of, as in **bacteriostatic,** which is said of something that prevents the growth of bacteria.

G. Gram's stain method for differential staining of bacteria. Gram-positive bacteria stain a purple-black color, and gram-negative bacteria stain a pink color.

H. Nosocomial Infection: a hospital-acquired infection. Often caused by *Pseudomonas* species, *Staphylococcus* species, *Candida albicans,* or *Escherichia coli.*

II. CONDITIONS THAT INFLUENCE ANTIMICROBIAL ACTION

CRT Exam Content Matrix: IIB1
RRT Exam Content Matrix: IIB1

A. Chemical Concentration: The more concentrated a chemical is, the more rapid the action.

B. Intensity of the Physical Agent: The more intense a physical agent (e.g., heat), the more rapidly the organisms are killed.

C. Time: the longer the organisms are exposed to the agent, the greater the number killed.

D. Temperature: Increasing the temperature of a chemical agent shortens the exposure time required to kill the organisms.

E. Type of Organism: Vegetative forms of bacteria are more easily killed than spore-forming bacteria. Spores are more resistant to both chemical and physical agents.

F. Number of Organisms: The more organisms, the longer the exposure time required to kill them.

G. Nature of Material Bearing the Organism: The presence of blood, sputum, or other medium provides protection for the organisms. It is for this reason that **equipment must be thoroughly washed in soapy water and rinsed off before the decontamination process.**

III. THREE MAIN CLASSES OF BACTERIA

CRT Exam Content Matrix: IIB1
RRT Exam Content Matrix: IIB1

A. Cocci: Sphere-Shaped Bacteria

B. Spirillum: Spiral-Shaped Bacteria

C. Bacilli: Rod-Shaped Bacteria
1. Bacilli are the bacteria most frequently encountered on respiratory equipment.
2. They **are not** spore-forming bacteria.
3. Examples of bacilli (often causing pneumonia)
   a. *Klebsiella pneumoniae:* a gram-negative bacillus
   b. *Pseudomonas aeruginosa:* a gram-negative bacillus
   c. *Mycobacterium* species: a gram-positive bacillus and causative agent of TB
   d. *Legionella* species: gram-negative bacilli
   e. *Serratia marcescens:* a gram-negative bacillus and secondary invader in respiratory and burn patients.
   f. *Haemophilus influenzae:* a gram-negative bacillus

Exam Note

The aforementioned gram-negative organisms are often responsible for necrotizing forms of pneumonia.

IV. STERILIZATION AND DISINFECTION TECHNIQUES

CRT Exam Content Matrix: IIB1
RRT Exam Content Matrix: IIB1

A. **Physical Agents**
1. **Autoclave (steam under pressure)**
   a. Heat in the form of steam is one of the most dependable and practical methods for decontamination.
   b. **Normal operating levels are 15 min at 121° C and 15 psig (2 atm).**
   c. **Autoclaving sterilizes equipment.**
   d. Kills organisms by coagulation of the cell protein.
   e. Bacteria filters are commonly sterilized by this method, but any material made of rubber cannot withstand the intense heat.
   f. The tops of nebulizers and humidifiers should be attached loosely to allow exposure to all parts of the device.
   g. Equipment to be autoclaved must be thoroughly washed in soapy water, dried, and wrapped in muslin, cloth, or a paper bag.
   h. Written on the outside of the wrap should be information including the time and date of processing, what kind of equipment is inside the wrap, and who prepared the equipment for processing.

2. **Pasteurization**
   a. Equipment must be washed in soapy water and rinsed off before placement in the pasteurizing machine.
   b. Equipment is immersed in hot water at 60° to 70° C for 20 to 30 min.
   c. The hotter the water, the less time needed to clean the equipment.
   d. Pasteurization disinfects equipment, but spores are not killed.

B. **Chemical Agents**
1. **Ethylene oxide gas sterilization**
   a. Equipment must be washed in soapy water, rinsed, **dried completely,** and placed in a sealed plastic bag before being placed in the sterilization chamber.
   b. If equipment is not completely dry before the sterilization process, ethylene oxide combines with water to form ethylene glycol, an irritating substance found in antifreeze.
   c. Ethylene oxide kills all organisms including spores, therefore it **sterilizes equipment.**

d. It is a highly flammable gas, but when it is mixed with approximately 90% carbon dioxide or freon, the explosive danger is minimized.

e. Equipment may be processed in one of two ways.
   (1) Warm gas: 50° to 56° C for 4 h
   (2) Cold gas: 22° C (room temperature) for 6 to 12 h

f. After exposure to the gas, the equipment must be aerated for about 12 h at 50° to 60° C.

g. Most respiratory therapy equipment can be decontaminated by this method.

h. The recommended gas concentration is 800 to 1000 mg/L.

i. Because moisture enhances the action of ethylene oxide, it is recommended that the relative humidity within the sterilizing chamber be maintained at 50% or more.

j. Items placed in sealed plastic bags are suitable for use for up to 1 yr after gas sterilization, provided the bag is intact.

2. **Alcohols**
   a. Ethyl alcohol (95% concentration) and isopropyl alcohol (70% concentration) are the most commonly used in the clinical setting.
   b. Alcohols are bactericidal and fungicidal but not sporicidal; therefore, they disinfect (but do not sterilize) equipment.
   c. Alcohols kill organisms by destroying the cell protein.
   d. Action is decreased when diluted below 50%.
   e. Alcohol is used as a disinfectant to wipe down respiratory therapy equipment.

3. **Glutaraldehydes**
   a. Are related to formaldehyde.
   b. The most common glutaraldehyde product is Cidex, which is an alkaline glutaraldehyde solution.
   c. These agents are **bactericidal** in 10 to 15 min and sporicidal in 3 to 10 h, depending on the temperature of the solution.
   d. Glutaraldehydes are normally used to disinfect equipment but may be used to sterilize. Organisms are killed by coagulation of the cell protein.
   e. Equipment must be washed in soapy water and rinsed off before being placed in the solution bath.
   f. On removal from the solution bath (with gloves to prevent skin irritation), the equipment should be rinsed off and thoroughly dried before packaging.
   g. Cidex solution remains active for 28 days.

4. **Acetic acid (vinegar)**
   a. Kills vegetative bacteria but not spores; therefore, it **disinfects equipment.**
   b. It is very effective against *Pseudomonas* species.
   c. Acetic acid is used as a disinfectant for home care equipment and is often run through room humidifiers for cleaning purposes.
   d. It is not recommended for use on respiratory therapy equipment in the clinical setting, unless it is used in combination with more effective methods.

V. **IMPORTANT POINTS CONCERNING DECONTAMINATION OF EQUIPMENT**
   CRT Exam Content Matrix: IIB1
   RRT Exam Content Matrix: IIB1
   A. Use only sterile solutions in reservoirs.
   B. Solutions left in the reservoir should be discarded before adding fresh solution.
   C. Always date the container that holds the solution after it is opened; solutions should be discarded after 24 h. This reduces the possibility of filling a reservoir with contaminated solution.
   D. Condensation in the delivery tubing **should never be drained back into the reservoir.**
   E. Provide a method of routine surveillance to determine the effectiveness of the decontamination process. This is referred to as **quality control of equipment.**
      1. Processing indicators determine whether the disinfection or sterilization process was effective. There are two types of indicators.
         a. Biologic indicators: Strips of paper impregnated with bacterial spores are placed in a glass ampule that contains a growth medium. The ampule is then placed inside the sterilizer. After the sterilization process is complete, the ampule is broken and the spore strip is exposed to the growth medium. After an incubation period, if the spore strip changes color, bacteria are present and the sterilization process was ineffective.
         b. Chemical indicators are impregnated on packing tape and change color when exposed to certain conditions. Autoclave and ethylene oxide sterilization both use this type of indicator. These indicators show that the package went through the sterilization process but do not necessarily indicate that the equipment is sterile. Ensuring that the equipment is sterile is best accomplished with biologic indicators.
      2. Culture sampling: Equipment disinfected by chemical solutions, such as glutaraldehyde, or by pasteurization should be evaluated to determine whether the disinfection process was effective.

3. Swab sampling: A sterile swab is used to wipe an area of the equipment and is placed in a tube of sterile liquid broth to determine the presence of microorganisms.

F. Use of disposable equipment decreases the potential for cross-contamination. Because warm, moist humidifiers and nebulizers are ideal breeding grounds for bacteria, disposables are for single-patient use only.

G. The most cost-effective method of preventing cross-contamination of equipment among patients is by proper **HAND-WASHING** techniques (see *Universal Precautions* later in the chapter).

H. Disposable equipment should not be refilled or reused.

I. Equipment must be completely dry when packaged and stored to prevent new growth.

J. Handling of Contaminated Equipment:
1. All equipment and supplies taken from an isolation area must be double-bagged in nonporous plastic bags.
2. A person in isolation attire places the contaminated equipment into a bag while in the patient's room and then drops it in a bag held outside the room by a second person. The person dropping the bag of contaminated material into the second bag must be careful not to touch the second bag.
3. The person outside the room then ties off the second bag and takes it to the proper decontamination area.
4. The bag should be labeled to indicate that it is from an isolation area. Labeling should also identify the bag contents as well as the patient's name and room number. The labeling procedure may vary by institution.

VI. **INFECTION CONTROL AND STANDARD (UNIVERSAL) PRECAUTIONS**
CRT Exam Content Matrix: IIB4, IIB5
RRT Exam Content Matrix: IIB3, IIB4
A. **Standard (Universal) Precautions:** All health care providers should practice these precautions, regardless of the patient's diagnosis or presumed diagnosis. They apply to blood, body fluids, secretions, excretions, mucous membranes, and nonintact skin.
1. Hand washing: should be done for 15 s before and after visiting every patient, even if the examiner is wearing gloves. Alcohol-based hand sanitizers that do not require the use of water are preferred over soap and water because of their superior antimicrobial action. Hand sanitizers are also more convenient and reduce the potential of drying out the skin.
2. Gloves: should be worn when treating all patients.
3. Gown: should be worn when performing a task that may involve the splashing of fluids or spraying of blood.

4. Mask, eye goggles, face shield: should be worn when performing a task that may involve the splashing of fluids or spraying of blood.
5. Proper handling of needles and other sharp instruments: should be done as a precaution regardless of whether pathogens are thought to be present. Use extreme caution when handling needles and other sharp instruments.
a. Never recap used needles.
b. Used needles and syringes should be placed in puncture-resistant containers.
c. Never remove used needles by hand.

B. **Transmission-Based Precautions:** These precautions are used when working with patients who have contagious diseases for which standard precautions are inadequate. These precautions are implemented in addition to standard precautions. There are three types of transmission-based precautions.
1. **Precautions against contact**
a. Decrease the risk of transmission of microorganisms by direct or indirect contact.
b. Examples of diseases requiring these precautions include hepatitis, AIDS, venereal diseases, and staphylococcal infections.
c. In addition to standard precautions, placing the patient in a private room and discarding gloves and gowns before exiting the room is required.
2. **Precautions against airborne infections**
a. Decrease the risk of spread of infectious microorganisms through the air.
b. Diseases that may be transmitted by this route include tuberculosis, legionellosis, avian flu, and severe acute respiratory syndrome (SARS)
c. In addition to standard precautions, placing the patient in a private room with the door closed at all times is required; anyone entering the room should wear a HEPA mask.
d. To further aid in the reduction of airborne organisms, a special (negative pressure) ventilation system should be in place in the room so that air is safely discharged or recirculated in the room through a HEPA filter.
3. **Precautions against droplet spreading**
a. Decrease the risk of the transmission of infectious organisms via droplet spreading.
b. Examples of diseases transmitted by this route include *Haemophilus influenzae* infection, streptococcal pneumonia, epiglottitis, pertussis, meningitis, and adenovirus infections.
c. In addition to standard precautions, placing the patient in a private room and having anyone entering the room wear a mask is required.

⚠ If private rooms are not available for patients under these three types of special precautions, patients infected with the same organism may share a room. This is referred to as cohorting.

Exam Note

Both the CRT and RRT exam matrix list infectious disease protocols specific to avian influenza and SARS. These two respiratory disorders should be suspected in patients who exhibit respiratory symptoms and who have recently travelled to a country with avian flu or SARS activity. The aforementioned standard, contact, and airborne precautions should be used with patients given a diagnosis of or suspected of having avian flu or SARS. Additionally, health care workers involved in the care of patients with documented or suspected avian flu should receive the human influenza vaccine. Vaccination will not only provide protection against the current seasonal flu but may reduce the potential of the health care worker becoming infected with both human and avian strains.

POSTCHAPTER STUDY QUESTIONS

1. List four diseases that are spread by airborne pathogens.
2. What device should be used in the ventilation system through which air is discharged safely from the room of a patient with a disease caused by an airborne pathogen?
3. List three methods that may be used to sterilize respiratory therapy equipment.
4. List three diseases transmitted by the spread of droplets.
5. What is a nosocomial infection?
6. List four gram-negative organisms that may result in necrotizing pneumonia.
7. What methods are used to determine the effectiveness of the decontamination process?

See answers at the back of the text.

BIBLIOGRAPHY

Hess D and others, *Respiratory care principles and practice*, Philadelphia, 2002, Saunders.

Wilkins RL, Stoller JK, Kacmarek R, *Egan's fundamentals of respiratory care*, ed 9, St Louis, 2009, Mosby.

White G, *Basic clinical lab competencies for respiratory care: an integrated approach*, ed 4, Clifton Park, NY, 2003, Delmar.

ENTRY LEVEL CERTIFICATION EXAM: PRACTICE TEST

TIME LIMIT: 3 HOURS

> **Exam Note**
>
> The NBRC Entry-Level CRT Exam comprises 160 questions, 20 of which do not figure into the final score. The final score is based on 140 questions. The minimum passing score for the CRT Examination is 75%. To simulate the length of the CRT Exam, this practice test consists of 160 questions and all questions figure into your final score.

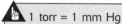

1 torr = 1 mm Hg

Directions: Each of the questions or incomplete statements in this test is followed by four suggested answers or completions. Choose the best answer and circle it on the test.

1. The physician orders a 35% aerosol mask to be set up for a patient who requires an inspiratory flow of 42 L/min. What is the minimum flow rate to which the flowmeter must be set to meet this patient's inspiratory flow demands?

   A. 6 L/min
   B. 8 L/min
   C. 10 L/min
   D. 12 L/min

2. A premature infant is receiving O_2 via a 50% O_2 hood and has a PaO_2 of 43 torr and a $PaCO_2$ of 40 torr. The respiratory therapist should recommend which of the following?

   A. Increase the O_2 to 70%.
   B. Intubate and institute mechanical ventilation.
   C. Initiate CPAP of 4 cm H_2O and 50% O_2.
   D. Increase the O_2 to 100%.

3. A patient arrives in the emergency department after being pulled from a burning house. The respiratory therapist should recommend obtaining which of the following measurements to best determine the severity of the patient's smoke inhalation?

   A. SpO_2
   B. HbCO
   C. PaO_2
   D. Hb

4. The physician has ordered 40% O_2 to be administered to an active 3 year old. Which of the following delivery devices would you recommend for this patient?

   A. O_2 tent
   B. Air entrainment mask
   C. Simple O_2 mask
   D. O_2 hood

5. The ability of the patient to follow instructions would be indicated by which of the following?

   A. Orientation to person
   B. Performance of tasks when asked
   C. Ability to feed himself
   D. Awareness of time

6. You suspect a patient may have a pulmonary embolism. Which of the following would be the most appropriate recommendation for diagnosis of this condition?

   A. Bronchoscopy
   B. V/Q lung scan
   C. Coagulation studies
   D. Shunt study

7. To most effectively increase a patient's alveolar minute ventilation while the patient is using a ventilator in the control mode, you would recommend increasing which of the following?

   A. Sigh rate
   B. Inspiratory flow
   C. VT
   D. Ventilator rate

8. Failure to hyperoxygenate a patient on a ventilator before ET suctioning may result in

   1. **Hypocarbia**
   2. **Hypoxemia**
   3. **Hypertension**
   4. **Bradycardia**

   A. 1 only
   B. 1 and 2 only
   C. 2 and 3 only
   D. 2 and 4 only

9. The most reliable method of determining whether the lungs of a patient receiving mechanical ventilation are getting stiffer and harder to ventilate is by measuring the

   A. Static lung compliance
   B. Dynamic lung compliance
   C. Spontaneous VT
   D. PaO_2

10. A 60-kg (132-lb), 52-year-old man is admitted to the ICU for the treatment of refractory hypoxemia. He is currently using a ventilator in the pressure support mode at 10 cm H_2O and an FiO_2 of 0.60. Other pertinent data are below

ABGs		
	pH	7.49
	$PaCO_2$	30 torr
	PaO_2	59 torr
Heart rate	120/min	
Respiratory rate	26/min	

    Which of the following should the respiratory therapist recommend at this time?

    A. Increase the pressure support level to 15 cm H_2O.
    B. Institute 5 cm H_2O PEEP.
    C. Increase the FiO_2 to 0.75.
    D. Initiate SIMV with the following variables: rate, 10; VT, 600 mL; FiO_2, 0.60.

11. If not cleaned properly, which one of the following devices is most likely to contaminate a patient's airways with bacteria?

    A. Bubble humidifier
    B. Heated wick humidifier
    C. Hydrosphere
    D. Heated jet nebulizer

12. A 70-kg (154-lb) patient is receiving mechanical ventilation. The respiratory therapist notes the patient's SpO_2 drops from 97% to 86%. The right lung is expanding more than the left, with clear breath sounds on the right but diminished ones on the left. The patient's endotracheal tube is taped at the 29-cm mark at the lip. Which of the following should the respiratory therapist do at this time?

    A. Withdraw the tube to the 24-cm mark.
    B. Recommend a stat chest x-ray film.
    C. Advance the endotracheal tube 2 cm.
    D. Obtain stat arterial blood gas levels.

13. Which one of the following sets of ABG measurements would be indicative of a renal compensated respiratory acidosis?

    A. pH 7.26, PCO_2 60 torr, PO_2 68 torr, HCO_3^- 24 mEq/L, BE 0
    B. pH 7.42, PCO_2 39 torr, PO_2 87 torr, HCO_3^- 22 mEq/L, BE −1
    C. pH 7.25, PCO_2 61 torr, PO_2 75 torr, HCO_3^- 26 mEq/L, BE +1
    D. pH 7.37, PCO_2 58 torr, PO_2 60 torr, HCO_3^- 31 mEq/L, BE +8

14. The following data have been collected for a patient receiving mechanical ventilation with a volume ventilator:

VT	750 mL	pH	7.29
Mode	SIMV	$PaCO_2$	50 torr
Ventilator rate	4/min	PaO_2	72 torr
Spontaneous rate	12/min	HCO_3^-	26 mEq/L
FiO_2	0.35	BE	+1

    On the basis of these data, which of the following should the respiratory therapist recommend?

    A. Increase the VT to 850 mL.
    B. Increase the FiO_2 to 0.40.
    C. Increase the ventilator rate to 8/min.
    D. Change to assist/control mode at a rate of 15/min.

15. Advantages of low-pressure, high-volume ET tube cuffs include

    1. **Easier insertion into the airway**
    2. **Less occlusion to tracheal blood flow**
    3. **Improved distribution of alveolar air**

    A. 1 only
    B. 2 only
    C. 1 and 2 only
    D. 2 and 3 only

16. Tracheal secretions tend to dry out in an intubated patient when inspired air has which of the following characteristics?

    1. **An absolute humidity of 24 mg/L of gas**
    2. **A water vapor pressure of 47 mm Hg**
    3. **50 mg of particulate water per liter of gas**
    4. **A relative humidity of 100% at 25°C**

    A. 2 only
    B. 1 and 3 only
    C. 1 and 4 only
    D. 2 and 3 only

17. It is important to monitor airway pressure in a patient receiving mechanical ventilation because it best reflects

    A. Lung compliance
    B. PaO_2
    C. $PaCO_2$
    D. ICP

18. When a patient is receiving ventilation in the control mode, how may the $PaCO_2$ best be raised?

    A. Increase the VT.
    B. Increase the FiO_2.
    C. Decrease the mechanical dead space.
    D. Decrease the respiratory rate.

19. A patient is receiving ventilation with a volume-cycled ventilator, and the low-pressure alarm suddenly sounds. The corrective action would be to

    A. Suction the patient.
    B. Begin manual resuscitation.
    C. Increase the flow.
    D. Determine whether the patient is disconnected from the ventilator.

20. After a patient has received bronchodilator therapy, the respiratory therapist attempts to perform nasotracheal suction on the patient. As the catheter enters the oropharynx, the following ECG waveform is seen on the oscilloscope monitor.

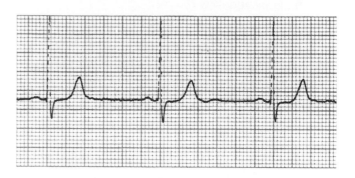

This ECG pattern is most likely the result of which of the following?

    A. Excessive suction pressure
    B. Hypoxemia
    C. Vagal nerve stimulation
    D. Hypercarbia

21. A 6-day-old premature infant of 30 weeks' gestational age is experiencing frequent periods of apnea with desaturation. Which of the following medications should the respiratory therapist recommend?

    A. Surfactant (Survanta)
    B. Albuterol (Proventil)
    C. Theophylline
    D. Naloxone (Narcan)

22. To prevent the obstruction of venous blood flow from the trachea, ET tube cuff pressure should not exceed

    A. 5 mm Hg
    B. 10 mm Hg
    C. 20 mm Hg
    D. 25 mm Hg

23. A postoperative 46-year-old, 80-kg (176-lb) patient is breathing spontaneously at a rate of 30/min with an FiO_2 of 0.50. The following ABG results are obtained:

pH	7.29
$PaCO_2$	62 torr
PaO_2	64 torr
HCO_3^-	29 mEq/L
BE	+4

    Mechanical ventilation is instituted with a VT of 800 mL and a FiO_2 of 0.5. The SIMV rate should be set on

    A. 4/min
    B. 6/min
    C. 12/min
    D. 16/min

24. The respiratory therapist is asked to deliver a medication to a patient with cystic fibrosis via nonpressurized aerosol that will improve the mobilization of sputum. Which of the following should be recommended?

    A. Acetylcysteine (Mucomyst)
    B. Propylene glycol
    C. Racemic epinephrine
    D. Dexamethasone (Decadron)

25. The therapeutic use of O_2 may aid in accomplishing which of the following?

    1. **Decrease the work of breathing**
    2. **Decrease myocardial work**
    3. **Prevent ARDS**
    4. **Increase the patient's respiratory rate**

    A. 1 only
    B. 1 and 2 only
    C. 2 and 3 only
    D. 1, 2, and 4 only

26. Inspiratory stridor is the major clinical sign of

    A. Tracheal malacia
    B. Tracheal stenosis
    C. Glottic edema
    D. Laryngotracheal web

27. A patient receiving mechanical ventilation with a volume ventilator is ordered to have PEEP initiated. Observation of which of the following values will *best* determine the optimal level of PEEP?

    A. Cardiac output
    B. PaO_2
    C. $PaCO_2$
    D. VD/VT

28. An 8-day-old neonate is receiving pressure-limited, time-cycled mechanical ventilation. Over the past 36 hours, the neonate's PaO_2 has decreased from 58 torr to 47 torr. The physician wants to increase the mean airway pressure. Which of the following should the respiratory therapist recommend increasing?

    1. **Inspiratory pressure limit**
    2. **Expiratory time**
    3. **Inspiratory time**

    A. 1 only
    B. 3 only
    C. 1 and 3 only
    D. 2 and 3 only

29. While assessing a patient with chest trauma in the ICU, the respiratory therapist observes that the patient's chest tube, which is connected to an underwater seal drainage system, is outside the chest wall. Which of the following statements are correct about this situation?

    A. The tube should be clamped immediately.
    B. A complete pneumothorax is possible.
    C. The tube should be disconnected from suction.
    D. Suction pressure should be increased.

30. Administration of high O_2 concentrations to a neonate for a prolonged period of time may result in which of the following?

    1. **Atelectasis**
    2. **Retinopathy of prematurity**
    3. **Pneumothorax**
    4. **Persistent pulmonary hypertension of the newborn**

    A. 2 and 4 only
    B. 1 and 2 only
    C. 1 and 3 only
    D. 1, 2, and 4

31. The data below pertain to an adult receiving mechanical ventilation:

Peak inspiratory pressure	50 cm H_2O
Plateau pressure	40 cm H_2O
VT	800 mL (0.8 L)
PEEP	10 cm H_2O

    On the basis of this information, this patient's static lung compliance is approximately which of the following?

    A. 16 mL/cm H_2O
    B. 20 mL/cm H_2O
    C. 27 mL/cm H_2O
    D. 37 mL/cm H_2O

32. A patient recovering postoperatively is receiving ventilation in the SIMV mode. The patient has normal ABG levels with the use of 35% O_2 but is still drowsy. The respiratory therapist should recommend decreasing the

    A. SIMV rate
    B. Inspiratory time
    C. VT
    D. Sigh volume

33. The respiratory therapist is transporting a patient with a nasal cannula running at 6 L/min. For the "E" cylinder to last at least 1 h, what is the minimum amount of pressure it must contain?

    A. 1000 psig
    B. 1200 psig
    C. 1400 psig
    D. 1600 psig

34. An 80-kg (176-lb) patient with ARDS is intubated and is receiving mechanical ventilation with the following settings:

Mode	SIMV
Rate	10
Tidal volume	700 mL
PEEP	10 cm H_2O

    The respiratory therapist notes that the patient's SpO_2 has dropped from 98% to 85% over the past 2 h. The therapist notes the PIP has increased from 36 cm H_2O to 46 cm H_2O, and the plateau pressure has increased from 28 cm H_2O to 38 cm H_2O. Which of the following should the therapist recommend?

    A. Increase the FiO_2 to 1.0.
    B. Suction the patient.
    C. Increase the PEEP to 12 cm H_2O.
    D. Administer aerosolized albuterol.

35. Which one of these drugs would be best to use to temporarily paralyze a patient to facilitate tracheal intubation?

    A. Atropine sulfate
    B. Succinylcholine (Anectine)
    C. Midazolam (Versed)
    D. Pancuronium bromide (Pavulon)

36. To begin the weaning process from the ventilator, a patient should be able to obtain an MIP of at least

    A. −10 cm H_2O
    B. −20 cm H_2O
    C. −30 cm H_2O
    D. −40 cm H_2O

37. While making O_2 rounds, you discover that the 6-inch reservoir tubing on a T-piece (Briggs adapter) setup has fallen off. What may result from this?

    1. **Delivered FiO_2 would decrease.**
    2. **Delivered FiO_2 would increase.**
    3. **The patient would entrain room air during inspiration.**
    4. **The total flow from the nebulizer would decrease.**

    A. 1 and 4 only
    B. 2 only
    C. 1 and 3 only
    D. 2 and 3 only

38. A patient has been paralyzed with vecuronium (Norcuron) and is receiving mechanical ventilation. Which of the following ventilator monitoring alarms would be the most important?

    A. Low pressure
    B. High pressure
    C. Inspired gas temperature
    D. I : E time

39. The use of the inspiratory plateau setting on a ventilator results in

    1. **Decreasing mean intrathoracic pressure**
    2. **Increasing diffusion of gases**
    3. **Decreasing atelectasis**

    A. 1 only
    B. 2 only
    C. 1 and 2 only
    D. 2 and 3 only

40. A patient with COPD is in the emergency department and is complaining of shortness of breath. ABG results with the patient breathing room air are below:

pH	7.31
$PaCO_2$	62 torr
PaO_2	44 torr
HCO_3^-	34 mEq/L
BE	+10

    The most appropriate recommendation for O_2 therapy is which of the following?

    A. Simple mask at 10 L/min.
    B. Nasal cannula at 6 L/min.
    C. Air entrainment mask at 28%.
    D. Aerosol mask at 40%.

41. During CPR, the physician is preparing to administer lidocaine intravenously and discovers that the IV is infiltrated. The most appropriate action to take at this time is to

    A. Instill the lidocaine down the ET tube.
    B. Administer the lidocaine using a handheld nebulizer.
    C. Place a new IV line and administer the lidocaine.
    D. Administer the lidocaine sublingually.

42. Which of following medications would be most indicated in the treatment of a patient with large amounts of thick secretions?

    A. Salmeterol
    B. Hypotonic saline
    C. Acetylcysteine
    D. Albuterol

43. Which of these devices is not a low-flow device?

    A. Nasal cannula
    B. Venturi mask
    C. Partial rebreathing mask
    D. Simple O_2 mask

44. You are instructing a patient about the proper procedure for using an MDI. You would instruct the patient to activate the medication in the inhaler

    A. Just before inspiration.
    B. Just after inspiration has begun.
    C. At the end of exhalation.
    D. After inhaling as deeply as possible.

45. After the intubation of a patient, the respiratory therapist is assessing the chest x-ray films for proper tube placement. The tip of the tube is at the level of the fourth rib. This indicates which of the following?

    A. The tube position is too low.
    B. The tube is too high.
    C. The tube is in the esophagus.
    D. The tube is in proper position in the midtrachea.

46. While suctioning through a patient's ET tube, the respiratory therapist begins having difficulty removing the thick secretions. Which of the following is the appropriate measure to take?

    A. Increase the suction pressure to −160 torr.
    B. Use a larger suction catheter.
    C. Apply continuous suction while withdrawing the catheter.
    D. Instill saline down the ET tube before suctioning.

47. The following ABG levels are collected from a patient using a 50% Venturi mask:

pH	7.37
PaCO$_2$	40 torr
PaO$_2$	70 torr

If the barometric pressure is 747 torr, which of the following represents this patient's P(A–a)O$_2$?

A. 170 torr
B. 230 torr
C. 300 torr
D. 350 torr

48. A patient has just been intubated and the CO$_2$ detector on the proximal end of the ET tube reads near zero. Which statement is true regarding this situation?

A. The tube is in the trachea.
B. The tube is in the esophagus.
C. The tube should be withdrawn 2 cm.
D. The tube is in the right mainstem bronchus.

49. The following data are collected for a neonate receiving mechanical ventilation with a pressure ventilator:

Mode	IMV	pH	7.41
Ventilator rate	40/min	PaCO$_2$	43 torr
Inspiratory pressure	28 cm H$_2$O	PaO$_2$	41 torr
FiO$_2$	0.70	HCO$_3^-$	23 mEq/L
PEEP	4 cm H$_2$O	BE	0

On the basis of these data, the respiratory therapist should recommend which of the following?

A. Increase the ventilator rate to 45/min.
B. Increase PEEP to 6 cm H$_2$O.
C. Increase inspiratory pressure to 32 cm H$_2$O.
D. Increase FiO$_2$ to 0.80.

50. Heavy smokers commonly have HbCO levels as high as

A. 10%
B. 20%
C. 30%
D. 40%

51. The following data have been collected from a 70-kg (154-lb) patient receiving mechanical ventilation with a volume ventilator:

Mode	Assist/control	ABGs:	
Ventilator rate	12/min	pH	7.37
		PaCO$_2$	42 torr
VT	750 mL	PaO$_2$	161 torr
FiO$_2$	0.80	HCO$_3^-$	25 mEq/L
PEEP	10 cm H$_2$O	BE	0

On the basis of these data, which of the following ventilator setting changes should the respiratory therapist recommend?

A. Decrease VT to 700 mL.
B. Decrease PEEP to 8 cm H$_2$O.
C. Increase the ventilator rate to 15/min.
D. Decrease FiO$_2$ to 0.70.

52. You are assisting the physician with cardioversion on a patient exhibiting atrial fibrillation. You should recommend which of the following levels of energy to conduct this procedure?

A. 50 J
B. 150 J
C. 200 J
D. 350 J

53. A 75-kg (165-lb) male patient is receiving mechanical ventilation in the SIMV mode and has the following ABGs:

pH	7.29
PaCO$_2$	59 torr
PaO$_2$	75 torr
HCO$_3^-$	27 mEq/L
BE	+2

The ventilator settings are as follows

FiO$_2$	0.35
SIMV rate	8/min
Spontaneous rate	24/min
VT	600 mL

Which of the following could be *increased* to correct this acid–base abnormality?

1. **Inspiratory flow**
2. **SIMV rate**
3. **VT**
4. **FiO$_2$**

A. 1 and 2
B. 2 and 3
C. 1 and 3
D. 2 and 4

54. The following ABG results are obtained from a patient recently pulled from a house fire. The blood is drawn with the patient using a non-rebreathing mask.

pH	7.23
PaCO$_2$	25 torr
PaO$_2$	250 torr
HCO$_3^-$	15 mEq/L
BE	−10
SaO$_2$	65%

This patient's acidemia is most likely the result of

A. Severe hypoxia
B. Hyperventilation
C. Hypocapnia
D. Airway obstruction

55. An oral ET tube is inserted into an adult patient. A leak is still heard after a large amount of air is placed in the cuff. This problem could be caused by which of the following?

A. The ET tube is too short.
B. The ET tube is too long.
C. The internal diameter of the ET tube is too large.
D. The outside diameter of the ET tube is too small.

56. What is the most negative pressure that should supply the suction catheter when suctioning an adult?

A. −60 mm Hg
B. −80 mm Hg
C. −120 mm Hg
D. −160 mm Hg

57. The following spontaneous ventilation variables are collected from a 68-kg (150-lb) patient with a 2-L/min nasal cannula:

VT	500 mL
Respiratory rate	10/min

This patient's alveolar minute ventilation is which of the following?

A. 2.8 L
B. 3.5 L
C. 4.3 L
D. 5.0 L

58. While performing postural drainage and percussion, the respiratory therapist palpates subcutaneous emphysema in the patient. The practitioner should postpone the therapy and recommend which of the following?

A. Measure ABG levels
B. Initiate IPPB therapy
C. Obtain chest x-ray films
D. Do bedside spirometry

59. A patient's PaO$_2$ increases after mechanical ventilation is initiated at 21% O$_2$. What accounts for the improved oxygenation status?

1. **Increased distribution of ventilation**
2. **Increased VD/VT ratio**
3. **Decreased venous return to the heart**
4. **Increased P(A−a)O$_2$ gradient**

A. 1 only
B. 1 and 4 only
C. 1, 2, and 3 only
D. 1, 3, and 4 only

60. You enter a patient's room to administer a treatment and the patient is unresponsive. After opening the airway, what is the next appropriate measure to take?

A. Give two breaths.
B. Check for a pulse.
C. Deliver six abdominal thrusts.
D. Determine whether the patient is breathing.

61. The following data are collected from a patient receiving mechanical ventilation with a volume ventilator:

PEEP level	PaO$_2$	PvO$_2$	VT
6 cm H$_2$O	64 torr	35 torr	800 mL
8 cm H$_2$O	70 torr	38 torr	800 mL
10 cm H$_2$O	75 torr	43 torr	800 mL
12 cm H$_2$O	80 torr	37 torr	800 mL

Which of the following represents optimal PEEP?

A. 6 cm H_2O
B. 8 cm H_2O
C. 10 cm H_2O
D. 12 cm H_2O

62. During the administration of IPPB, the respiratory therapist notices that the machine repeatedly cycles on shortly after the patient has begun expiration. To correct this problem, the practitioner should check which one of the following controls?

A. Flow control
B. Peak pressure control
C. Sensitivity control
D. Air mix control

63. Which of the following are advantages of a nasopharyngeal airway?

1. **It assures lower airway patency during mechanical ventilation.**
2. **It provides an adequate route for nasotracheal suctioning.**
3. **It is well tolerated by the semicomatose patient.**

A. 1 only
B. 2 only
C. 1 and 2 only
D. 2 and 3 only

64. If the respiratory therapist chooses an "E" cylinder to transport a patient within the hospital and it contains 650 psig of O_2, how long will the cylinder last if the flow is run at 10 L/min?

A. 18 min
B. 35 min
C. 56 min
D. 1 h, 45 min

65. Which of these airway changes will affect the delivered VT on a pressure-limited ventilator?

1. **Decreased lung compliance**
2. **Increased lung compliance**
3. **Increased airway resistance**

A. 1 only
B. 1 and 2 only
C. 2 and 3 only
D. 1, 2, and 3

66. Which of the following should be recommended first for a patient with a tension pneumothorax?

A. Obtain a stat chest x-ray film.
B. Obtain stat ABG levels.
C. Administer an IPPB treatment.
D. Release air from the pleural space.

67. A patient with COPD using a 50% air entrainment mask becomes drowsy and unresponsive. The patient's reaction most likely is the result of

A. Insufficient oxygenation
B. Decreased venous return
C. Increased $PaCO_2$
D. Excessive ventilation

68. While performing chest physical therapy on a ventilator patient, the respiratory therapist percusses an area of hyperresonance. This assessment is consistent with which of the following conditions?

A. Pleural effusion
B. Pneumothorax
C. Atelectasis
D. Consolidation

69. A patient's pulse drops from 92 to 54 beats/min when a suction catheter is inserted into the oropharynx. The most likely cause is

A. Hypoxia
B. Vagal stimulation
C. Hypocarbia
D. Coughing

70. After setting up a simple O_2 mask, you kink the O_2 tubing and the humidifier produces a high-pitched whistling sound. This indicates which of the following?

A. There are no leaks in the setup.
B. The O_2 flow to the mask is too low.
C. There may be a crack in the O_2 tubing.
D. The capillary tube in the humidifier may be loose.

71. The following pulmonary function results are obtained for a patient:

FEV_1/FVC	90% of predicted
FVC	55% of predicted

On the basis of these data, the patient most likely has which of the following?

A. Emphysema
B. Cystic fibrosis
C. Chronic bronchitis
D. Pulmonary fibrosis

72. You are asked to deliver a low percentage of O_2 to a patient whose respiratory rate is 30/min with an irregular breathing pattern. Which device would be the best choice?

    A. Nasal cannula at 2 L/min
    B. Venturi mask at 28%
    C. Simple O_2 mask at 5 L/min
    D. Partial rebreathing mask at 8 L/min

73. Which of the following ABG results would be considered normal in a patient with severe COPD?

    A. pH 7.50, PCO_2 40 torr, PO_2 56 torr, HCO_3^- 30 mEq/L, BE +4
    B. pH 7.29, PCO_2 54 torr. PO_2 70 torr, HCO_3^- 23 mEq/L, BE 0
    C. pH 7.36, PCO_2 40 torr, PO_2 85 torr, HCO_3^- 24 mEq/L, BE +1
    D. pH 7.38, PCO_2 60 torr, PO_2 57 torr, HCO_3^- 33 mEq/L, BE +10

74. The following data are collected for a patient receiving mechanical ventilation with a volume ventilator:

Mode	Control
VT	800 mL
Ventilator rate	10/min
FiO_2	0.40
Inspiratory flow	40 L/min

    The I:E ratio with the use of these ventilator settings is which of the following?

    A. 1:1
    B. 1:2
    C. 1:3
    D. 1:4

75. Which of the following is not a hazard of IPPB?

    A. Decreased cardiac output
    B. Increased venous blood return
    C. Excessive ventilation
    D. Gastric insufflation

76. Initiation of an inspiratory pause during mechanical ventilation may be contraindicated in patients with which of the following conditions?

    A. Pulmonary edema
    B. Hypotension
    C. Atelectasis
    D. Hypoxemia

77. What is the most appropriate ventilator VT setting on a 75-kg (165-lb) patient?

    A. 400 mL
    B. 500 mL
    C. 700 mL
    D. 900 mL

78. Which of the following variables, when changed, will alter the inspiratory time on a volume-limited ventilator?

    1. **Rate control**
    2. **Flow control**
    3. **VT control**
    4. **Expiratory resistance control**

    A. 1 and 2 only
    B. 2 and 3 only
    C. 2 and 4 only
    D. 1, 2, and 3

79. Which of the following situations would result in the high-pressure alarm being activated on a volume-limited ventilator?

    1. **Leak in the circuit**
    2. **Patient disconnected from the ventilator**
    3. **Patient coughing**
    4. **Water in the tubing**

    A. 1 and 3 only
    B. 2 and 4 only
    C. 3 and 4 only
    D. 1, 3, and 4 only

80. Which statement concerning the inspiratory hold control on a volume ventilator is *FALSE?*

    A. It may be used to improve oxygenation.
    B. It will increase intrathoracic pressure.
    C. It should result in a decreased $P(A–a)O_2$ gradient.
    D. It is used to calculate tubing compliance.

81. While making O_2 rounds, the respiratory therapist notices that the mist coming from the exhalation ports of a patient's aerosol mask completely disappears as the patient inhales. The therapist should recommend which of the following?

   A. Add a heater to the nebulizer.
   B. Decrease the flow.
   C. Analyze the FiO_2.
   D. Increase the flow.

82. A diabetic patient enters the emergency department breathing deeply at a respiratory rate of 26/min. This type of breathing pattern is referred to as

   A. Kussmaul respiration
   B. Biot respiration
   C. Cheyne-Stokes respiration
   D. Hypopnea

83. The bacterial filter on a ventilator needs to be cleaned. Which of the following cleaning methods would be most appropriate to recommend?

   A. Soaking in glutaraldehyde solution for 20 min
   B. Ethylene oxide gas sterilization
   C. Autoclaving
   D. Pasteurization

84. The following data are obtained from a 32-year-old patient with pneumonia in the ICU using a 60% aerosol mask:

Respiratory rate	28/min	ABGs:	
		pH	7.47
Pulse	108/min	$PaCO_2$	32 torr
		PaO_2	55 torr

   Which of the following would you recommend at this time?

   A. Intubate and institute mechanical ventilation.
   B. Initiate CPAP.
   C. Increase to 70% aerosol mask.
   D. Change to a non-rebreathing mask at 15 L/min.

85. The polarographic O_2 analyzer you are using to analyze a patient's aerosol mask is reading inaccurately. Which of the following would not result in this inaccurate reading?

   A. No electrolyte gel
   B. Torn membrane
   C. Water on the membrane
   D. Dead fuel cell

86. Which of the following processes or agents can sterilize equipment?

   1. **Autoclave**
   2. **Ethylene oxide**
   3. **Glutaraldehyde**
   4. **Alcohol**

   A. 1 and 2 only
   B. 2 and 3 only
   C. 1 and 4 only
   D. 1, 2, and 3

87. If a patient has an ideal breathing pattern, what is the approximate percentage of O_2 delivered with a nasal cannula at 5 L/min?

   A. 28%
   B. 36%
   C. 40%
   D. 45%

88. Which of the following devices delivers the highest percent body humidity?

   A. Pass-over humidifier
   B. Bubble humidifier
   C. Heated wick humidifier
   D. Jet humidifier

89. After turning the O_2 flowmeter completely off, you notice the water in the humidifier is still slightly bubbling. What is the most likely reason for this?

   A. The humidifier lid is not tight.
   B. There is a crack in the humidifier jar.
   C. The wall outlet is loose.
   D. There is a faulty valve seat in the flowmeter.

90. The following data are collected from a patient receiving mechanical ventilation with a volume ventilator:

Mode	Assist/control	ABGs:	
Ventilator rate	12	pH	7.29
		$PaCO_2$	55 torr
VT	750 mL	PaO_2	68 torr
FiO_2	0.40	HCO_3^-	25 mEq/L
		BE	−1

Based on this information, the most appropriate recommendation is which of the following?

A. Increase the FiO_2.
B. Add PEEP.
C. Increase the VT.
D. Decrease the ventilator rate.

91. A 26-year-old patient has been experiencing a moderate asthmatic attack for 30 min. Which of the following ABG results would you expect to observe if the patient was breathing room air?

	pH	$PaCO_2$ (torr)	PaO_2 (torr)
A.	7.42	44	81
B.	7.08	24	50
C.	7.51	27	60
D.	7.27	52	63

92. The respiratory therapist is performing a leak test on a volume ventilator. Which adjustment should the therapist make to the ventilator?

A. Set the high-pressure limit to its maximal level.
B. Set the rate control to its maximal level.
C. Set the flow control to its maximal level.
D. Remove the test lung from the circuit.

93. If a patient's $PaCO_2$ decreases to 27 torr, all of the following could have increased *EXCEPT*

A. Physiologic dead space
B. Alveolar ventilation
C. Respiratory rate
D. VT

94. Which of the following oxygen delivery devices should be recommended for a patient brought into the emergency department with a smoke inhalation injury?

A. Venturi mask
B. Nasal cannula
C. Simple O_2 mask
D. Non-rebreathing mask

95. Hazards associated with aerosol therapy include all of the following *EXCEPT*

A. Fluid overload in infants
B. Bronchospasm
C. Swelling of dried, retained secretions
D. Bradycardia

96. If a small hole is present in the exhalation valve diaphragm of an IPPB circuit, the machine

A. Automatically cycles into exhalation
B. Cycles into exhalation prematurely on each breath
C. Delivers an increased inspiratory pressure to the patient
D. Does not cycle into exhalation

97. Which of the following organisms is most frequently cultured from heated nebulizers and humidifiers?

A. *Staphylococcus aureus*
B. *Pseudomonas aeruginosa*
C. *Mycobacterium tuberculosis*
D. *Serratia marcescens*

98. The following data are obtained from a 36-week-old infant who is receiving mechanical ventilation with a pressure ventilator in the neonatal ICU:

Mode	IMV	ABGs:	
Inspiratory pressure	26 cm H_2O	pH	7.45
		$PaCO_2$	36 torr
FiO_2	0.60	PaO_2	98 torr
PEEP	8 cm H_2O		
Ventilator rate	35/min		

Which of the following should the respiratory therapist recommend at this time?

A. Decrease PIP to 20 cm H_2O.
B. Decrease PEEP to 6 cm H_2O.
C. Increase the ventilator rate to 40/min.
D. Decrease FiO_2 to 0.50.

99. The following arterial blood gas result is obtained from a patient breathing room air:

pH	7.38
$PaCO_2$	64 torr
PaO_2	55 torr
HCO_3^-	36 mEq/L
BE	+10

These values are consistent with which of the following conditions?

A. Chronic respiratory acidemia
B. Chronic metabolic alkalemia
C. Acute respiratory acidemia
D. Acute metabolic alkalemia

100. The respiratory therapist is administering IPPB therapy to a postoperative patient using a mouthpiece. During the treatment, the patient is unable to cycle the machine off. What could be done to correct this problem?

1. **Check for a leak in the system.**
2. **Check the exhalation valve function.**
3. **Decrease the cycling pressure to 10 cm H_2O.**
4. **Adjust the sensitivity.**

A. 1 only
B. 3 only
C. 1 and 2 only
D. 2 and 4 only

101. While delivering a bronchodilating agent to a patient using a handheld nebulizer, you note the pulse increases from 72/min to 88/min over the first 5 min of therapy. Which of the following is the most appropriate action to take?

A. Stop the treatment immediately and notify the physician.
B. Continue the treatment as ordered.
C. Increase the inspiratory pressure for the remainder of the treatment.
D. Give the remainder of the treatment with saline only.

102. A postoperative patient is to be treated for the prevention of atelectasis. The patient is still heavily sedated. Which type of therapy should be recommended?

A. Flutter valve
B. Incentive spirometry
C. PEP
D. IPPB

103. Which of the following can be determined from a forced expiratory spirogram?

1. **FEV_1**
2. **$FEF_{200-1200}$**
3. **FRC**
4. **Diffusion capacity**

A. 1 only
B. 1 and 2 only
C. 3 and 4 only
D. 1, 2, and 4

104. A patient with COPD is admitted because of a fever, coughing, and mild confusion. O_2 is administered via a nasal cannula at 5 L/min. One-half hour later the patient is less alert. ABG analysis is as follows

	On admission (room air)	**With nasal cannula (5 L/min)**
pH	7.30	7.23
$PaCO_2$	65 torr	76 torr
PaO_2	36 torr	46 torr
HCO_3^-	34 mEq/L	34 mEq/L
BE	+9	+9

The most appropriate change in the patient's treatment would be to

A. Use a 28% Venturi mask
B. Decrease the O_2 flow to 2 L/min
C. Use a non-rebreathing mask at 10 L/min
D. Institute mechanical ventilation with an FiO_2 of 0.40

105. A nebulizer is set on the 40% dilution mode and connected to an O_2 flowmeter running at 12 L/min. What is the total flow output of this nebulizer?

A. 24 L/min
B. 36 L/min
C. 48 L/min
D. 54 L/min

106. A patient receiving mechanical ventilation has the following ABG values

pH	7.54
$PaCO_2$	26 torr
PaO_2	102 torr
HCO_3^-	24 mEq/L
BE	0

All of the following ventilator changes would help correct this *EXCEPT*

A. Increasing the respiratory rate
B. Decreasing the VT
C. Instituting SIMV
D. Adding mechanical dead space

107. A humidifier will not bubble if

A. The capillary tube is plugged
B. The pop-off valve is open
C. The O_2 tubing is cracked
D. The reservoir jar is loose

108. A patient has a VT of 450 mL and a respiratory rate that fluctuates between 15/min and 25/min. Which of the following is the best device for the administration of a controlled O_2 percentage?

A. Partial rebreathing mask
B. Simple O_2 mask
C. Venturi mask
D. Nasal cannula

109. A patient begins using a non-rebreathing mask at 15 L/min. An ABG analysis reveals a PaO_2 of 580 torr. The respiratory therapist should recommend which of the following?

A. Decrease the flow rate to 10 L/min.
B. Change to a partial rebreathing mask at 10 L/min.
C. Change to simple O_2 mask at 8 L/min.
D. Discontinue O_2 therapy.

110. A patient with bronchiectasis has been receiving postural drainage and percussion for 2 days. The patient's chest radiograph has not shown improvement, and he still is having difficulty expectorating sputum. Which of the following therapies may be of benefit in the treatment of this patient?

1. **Intrapulmonary percussive ventilation (IPV)**
2. **Flutter valve device**
3. **PEP therapy**

A. 1 only
B. 1 and 2 only
C. 2 and 3 only
D. 1, 2, and 3

111. While preparing to analyze the O_2 concentration on a patient's aerosol mask, you notice water in the aerosol tubing. What effect does this have on the operation of this device?

A. Decreases the FiO_2
B. Increases the FiO_2
C. Increases air entrainment into the nebulizer
D. Increases gas flow to the patient

112. The following data are obtained from an infant in the neonatal ICU receiving mechanical ventilation with a pressure ventilator:

Mode	IMV	ABGs:	
PIP	20 cm H_2O	pH	7.29
Ventilator rate	40/min	$PaCO_2$	51 torr
		PaO_2	53 torr
FiO_2	0.40	HCO_3^-	22 mEq/L
PEEP	5 cm H_2O	BE	+1

On the basis of these data, which of the following would you recommend at this time?

A. Increase FiO_2 to 0.60.
B. Decrease the ventilator rate to 35/min.
C. Increase PEEP to 8 cm H_2O.
D. Increase PIP to 24 cm H_2O.

113. To minimize an increased airway resistance produced by high-density aerosol inhalation, the respiratory therapist should

A. Use a bronchodilator in conjunction with the aerosol
B. Instruct the patient to breathe through the nose
C. Use a heated aerosol
D. Perform chest physical therapy after the aerosol treatment

114. A patient's heated nebulizer is delivering 41 mg H_2O per liter of gas. The percentage of body humidity delivered by this device is

A. 32%
B. 41%
C. 64%
D. 93%

115. A patient arrives in the emergency department after being pulled from a burning house. The respiratory therapist places a pulse oximeter on the patient's earlobe and obtains an SpO_2 reading of 98%. Blood for ABG analysis is drawn, and the SaO_2 analyzed by co-oximetry is 76%. Which of the following is the most likely reason for the discrepancy in the two saturation readings?

    A. The oximeter needs to be calibrated.
    B. The co-oximeter electrode is out of calibration.
    C. There is an elevated HbCO level.
    D. The pulse oximeter probe is loose.

116. The respiratory therapist is monitoring the hemodynamic status of a patient who has just been transfused with packed red blood cells. Following the transfusion, the patient's PvO_2 increases from 31 torr to 36 torr. The therapist should conclude which of the following has occurred?

    A. Intrapulmonary shunting has increased.
    B. Cardiac output has decreased.
    C. V/Q mismatching has increased.
    D. Oxygen delivery to the tissues has increased.

117. A patient with a broken nose and cheekbone is ordered to have 40% O_2 initiated. The patient's secretions are thick. On the basis of this information, which O_2 delivery device would be indicated?

    A. Nasal cannula at 5 L/min
    B. Face tent
    C. Simple O_2 mask at 8 L/min
    D. Aerosol mask

118. The following pulmonary function data are obtained from a patient before and after bronchodilator therapy:

	Before	After
FVC	37% of predicted	53% of predicted
FEV_1	42% of predicted	56% of predicted
FEV_1/FVC	40%	55%

    Which of the following is the correct interpretation of these results?

    A. Severe obstructive disease, significant bronchodilator response
    B. Severe restrictive disease, no bronchodilator response
    C. Moderate obstructive disease, no bronchodilator response
    D. Severe restrictive disease, significant bronchodilator response

119. The respiratory therapist reviews a ventilator flow sheet and observes that the peak inspiratory pressure has been gradually increasing over the past several hours with no change in the static pressure. Which of the following should the therapist conclude?

    A. The lungs are becoming harder to ventilate.
    B. Lung compliance is decreasing.
    C. Atelectasis is most likely developing.
    D. Airway resistance is increasing.

120. Which device is not connected to a humidifier.

    A. Simple O_2 mask at 8 L/min
    B. T-piece (Briggs adapter)
    C. Partial rebreathing mask at 12 L/min
    D. Nasal cannula at 6 L/min

121. Which of the following respiratory medications is not considered a bronchodilating agent?

    A. Metaproterenol (Alupent)
    B. Ipratropium bromide (Atrovent)
    C. Terbutaline sulfate (Brethine)
    D. Acetylcysteine (Mucomyst)

122. A patient is breathing 16 times per minute and has a VT of 450 mL. What is this patient's minute ventilation?

    A. 4.2 L
    B. 6.1 L
    C. 7.2 L
    D. 8.6 L

123. A patient is breathing spontaneously using a 50% aerosol mask with the following ABG results

pH	7.36
$PaCO_2$	43 torr
PaO_2	48 torr
HCO_3^-	24 mEq/L

    Based on this information, the most appropriate recommendation is which of the following?

    A. Initiate CPAP.
    B. Increase the O_2 percentage to 70%.
    C. Have the patient begin using a non-rebreathing mask.
    D. Have the patient begin using a simple O_2 mask at 10 L/min.

124. A patient is receiving mechanical ventilation with the following settings:

VT	750 mL
Respiratory rate	12/min
Mode	Assist/control
PEEP	10 cm H_2O
FiO_2	0.60

ABG results on these settings are as follows:

pH	7.41
$PaCO_2$	38 torr
PaO_2	174 torr

Based on this information, what would be the appropriate ventilator change?

A. Decrease PEEP to 8 cm H_2O.
B. Decrease FiO_2 to 0.50.
C. Decrease VT to 650 mL.
D. Increase inspiratory flow.

125. The reduction in urinary output caused by mechanical ventilation may be the result of

1. **Decreased renal blood flow**
2. **Decreased production of ADH**
3. **Increased renal blood flow**
4. **Increased production of ADH**

A. 1 only
B. 1 and 4 only
C. 2 and 3 only
D. 3 and 4 only

126. Which values indicate that a patient is ready to be weaned from mechanical ventilation?

1. **VD/VT ratio of .45**
2. **MIP of −31 cm H_2O**
3. **P(A−a)O_2 of 460 mm Hg with the use of 100% O_2**
4. **Vital capacity of 8 mL/kg of body weight**

A. 1 and 2 only
B. 2 and 3 only
C. 1, 2, and 4 only
D. 2, 3, and 4 only

127. A patient is using a volume ventilator set on a tidal volume of 800 mL, but the exhaled volume display is reading 500 mL. The respiratory therapist wants to determine the volume that the ventilator is actually delivering. To most accurately measure this volume, the therapist should place a respirometer

A. At the exhalation valve.
B. At the patient wye connector.
C. At the ventilator outlet.
D. At the humidifier outlet.

128. A patient is receiving mechanical ventilation with a volume ventilator in the control mode. The low-pressure alarm is sounding. Which of the following may be the cause of the alarm activation?

A. Water in the tubing
B. Patient disconnected from the ventilator
C. Secretions in the patient's airway
D. Kink in the ventilator tubing

129. The respiratory therapist is preparing to suction an intubated patient. Which of the following steps in the procedure is most important?

A. Lubricate the catheter with a water-soluble gel before suctioning.
B. Oxygenate the patient before and after the procedure.
C. Instill normal saline down the ET tube before suctioning.
D. Suction the oropharynx after ET tube suctioning.

130. You have just obtained blood from the patient's radial artery to determine ABG results. As you run the blood through the blood gas analyzer, you notice you failed to remove an air bubble from the sample. The blood gas results will most likely reflect values with a

A. High pH and low PO_2
B. Low PCO_2 and low PO_2
C. Low PCO_2 and high PO_2
D. High PCO_2 and high PO_2

131. You are monitoring a patient with Guillain-Barré syndrome for signs of respiratory impairment. Which one of the following variables would signal the earliest indication?

A. PaO_2
B. $PaCO_2$
C. MIP
D. VT

Questions 132–134 relate to the following situation:

A 36-year-old, 65-kg (143-lb) unconscious man is admitted to the emergency department. His breathing rate is 8/min and very shallow. A drug overdose is suspected.

132. To maintain a patent airway, what type of device should be employed?

    A. Bite block
    B. Oropharyngeal airway
    C. Tongue depressor
    D. Esophageal obturator airway

133. The patient becomes apneic and mechanical ventilatory support is required. How would the airway best be maintained at this time?

    A. CPAP mask
    B. Cuffed ET tube
    C. Uncuffed ET tube
    D. Fenestrated tracheostomy tube

134. The most appropriate ventilator settings would be which of the following?

    A. VT 600 mL, rate 8, control mode
    B. VT 800 mL, rate 6, control mode
    C. VT 700 mL, rate 12, assist/control mode
    D. VT 1000 mL, rate 14, assist/control mode

Questions 135–137 relate to the following situation:

A 48-year-old, 75-kg (165-lb) woman is in the ICU after coronary bypass surgery. The patient is to receive mechanical ventilation.

135. As you connect the patient to the ventilator, you notice the peak inspiratory pressure is registering only 10 cm H_2O on the manometer and the exhaled volume display is showing 300 mL less than the ventilator volume setting. Which of the following could be causing this problem?

    1. There is a leak around the humidifier.
    2. The medication nebulizer is not connected tightly.
    3. There is no water in the humidifier.

    A. 1 only
    B. 2 only
    C. 1 and 2 only
    D. 2 and 3 only

136. During ventilator checks 6 h later, you notice the peak inspiratory pressure has been gradually increasing. What could be the cause of this occurrence?

    1. Bronchospasm
    2. Accumulation of secretions
    3. Increasing pulmonary compliance
    4. Decreasing airway resistance

    A. 1 and 2 only
    B. 2 and 3 only
    C. 3 and 4 only
    D. 1, 2, and 3 only

137. The following day, the patient begins T-tube flow-by for weaning purposes. During this time, the patient's respiratory rate increases to 30/min and her blood pressure begins to drop. What is the appropriate measure to take at this time?

    A. Initiate SIMV at a rate of 10/min.
    B. Obtain a stat chest film.
    C. Initiate CPAP.
    D. Institute control mode at a rate of 10/min.

Questions 138–140 relate to the following situation:

A 17-year-old boy with multiple rib fractures is admitted to the emergency department after a motor vehicle accident. An ABG analysis reveals the following results with the patient breathing room air:

pH	7.50
$PaCO_2$	30 torr
PaO_2	44 torr
HCO_3^-	25 mEq/L
BE	+1

138. These data indicate which of the following?

    1. Decreased $P(A-a)O_2$
    2. Hyperventilation
    3. Respiratory acidosis

    A. 1 only
    B. 2 only
    C. 1 and 2 only
    D. 2 and 3 only

139. The patient's condition has deteriorated and mechanical ventilation is initiated. What variables should the respiratory therapist determine at this time?

    1. **VT required by patient**
    2. **Patient's FVC**
    3. **Patient's MIP**
    4. **Minute ventilation required by patient**

    A. 1 and 2 only
    B. 2 and 3 only
    C. 1 and 4 only
    D. 1, 2, and 3 only

140. Six days later, the physician is considering weaning this patient from the ventilator. The following data are collected

MIP	-30 cm H_2O
VC	3.0 L
Mode	Assist/control
Ventilator rate	12/min
VT	650 mL
FiO$_2$	0.35
pH	7.38
PaCO$_2$	41 torr
PaO$_2$	86 torr
HCO$_3^-$	24 mEq/L
BE	0

    On the basis of this information, the therapist should recommend which of the following?

    A. Institute SIMV.
    B. Continue mechanical ventilation on assist/control.
    C. Increase the VT.
    D. Add PEEP of 4 cm H_2O.

141. After PEEP is initiated for a patient, the respiratory therapist should expect which of the following to occur?

    1. **Increased FRC**
    2. **Increased plateau pressure**
    3. **Increased lung compliance**
    4. **Decreased A–a gradient**

    A. 1 and 2 only
    B. 3 and 4 only
    C. 1, 3, and 4 only
    D. 2, 3, and 4 only

142. A 70-kg (154-lb) patient in the ICU is receiving mechanical ventilation with a volume ventilator in the assist/control mode, rate of 10/min, tidal volume of 700 mL, PEEP of 5 cm H_2O, and 50% oxygen. Arterial blood gas levels are as follows:

pH	7.52
PaCO$_2$	31 torr
PaO$_2$	57 torr
HCO$_3^-$	23 mEq/L
BE	-1

    Which of the following ventilator changes is most appropriate at this time?

    A. Increase the oxygen to 60%.
    B. Decrease the tidal volume to 600 mL.
    C. Increase the PEEP to 10 cm H_2O.
    D. Decrease the ventilator rate to 8/min.

143. A patient has a pH of 7.18 and a PaCO$_2$ of 24 torr. Which of the following can be concluded regarding this blood gas data?

    A. Respiratory acidosis is present.
    B. The patient is hypoventilating.
    C. Metabolic acidosis is present.
    D. The base excess must be increased.

144. An alert, spontaneously breathing patient has a PaCO$_2$ of 33 torr and a PaO$_2$ of 55 torr while receiving an FiO$_2$ of 0.70. Which of the following is the most appropriate way to increase the patient's PaO$_2$?

    A. Increase the FiO$_2$ only.
    B. Intubate and increase the FiO$_2$.
    C. Apply CPAP at 60% oxygen.
    D. Apply CPAP at 100% oxygen.

145. The respiratory therapist is assessing the patient's spontaneous ventilatory variables. The PaCO$_2$ is 50 mm Hg, the PETCO$_2$ is 30 mm Hg, and the tidal volume is 600 mL. What is the patient's dead space volume?

    A. 150 mL
    B. 240 mL
    C. 360 mL
    D. 480 mL

146. The following data have been collected from a patient receiving mechanical ventilation with a volume ventilator:

		ABGs:	
VT	650 mL		
		pH	7.37
Mode	SIMV	PaCO$_2$	38 torr
Ventilator rate	10/min	HCO$_3^-$	26 mEq/L
		BE	+2
PaO$_2$	148 torr		
FiO$_2$	0.75		
PEEP	12 cm H$_2$O		

Based on this data, the most appropriate recommendation is which of the following?

A. Decrease PEEP to 8 cm H$_2$O.
B. Decrease SIMV rate to 8/min.
C. Decrease VT to 600 mL.
D. Decrease FiO$_2$ to 0.65.

147. The high-pressure alarm on a volume-cycled ventilator should be set approximately 10 cm H$_2$O pressure above which of the following?

A. PEEP level
B. Plateau pressure
C. Mean airway pressure
D. Peak airway pressure

148. A chest x-ray film reveals that the tip of the patient's ET tube is located at the level of the fourth rib. The respiratory therapist observes that the tube is taped at the teeth at the 27-cm mark. What is the most appropriate action to take?

A. Withdraw the tube to the 23-cm mark.
B. Advance the tube 2 cm.
C. Make no changes to the tube position.
D. Withdraw the tube to the 18-cm mark.

149. While assessing a patient's chest radiograph, you observe an area of hyperlucency. This may be the result of which of the following?

1. **Hyperinflation**
2. **Atelectasis**
3. **Emphysema**
4. **Pneumothorax**

A. 1 and 3 only
B. 2 and 3 only
C. 1, 3, and 4 only
D. 2, 3, and 4 only

150. The respiratory therapist is called to a patient's room to check the oxygen setup. The flow to the patient's mask is supplied by an air flowmeter running at 10 L/min and an O$_2$ flowmeter running at 10 L/min. The delivered oxygen percentage from this device is

A. 24%
B. 35%
C. 40%
D. 60%

151. A patient with severe COPD is using a 28% air entrainment mask and has a PaO$_2$ of 61 torr. Which of the following should the respiratory therapist recommend at this time?

A. Initiate CPAP.
B. No changes are required at this time.
C. Increase O$_2$ to 40%.
D. Have the patient begin using a non-rebreathing mask.

152. The respiratory therapist is called to the pediatric ICU to suction an 8-year-old ventilator patient with pneumonia who is intubated with a 6.0 ET tube. Which of the following represents the most appropriate catheter size and suction pressure to use on this patient?

A. 8 Fr catheter, −100 mm Hg
B. 10 Fr catheter, −60 mm Hg
C. 8 Fr catheter, −80 mm Hg
D. 10 Fr catheter, −100 mm Hg

153. The respiratory therapist has received an order for postural drainage and percussion for a 34-year-old patient whose chest x-ray film indicates atelectasis of the posterior basal segment of the right lower lobe. The patient should be placed in which of the following positions to help drain this segment?

A. Lying on left side with bed flat
B. Prone, with head of bed down
C. Lying on left side with head of bed down
D. Supine, with head of bed down

154. The respiratory therapist is performing bag-mask ventilation on a patient with severe COPD during CPR. Which of the following describes the best method for ventilating the lungs of this patient?

   A. The bag should be connected to an air flowmeter.
   B. The flow to the bag should be 10 L/min with no reservoir attachment.
   C. The bag should be connected to an O_2 blender set at 30%.
   D. The bag should have a reservoir attachment and a flow of 15 L/min.

155. A patient is brought into the emergency department after being pulled from a burning house. The patient's ABG results with a non-rebreathing mask are as follows: pH, 7.23; $PaCO_2$, 21 torr; PaO_2, 197 torr; HCO_3^-, 10 mEq/L; SaO_2, 65%. From this information, which of the following statements are true?

   1. The patient should begin using a simple O_2 mask at 10 L/min.
   2. The SpO_2 should be measured because of the discrepancy in the PaO_2 and SaO_2.
   3. The patient is hyperventilating because of severe hypoxia.
   4. The blood gas levels reveal a partially compensated respiratory acidemia.

   A. 3 only
   B. 1 and 4 only
   C. 3 and 4 only
   D. 2, 3, and 4 only

156. Neonatal retinopathy can be prevented if the PaO_2 does not exceed what level?

   A. 50 torr
   B. 60 torr
   C. 70 torr
   D. 80 torr

157. After administering a bland aerosol treatment to a patient, the respiratory therapist auscultates bilateral rhonchi. The therapist should recommend which of the following?

   A. Discontinue the treatment and initiate IPPB therapy.
   B. Encourage the patient to deep breath and cough.
   C. Initiate bronchodilator therapy.
   D. Discontinue the therapy.

158. While ventilating the lungs of an intubated apneic patient with a manual resuscitator, you notice very little resistance when the bag is compressed and the patient's chest rises only minimally. Which of the following may be the cause of this problem?

   A. Excessive ET tube cuff pressure.
   B. The exhalation valve is jammed in the closed position.
   C. The patient's lung compliance is decreased.
   D. Inadequate ET tube cuff pressure.

159. The respiratory therapist is called to the emergency department to assess a 3-year-old child who was pulled from the bottom of a swimming pool. He is unresponsive and pale and has peripheral cyanosis. Vital signs are as follows

Heart rate	50/min
Blood pressure	58/26 mm Hg
Respiratory rate	10/min with intercostal retractions
Temperature	33° C (91.4° F)

   Which of the following treatments are appropriate?

   1. Endotracheal intubation
   2. Heated aerosol mask at 100% O_2
   3. Manual ventilation with 100% O_2
   4. Chest compressions

   A. 1 and 3 only
   B. 2 and 4 only
   C. 1 and 4 only
   D. 1, 3, and 4 only

160. The following data are collected from a 75-kg (165-lb) patient using a 40% aerosol mask:

VT	500 mL
Respiratory rate	12

   This patient's alveolar minute ventilation is which of the following?

   A. 4.0 L
   B. 5.0 L
   C. 6.0 L
   D. 7.0 L

END OF ENTRY LEVEL PRACTICE EXAM.
FOR ANSWER KEY/RATIONALES, GO TO
THIS SECTION ON EVOLVE EXAM REVIEW.

ADVANCED PRACTITIONER WRITTEN REGISTRY EXAM: PRACTICE TEST

TIME LIMIT: 2 HOURS

Exam Note

The NBRC Advanced Practitioner Written Registry Exam comprises 115 questions, 15 of which do not figure into the final score. The final score is based on 100 questions. The minimum passing score for the RRT Examination is 70%. To simulate the length of the RRT Exam, this practice test consists of 115 questions and all questions figure into your final score.

 1 torr = 1 mm Hg

Directions: Each of the questions or incomplete statements below is followed by four suggested answers or completions. Select the best answer.

1. While evaluating a patient's cardiopulmonary status, the respiratory therapist determines that the patient has a 6-s capillary refill time. This reflects which of the following conditions?

   A. Increased QT
   B. Decreased peripheral perfusion
   C. Hypertension
   D. Sufficient perfusion to the extremities

2. While making O_2 rounds, the respiratory therapist notices that the reservoir bag on the patient's non-rebreathing mask completely deflates as the patient inspires. Which of the following should the therapist recommend at this time?

   A. Change to partial rebreathing mask.
   B. Instruct the patient to take more shallow breaths.
   C. Increase flow to the mask.
   D. Remove the one-way valve between the bag and the mask.

3. Continuous monitoring of a neonate's PaO_2 is best achieved by the use of which of the following methods?

   A. Transcutaneous monitoring
   B. Pulse oximetry
   C. Capnography
   D. Pulmonary artery catheter

4. The respiratory therapist palpates no pulse on a patient, but the ECG oscilloscope monitor shows QRS complexes on the tracing. The therapist should

   A. Get stat ABG studies
   B. Administer a stat IPPB treatment with atropine
   C. Begin cardiac compressions
   D. Recommend a stat chest radiograph

5. A patient is being administered CPAP via mask at 8 cm H_2O. The low-pressure alarm is sounding, and the manometer is reading 2 cm H_2O. Which of the following may be causing this situation?

   1. **Excessive flow**
   2. **Loose-fitting mask**
   3. **Leak around tubing connection**
   4. **Inappropriate low-pressure alarm setting**

   A. 1 and 2 only
   B. 2 and 3 only
   C. 2 and 4 only
   D. 2, 3, and 4 only

6. Which of the following statements regarding a pulse-dose O_2 system is true?

   A. O_2 is delivered to the patient only as the patient inspires.
   B. Higher flows are required for equivalent O_2 concentrations.
   C. A nasal cannula cannot be used as an O_2 delivery device with this system.
   D. The system cannot be incorporated with O_2 cylinders.

7. The respiratory therapist is setting up a portable liquid oxygen system for a patient with a chronic lung condition who attends church each week. The patient is using a 2 L/min nasal cannula, and the portable oxygen container holds 4 lb of oxygen. The therapist should explain to the patient that the oxygen supply will last for approximately what length of time?

   A. 4.5 h
   B. 8 h
   C. 11.5 h
   D. 14 h

8. While reviewing a patient's chart, the respiratory therapist notices that the patient's Hb level is 20 g/dL and SpO_2 is 80%. Which of the following is *true* regarding this situation?

   A. The patient is most likely cyanotic.
   B. The patient is hypoxic.
   C. The patient is hyperventilating.
   D. The patient has a normal HbO_2 level.

9. A patient enters the emergency department after a motor vehicle accident in mild respiratory distress and complaining of soreness on the left side of the chest. Auscultation of breath sounds reveals diminished breath sounds in the left lung. After administering O_2 to the patient, the respiratory therapist should recommend which of the following first?

   A. IPPB with a bronchodilator
   B. Stat chest radiograph
   C. CBC
   D. CPAP at 4 cm H_2O

10. A patient is using a 30% air entrainment mask with an O_2 flow of 4 L/min. The total flow being delivered by this O_2 setup is which of the following?

    A. 16 L/min
    B. 24 L/min
    C. 36 L/min
    D. 44 L/min

11. A patient is having difficulty cycling the IPPB machine into the inspiratory phase. The respiratory therapist should adjust which of the following controls?

    A. Sensitivity
    B. Flow rate
    C. Inspiratory pressure
    D. Air dilution

12. The following ABG results are obtained from an adult patient using a 50% aerosol mask:

pH	7.45
$PaCO_2$	34 torr
PaO_2	57 torr
HCO_3^-	25 mEq/L
BE	+2

    On the basis of these data, the respiratory therapist should recommend which of the following?

    A. Administer a stat IPPB treatment.
    B. Increase O_2 to 70%.
    C. Institute CPAP mask.
    D. Have the patient begin using a 100% non-rebreathing mask.

13. A 58-year-old patient with emphysema enters the emergency department using a 2-L/min nasal cannula. Blood for ABG analysis is drawn, and after the results are evaluated, the O_2 flow is increased to 5 L/min. Below are ABG results for both flow rates:

	(2 L/min)	(5 L/min)
pH	7.34	7.28
$PaCO_2$	62 torr	77 torr
PaO_2	44 torr	52 torr
HCO_3^-	35 mEq/L	35 mEq/L
BE	+10	+10

    On the basis of these data, which of the following should the respiratory therapist recommend?

    A. Decrease the liter flow to 3 L/min.
    B. Initiate CPAP at 4 cm H_2O and 60% O_2.
    C. Increase the liter flow to 6 L/min.
    D. Institute noninvasive ventilation.

14. A 34-year-old female patient enters the emergency department complaining of severe chest pain. The patient is given a 50% air entrainment mask. Thirty minutes later, blood is drawn and the ABG results are as follows:

pH	7.50
$PaCO_2$	31 torr
PaO_2	253 torr
HCO_3^-	24 mEq/L
BE	−1

Which of the following is a true statement regarding these ABG results?

A. The results appear to be accurate and consistent with the FiO_2.
B. The PaO_2 is too high for the FiO_2.
C. The $PaCO_2$ is not consistent with the pH.
D. The results represent a metabolic alkalosis.

15. A patient in the cardiac ICU is intubated and is receiving mechanical ventilation with 40% O_2. The following data have been collected:

pH	7.41	HCO_3^-	23 mEq/L
$PaCO_2$	37 torr	$C(a–v)O_2$	8.1 vol%
PaO_2	81 torr	PCWP	2 mm Hg
		BE	−2

On the basis of these data, the respiratory therapist should recommend which of the following?

A. Administer a diuretic.
B. Institute PEEP at 5 cm H_2O.
C. Administer fluids.
D. Increase the FiO_2.

16. The physician wants to wean a patient from a ventilator. Which of the following variables obtained by the respiratory therapist indicate weaning will most likely be successful?

1. **MIP of −28 cm H_2O**
2. **P(A–a)O_2 of less than 200 torr with the use of 100% O_2**
3. **Vital capacity of 19 mL/kg body weight**

A. 1 only
B. 1 and 3 only
C. 2 and 3 only
D. 1, 2, and 3

17. The respiratory therapist is calibrating a helium analyzer. When calibrated to room air, the analyzer should read

A. 0%
B. 21%
C. 79%
D. 100%

18. A 43-year-old patient in ICU is receiving 40% O_2 by air entrainment mask. His PaO_2 is 58 torr, and his shunt has been calculated to be 6%. Which of the following is most likely causing his hypoxemia?

A. Pulmonary edema
B. Lobar pneumonia
C. Pneumothorax
D. Hypoventilation

19. A V/Q scan is conducted on a patient in whom pulmonary embolism is suspected. The scan shows normal ventilation and the absence of perfusion in the left upper lobe. The respiratory therapist should estimate the V/Q ratio in this area to be which of the following?

A. Less than 0.5
B. 0.8
C. 1.0
D. More than 2.0

20. While making ventilator checks, the respiratory therapist measures the ET-tube cuff pressure to be 40 mm Hg. At peak inspiratory pressure, air is passing around the cuff. Which of the following actions should the therapist take at this time?

A. Decrease cuff pressure to 20 mm Hg.
B. Add more air to the cuff to stop the leak.
C. Recommend changing to a larger tube.
D. Maintain the cuff pressure at 40 mm Hg.

21. The respiratory therapist is asked to assess a 30-week gestational age infant with persistent pulmonary hypertension of the newborn (PPHN). Which of the following would you recommend to help treat this condition?

1. **Permissive hypercapnia**
2. **Nitric oxide**
3. **Pre- and postductal oxygenation study**
4. **Hyperventilation**

A. 1 only
B. 1 and 3 only
C. 2 and 4 only
D. 2, 3 and 4 only

22. The following data are collected from an infant receiving mechanical ventilation with a pressure ventilator:

Mode	IMV
Ventilator rate	35/min
Inspiratory pressure	26 cm H_2O
PEEP	6 cm H_2O
FiO_2	0.40
pH	7.27
$PaCO_2$	52 torr
PaO_2	47 torr
HCO_3^-	22 mEq/L

On the basis of these data, the respiratory therapist should recommend which of the following?

A. Decrease PEEP to 4 cm H_2O.
B. Increase the ventilator rate to 40/min.
C. Decrease inspiratory pressure to 22 cm H_2O.
D. Decrease the inspiratory flow.

23. After assisting the physician with a bronchoscopy, the respiratory therapist should disinfect the bronchoscope with which of the following techniques?

A. Wipe down with alcohol.
B. Wipe down with povidone-iodine (Betadine) solution.
C. Soak in glutaraldehyde for 15 to 20 min.
D. Steam autoclave for 15 min.

24. A patient with a peak inspiratory flow of 40 L/min is to be given O_2 with a 30% air entrainment mask. What is the minimum O_2 flow required to meet the patient's inspiratory flow demands?

A. 3 L/min
B. 5 L/min
C. 8 L/min
D. 10 L/min

25. The RCP is performing postural drainage and percussion on a patient with right lower lobe atelectasis and observes the tracing below on the cardiac monitor.

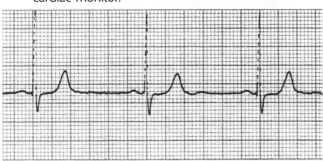

This heart rhythm is most likely the result of which of the following?

A. Vagal stimulation
B. Hypoxemia
C. Loose ECG lead
D. Artifact from patient movement

26. The respiratory therapist has just completed assisting the physician with a bronchoscopy on a ventilator patient and notices the high-pressure alarm is activated. This increased pressure could be the result of all of the following *EXCEPT*

A. Pneumothorax
B. Bronchospasm
C. Hypotension
D. Pulmonary hemorrhage

27. The following data have been collected from a patient in the cardiac ICU:

pH	7.42
$PaCO_2$	42 torr
PaO_2	70 torr
HCO_3^-	25 mEq/L
SaO_2	93%
PvO_2	34 torr
SvO_2	72%
$P(A-a)O_2$	100 torr
Hb	14 g/dL

Based on these data, which of the following represents this patient's intrapulmonary shunt?

A. 4%
B. 7%
C. 9%
D. 12%

28. After a cardiac arrest, a 48-year-old female begins receiving mechanical ventilation. A pulmonary artery catheter is in place. The following data are obtained

BP	94/52 mm Hg
Pulse	116/min
PCWP	6 mm Hg
PAP	40/22 mm Hg
QT	3.5 L/min

Based on these data, which of the following has increased?

A. Pulmonary vascular resistance
B. Left atrial pressure
C. Stroke volume
D. Systemic vascular resistance

29. A tall, thin, otherwise healthy 24-year-old man enters the emergency department complaining of chest pain with mild respiratory distress. A chest radiograph reveals a spontaneous pneumothorax of approximately 10%. Which of the following should the respiratory therapist recommend?

1. **O_2 therapy**
2. **Needle aspiration**
3. **Chest tube insertion**
4. **Continuous pulse oximetry**

A. 2 and 3 only
B. 1 and 4 only
C. 1, 2, and 3 only
D. 1, 3, and 4 only

30. The respiratory therapist is having difficulty intubating a patient who is in respiratory failure. In place of an ET tube, which of the following should be inserted to facilitate the most effective manual ventilation?

A. Esophageal tracheal Combitube
B. Nasopharyngeal airway
C. Oropharyngeal airway
D. Nasogastric airway

31. An infant has just been delivered at 30 weeks' gestation and appears cyanotic. While administering O_2, the respiratory therapist should recommend which of the following?

A. Obtain a chest x-ray film.
B. Determine the Apgar score of the infant.
C. Obtain ABG analysis.
D. Insert a UAC.

32. A patient with chest trauma is receiving mechanical ventilation with a volume ventilator. The VT is 800 mL, and the returned exhaled volume is 500 mL. Which of the following could be causing this problem?

A. Inadequate inspiratory flow
B. Leak around chest tube
C. Excessive ET-tube cuff pressure
D. Low humidifier H_2O level

33. The respiratory therapist is having difficulty calibrating a transcutaneous O_2 monitor to room air prior to attaching to an infant. This is most likely because of which of the following?

A. The membrane is torn.
B. The sensor will not stick to the infant's skin properly.
C. There is poor perfusion to the sensor site.
D. The infant is hemodynamically unstable.

34. After administration of 200 J with a defibrillator, ventricular fibrillation continues. Which of the following is the appropriate measure to recommend at this time?

A. Administer $NaHCO_3^-$.
B. Repeat defibrillation with 300 J.
C. Administer intracardiac epinephrine.
D. Repeat defibrillation at 400 J.

35. The following data have been recorded from a patient receiving mechanical ventilation with a volume ventilator:

Mode	Assist/control	pH	7.51
Ventilator rate	10/min	$PaCO_2$	30 torr
VT	750 mL	PaO_2	57 torr
FiO_2	0.60	HCO_3^-	25 mEq/L
PEEP	6 cm H_2O		

Based on this information, the respiratory therapist should recommend which of the following?

A. Increase PEEP to 8 cm H_2O.
B. Decrease the VT to 700 mL.
C. Decrease the rate to 8/min.
D. Increase the FiO_2 to 0.70.

36. The following data have been obtained from a patient receiving mechanical ventilation with a volume ventilator:

PEEP	Peak pressure	Plateau pressure	VT
4 cm H_2O	32 cm H_2O	24 cm H_2O	600 mL
6 cm H_2O	37 cm H_2O	24 cm H_2O	600 mL
8 cm H_2O	43 cm H_2O	28 cm H_2O	600 mL
10 cm H_2O	47 cm H_2O	31 cm H_2O	600 mL

Optimal PEEP is which of the following?

A. 4 cm H_2O
B. 6 cm H_2O
C. 8 cm H_2O
D. 10 cm H_2O

37. The respiratory therapist is assisting the physician in the insertion of a Swan-Ganz catheter. The patient is hemodynamically stable at the time. The therapist would know the catheter tip has entered the pulmonary artery when which of the following pressures is observed?

    A. 12/4 mm Hg
    B. 24/10 mm Hg
    C. 40/0 mm Hg
    D. 110/75 mm Hg

38. A postoperative patient is to be weaned from mechanical ventilation. The following ventilator settings are being used

Mode	SIMV
Ventilator rate	6/min
VT	700 mL
FiO$_2$	0.40
Pressure support	25 cm H$_2$O
ABGs:	
pH	7.44
PaCO$_2$	37 torr
PaO$_2$	97 torr

    Which of the following should the respiratory therapist recommend to begin weaning this patient?

    A. Decrease the FiO$_2$.
    B. Decrease pressure support.
    C. Decrease VT.
    D. Increase inspiratory flow.

39. A patient has the following pulmonary function results:

FVC	56% of predicted
FEV$_1$	53% of predicted
FEV$_1$/FVC	86%
TLC	75% of predicted
Peak flow	108% of predicted

    The most appropriate interpretation of these results is which of the following?

    A. Obstructive disease only
    B. Restrictive disease only
    C. Mixed obstructive and restrictive disease
    D. Normal pulmonary function results

40. A patient with severe COPD is using a 2-L/min nasal cannula. Blood for ABG results is drawn, and after interpretation of the results, the liter flow is increased to 5 L/min; another ABG sample is drawn 1 h later. The ABG results are:

	(2 L/min)	(5 L/min)
pH	7.34	7.28
PaCO$_2$	62 torr	81 torr
PaO$_2$	46 torr	84 torr
HCO$_3^-$	35 mEq/L	35 mEq/L
BE	+12	+12

    While using the 5-L/min cannula, the patient seems lethargic and drowsy. On the basis of this information, the respiratory therapist should recommend which of the following?

    A. Institute noninvasive ventilation.
    B. Give the patient a non-rebreathing mask at 12 L/min.
    C. Decrease liter flow to 3 L/min.
    D. Initiate CPAP at 4 cm H$_2$O with an FiO$_2$ of 0.40.

41. A patient with COPD is extubated after receiving mechanical ventilation for 2 wk. For several hours after extubation, the patient complains of progressively worsening shortness of breath while using a 2-L/min nasal cannula. His respiratory rate has increased from 16/min to 26/min. The most appropriate recommendation is which of the following?

    A. Initiate noninvasive positive pressure ventilation.
    B. Reintubate and begin mechanical ventilation.
    C. Give the patient a non-rebreathing mask.
    D. Begin postural drainage and percussion every 4 h.

42. Independent lung ventilation is indicated with which of the following conditions?

    1. **Unilateral bronchopulmonary fistula**
    2. **Single lung transplantation**
    3. **ARDS with pulmonary edema**

    A. 1 only
    B. 1 and 2 only
    C. 2 and 3 only
    D. 1, 2, and 3

43. After a ventilator patient's PEEP level is increased from 8 cm H_2O to 12 cm H_2O, the PvO_2 drops from 37 torr to 33 torr. This indicates which of the following?

    A. Venous return has increased.
    B. Tissue oxygenation has increased.
    C. Static CL has increased.
    D. QT has decreased.

44. A patient's pulmonary function study shows an FRC of 127% of predicted. The patient most likely has which of the following conditions?

    A. Pulmonary fibrosis
    B. Atelectasis
    C. Emphysema
    D. Pneumonia

45. The high-pressure alarm is activated on a patient's volume ventilator. Which of the following should the respiratory therapist do to help correct this problem?

    1. Add air to the ET-tube cuff.
    2. Suction the patient's ET tube.
    3. Make sure the expiratory drive line is connected.

    A. 1 only
    B. 2 only
    C. 2 and 3 only
    D. 1, 2, and 3

46. The following data are collected from a patient receiving mechanical ventilation

	8:00 PM	**11:00 PM**
PAP	24/12 mm Hg	42/20 mm Hg
PVR	2.1 mm Hg/L/min	4.2 mm Hg/L/min
PCWP	6 mm Hg	7 mm Hg

    On the basis of this information, these changes are most likely the result of which of the following?

    A. Pulmonary embolus
    B. Left ventricular failure
    C. Aortic stenosis
    D. Overhydration

47. Hyperbaric O_2 therapy is indicated in which of the following clinical conditions?

    A. Pulmonary embolism
    B. CO poisoning
    C. Bronchopleural fistula
    D. Tension pneumothorax

48. The following data are collected from a 43-year-old patient breathing room air at a PB of 747 torr:

pH	7.24
$PaCO_2$	68 torr
PaO_2	60 torr
HCO_3^-	26 mEq/L
BE	+1

    All of the following statements are true about this situation *EXCEPT*

    1. The patient is hypoventilating.
    2. The $P(A-a)O_2$ is increased.
    3. The patient has chronic hypoxemia.

    A. 2 only
    B. 3 only
    C. 1 and 2 only
    D. 2 and 3 only

49. A 5-ft 5-inch, 120-kg (264-lb) woman is brought to the emergency department and is receiving ventilation with a manual resuscitator and mask at 100% O_2. A drug overdose is suspected. After intubating the patient, the respiratory therapist is asked to recommend initial ventilator settings. What are the most appropriate settings for this patient's ventilator?

    A. SIMV; rate, 10/min; VT, 1.0 L; FiO_2, 1.0
    B. Assist/control; rate, 16/min; VT, 800 mL; FiO_2, 1.0
    C. Assist/control; rate, 12/min; VT, 1.2 L; FiO_2, 1.0
    D. SIMV; rate, 12/min; VT, 650 mL; FiO_2, 1.0

50. Below is a volume waveform from a patient receiving mechanical ventilation with a volume ventilator.

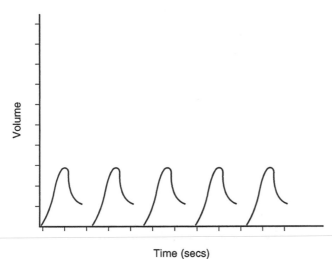

Time (secs)

This waveform indicates which of the following?

A. It represents a normal volume waveform.
B. The patient has obstructive lung disease.
C. There may be a leak around the ET-tube cuff.
D. The patient is coughing or agitated.

51. A patient with ARDS is receiving mechanical ventilation via a volume ventilator with a PEEP of 15 cm H_2O and an FiO_2 of 1.0 but remains hypoxemic. The peak inspiratory pressure is 53 cm H_2O. Which of the following ventilator modifications is the most appropriate recommendation at this time?

A. Increase the PEEP to 20 cm H_2O.
B. Initiate pressure control ventilation.
C. Sedate the patient and place the ventilator in the control mode.
D. Begin in-line bronchodilator therapy using an MDI.

52. The blood gas results below are for a 75-kg (165-lb) patient with COPD who is breathing room air:

pH	7.24
$PaCO_2$	78 torr
PaO_2	41 torr
HCO_3^-	36 mEq/L
BE	+12

Which of the following ventilator settings is most appropriate for this patient?

A. Tidal volume, 900 mL; rate, 10/min; FiO_2, 0.60
B. Tidal volume, 650 mL; rate, 12/min; FiO_2, 0.40
C. Tidal volume, 750 mL; rate, 15/min; FiO_2, 0.50
D. Tidal volume, 800 mL; rate, 8/min; FiO_2, 0.80

53. The following data are collected from a patient receiving mechanical ventilation with a volume ventilator:

PEEP	PaO_2	PvO_2
4 cm H_2O	68 torr	36 torr
6 cm H_2O	73 torr	38 torr
8 cm H_2O	77 torr	34 torr
10 cm H_2O	80 torr	32 torr

Optimal PEEP is which of the following?

A. 4 cm H_2O
B. 6 cm H_2O
C. 8 cm H_2O
D. 10 cm H_2O

54. The respiratory therapist has just completed assisting the physician with a thoracentesis when the patient becomes anxious and complains of shortness of breath. The therapist finds that the patient also has tachycardia. Which of the following should the therapist recommend at this time?

A. Chest radiograph
B. V/Q scan
C. Bronchoscopy
D. Echocardiogram

55. The following ABG results are recorded for a patient receiving mechanical ventilation with a volume ventilator:

pH	7.26
$PaCO_2$	25 torr
PaO_2	89 torr
HCO_3^-	27 mEq/L
BE	+2

The respiratory therapist should recommend which of the following?

A. Decrease the ventilator VT.
B. Administer $NaHCO_3^-$.
C. Get another ABG sample for repeat analysis because this indicates a laboratory error.
D. Increase the ventilator rate.

56. A patient is receiving helium/O_2 therapy through a simple O_2 mask. The patient is experiencing shortness of breath. The respiratory therapist should

  A. Increase flow to the mask
  B. Discontinue the treatment
  C. Instruct the patient to take deeper breaths
  D. Change to a non-rebreathing mask

57. The following data are collected from a patient using a 60% aerosol mask:

pH	7.42
$PaCO_2$	45 torr
PaO_2	90 torr
HCO_3^-	25 mEq/L

  If the PB is 747 torr, this patient's $P(A-a)O_2$ is approximately which of the following?

  A. 150 torr
  B. 275 torr
  C. 305 torr
  D. 365 torr

58. Which of the following indicates that the patient should not be extubated?

  A. VC, 18 mL/kg; MIP, −37 cm H_2O; VD/VT, 28%
  B. VC, 15 mL/kg; MIP, −25 cm H_2O; VD/VT, 40%
  C. VC, 16 mL/kg; MIP, −15 cm H_2O; VD/VT, 50%
  D. VC, 20 mL/kg; MIP, −24 cm H_2O; VD/VT, 35%

59. The following pulmonary function data were obtained from a 51-year-old man with a height of 5 ft 10 inches and a weight of 77 kg (169 lb)

FVC	2.7 L
FEV_1	2.3 L
FEV_1/FVC	85%
DLCO	44% of predicted

  This patient most likely has which of the following conditions?

  A. Bronchiectasis
  B. Pulmonary fibrosis
  C. Emphysema
  D. Chronic bronchitis

60. The lungs of a 2-week-old infant are being ventilated with a pressure-limited, time-cycled ventilator. The peak inspiratory pressure is 24 cm H_2O, inspiratory time is 0.5 s, and the mean airway pressure (MAP) is 14 cm H_2O. If the inspiratory time is increased to 0.8 s, which of the following responses will most likely occur?

  A. MAP will increase.
  B. Peak inspiratory pressure will increase.
  C. VT will decrease.
  D. FiO_2 will increase.

61. The patient is having difficulty cycling the IPPB machine into the inspiratory phase. Which of the following modifications should the respiratory therapist make to correct this problem?

  1. **Increase the sensitivity.**
  2. **Make sure the patient's lips are sealed tight around the mouthpiece.**
  3. **Make sure all tubing connections are tight.**

  A. 1 only
  B. 1 and 2 only
  C. 2 and 3 only
  D. 1, 2, and 3

62. The respiratory therapist notes that the patient's $C(a-v)O_2$ increases from 4.0 vol% to 8.5 vol% after increasing the PEEP level from 5 to 10 cm H_2O. This suggests that which of the following has occurred?

  A. Static CL increased.
  B. R_{AW} decreased.
  C. QT decreased.
  D. MAP decreased.

63. The respiratory therapist has just intubated the patient, and the CO_2 detector on the proximal end of the ET tube reads 6%. This indicates which of the following?

  A. The tube is in the airway.
  B. The patient is hyperventilating.
  C. The tube is in the esophagus.
  D. The patient's VT is not adequate.

64. The following data are obtained from a patient receiving mechanical ventilation with a volume ventilator

Mode	SIMV	pH	7.44
Ventilator rate	6/min	$PaCO_2$	34 torr
VT	700 mL	PaO_2	89 torr
FiO_2	0.35	HCO_3^-	23 mEq/L
		BE	−1

On the basis of this information, the respiratory therapist should recommend which of the following?

A. Administer $NaHCO_3^-$.
B. Add mechanical VD.
C. Extubate and have the patient begin using a 35% Venturi mask.
D. Decrease the ventilator rate to 4/min.

65. While making O_2 rounds, the respiratory therapist notices that the reservoir tubing on a patient's T-piece setup has fallen off. How could this affect the operation of this device?

A. The total flow will increase.
B. The FiO_2 will decrease.
C. Less room air will be entrained.
D. The temperature of the inspired air will increase.

66. The lungs of a 2-month-old infant are being mechanically ventilated by a pressure-limited, time-cycled ventilator. The ventilator rate is 30/min, and the I:E time is 1:3. On the basis of this information, the inspiratory time is which of the following?

A. 0.3 s
B. 0.5 s
C. 0.8 s
D. 1.0 s

67. The following ECG strip appears on the cardiac monitor.

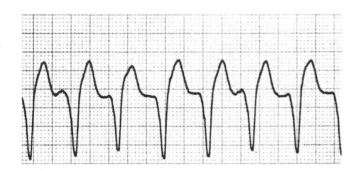

Which of the following should be done *first*?

A. Defibrillate the patient.
B. Order a stat chest radiograph.
C. Order serum electrolyte studies.
D. Obtain an ABG sample.

68. A patient has an arterial catheter in place, and a "damped" pressure tracing appears on the monitor. Which of the following should the respiratory therapist recommend at this time?

1. **Reposition the catheter.**
2. **Flush the line with heparinized saline solution.**
3. **Disconnect the transducer and flush out any air bubbles.**

A. 1 only
B. 1 and 2 only
C. 2 and 3 only
D. 1, 2, and 3

69. A 75-kg (165-lb) patient using a 2-L/min nasal cannula has a respiratory rate of 15/min and a VT of 550 mL. This patient's $\dot{V}_E$ is which of the following?

A. 5.8 L
B. 7.1 L
C. 8.3 L
D. 9.6 L

70. Obstructive sleep apnea is suspected in a patient. The respiratory therapist should recommend which of the following to help diagnose this condition?

A. ABG studies
B. Polysomnogram
C. V/Q scan
D. CT scan

71. Two hours after the insertion of a UAC in a 1-day old infant, cyanosis of the lower extremities is noted. The respiratory therapist should recommend which of the following?

A. Withdraw the catheter to the level of T8 on the radiograph.
B. Advance the catheter until the extremities turn pink.
C. Withdraw the catheter to the level of T2 on the radiograph.
D. Discontinue the UAC.

72. The respiratory therapist is ventilating the lungs of an intubated patient with a self-inflating manual resuscitator. When the bag is squeezed, little resistance is met and the patient's chest does not rise. Which of the following should the therapist do at this time?

   A. Check the bag intake valve for proper function.
   B. Make sure the reservoir is attached to the bag properly.
   C. Make sure the O_2 tubing has not fallen off the flowmeter.
   D. Increase the liter flow to the bag.

73. While a patient using a 4-L/min nasal cannula with an "E" cylinder is being transported, the cannula tubing becomes kinked between the mattress and the bed rail. The Bourdon gauge flowmeter device would

   A. Show a decreased liter flow.
   B. Continue to display an accurate flow reading.
   C. Show a higher flow reading than the patient is actually receiving.
   D. Show a lower flow than what the patient is actually receiving.

74. After setting up a 6-L/min cannula, the respiratory therapist kinks the cannula tubing and a high-pitched whistle is heard coming from the humidifier. The therapist should

   A. Replace the humidifier.
   B. Make sure the jar is connected tightly to the humidifier top.
   C. Decrease the liter flow.
   D. Place the cannula on the patient as ordered.

75. A patient's chest radiograph shows hyperinflation, right ventricular hypertrophy, and diffuse infiltrates. Which of the following would most likely be observed during a pulmonary assessment of this patient?

   1. **Pedal edema**
   2. **Paradoxical respirations**
   3. **Barrel chest**
   4. **Distended neck veins**

   A. 1 and 3 only
   B. 2 and 3 only
   C. 1, 3, and 4 only
   D. 1, 2, 3, and 4

76. A 34-year-old unconscious patient, admitted because of a drug overdose, is intubated and is receiving mechanical ventilation with a volume ventilator. The average peak inspiratory pressure is 30 cm H_2O. The high-pressure limit is set at 40 cm H_2O. One hour later, the patient becomes agitated and combative, and the high-pressure alarm sounds with each breath. The respiratory therapist should recommend

   A. Increasing the pressure limit to 50 cm H_2O.
   B. Decreasing the inspiratory flow.
   C. Increasing the VT.
   D. Administering pancuronium bromide (Pavulon).

77. A patient enters the emergency department using a 5-L/min nasal cannula. Although the patient is not cyanotic, ABG results reveal a PaO_2 of 45 torr and an SpO_2 of 98%. The respiratory therapist should recommend checking which of the following to better assess this patient's oxygenation status?

   A. Hb level
   B. VD/VT
   C. PvO_2
   D. $P(A-a)O_2$

78. While making O_2 rounds, the respiratory therapist observes H_2O bubbling in the aerosol tubing connected to a jet nebulizer set on 40%. Which of the following statements is true regarding this situation.

   A. Total flow will increase.
   B. FiO_2 will decrease.
   C. Air entrained into the nebulizer will increase.
   D. This is a heated nebulizer.

79. The lungs of a 2-week-old infant are being ventilated on a time-cycled, pressure-limited ventilator. The physician wants to increase the MAP. Which of the following could be increased to accomplish this?

   1. **PEEP**
   2. **PIP**
   3. **Inspiratory time**

   A. 1 only
   B. 2 only
   C. 2 and 3 only
   D. 1, 2, and 3

80. A 34-year-old, 80-kg (176-lb) man with a history of cardiac disease has been intubated, and the physician wants your recommendation for initial ventilator settings. Which of the following would be most beneficial in preventing cardiac side effects?

    A. SIMV mode; rate, 14/min; VT, 850 mL; FiO_2, 0.50
    B. Control mode; rate, 12/min; VT, 900 mL; FiO_2, 0.60
    C. Assist/control mode; rate, 14/min; VT, 800 mL; FiO_2, 0.50
    D. SIMV mode; rate, 10/min; VT, 800 mL; FiO_2, 0.50

81. The following data are obtained from a patient receiving mechanical ventilation with a volume ventilator; the VT is 750 mL:

	Peak pressure	Plateau pressure
2:00 PM	34 cm H_2O	16 cm H_2O
3:00 PM	38 cm H_2O	19 cm H_2O
4:00 PM	44 cm H_2O	23 cm H_2O

    On the basis of this information, the respiratory therapist should conclude which of the following?

    A. The patient is experiencing bronchospasms.
    B. R_{AW} is increasing.
    C. Static CL is decreasing.
    D. H_2O has accumulated in the ventilator tubing.

82. The most accurate method of determining how well the lungs of a patient with emphysema are being ventilated is by

    A. Measuring peak flow.
    B. Measuring FRC.
    C. Obtaining ABG samples.
    D. Measuring SpO_2.

83. After repeated attempts to wean a patient from mechanical ventilation without success, the respiratory therapist should recommend obtaining which of the following values?

    A. Serum electrolytes
    B. Peak flow studies
    C. Cardiac enzymes
    D. BUN level

84. A ventilator patient is receiving PEEP at 8 cm H_2O and an FiO_2 of 0.50. After the PEEP is increased to 10 cm H_2O, his QT drops from 4.8 L/min to 3.3 L/min. The respiratory therapist should recommend which of the following?

    A. Increase the PEEP to 12 cm H_2O.
    B. Decrease the PEEP to 8 cm H_2O, and increase the FiO_2 to 0.60.
    C. Discontinue PEEP.
    D. Maintain the PEEP at 10 cm H_2O, and increase the FiO_2 to 0.60.

85. Which of the following could cause an increase in peak inspiratory pressure on a volume ventilator?

    1. **Decreased CL**
    2. **Decreased R_{AW}**
    3. **Partially occluded ET tube**
    4. **High inspiratory flow setting**

    A. 1 and 2 only
    B. 2 and 3 only
    C. 1, 3, and 4 only
    D. 1, 2, 3, and 4

86. Before administering IPPB, the respiratory therapist notes subcutaneous emphysema around the neck tissues of the patient. Which of the following should the therapist do at this time?

    A. Administer the IPPB and recommend a chest radiograph.
    B. Measure the patient's SpO_2.
    C. Administer the IPPB using a lower inspiratory pressure.
    D. Withhold the IPPB and recommend a chest radiograph.

87. The following ventilator settings are recorded for a patient:

Mode	Control
Ventilator rate	10/min
VT	800 mL
FiO_2	0.40
PEEP	6 cm H_2O
Inspiratory flow rate	40 L/min

    On the basis of this information, the I:E is which of the following?

    A. 1:1
    B. 1:2
    C. 1:3
    D. 1:4

88. The I:E ratio alarm is sounding on a volume ventilator. Which of the following is the most appropriate ventilator setting change to correct this problem?

   A. Increase the flow rate.
   B. Decrease the VT.
   C. Add a 1-s inspiratory hold.
   D. Increase the ventilator rate.

89. The following data have been recorded for a patient receiving mechanical ventilation with a volume ventilator:

CVP	10 mm Hg
PAP	48/26 mm Hg
PCWP	10 mm Hg
QT	5.8 L/min

   On the basis of these data, the patient most likely has

   A. Pulmonary hypertension.
   B. Mitral valve regurgitation.
   C. Aortic stenosis.
   D. Right ventricular failure.

90. Which of the following indicates that a ventilator patient is most likely ready to be weaned?

   1. **VD/VT of 0.65**
   2. **MIP of −28 cm H_2O**
   3. **VC of 17 mL/kg of body weight**

   A. 2 only
   B. 1 and 2 only
   C. 2 and 3 only
   D. 1, 2, and 3

91. A ventilator patient suddenly becomes tachycardic and agitated, and the high-pressure alarm begins sounding. The respiratory therapist auscultates diminished breath sounds in the right lung and palpates the trachea left of midline. Which of the following should the therapist recommend at this time?

   A. Get a stat chest radiograph.
   B. Increase the ventilator rate.
   C. Insert a needle into the second intercostal space.
   D. Suction the patient's ET tube.

92. The H_2O in the water-seal bottle of a chest-tube drainage system fluctuates 5 to 10 cm H_2O as the patient is breathing. This is most likely the result of which of the following?

   A. A leak in the system.
   B. A clot in the tubing.
   C. The chest tube has slipped out of the pleural space.
   D. This is a normal occurrence with chest-tube drainage systems.

93. A patient enters the emergency department complaining of shortness of breath with a respiratory rate of 32/min and a VT that fluctuates between 350 mL and 500 mL. Which of the following is the most appropriate device to deliver approximately 40% O_2 to this patient?

   A. Nasal cannula at 5 L/min
   B. Simple O_2 mask at 6 L/min
   C. Partial rebreathing mask at 8 L/min
   D. Air entrainment mask

94. A patient is receiving mechanical ventilation with a volume ventilator that has an HME. Over the past 4 h, the respiratory therapist notes that the patient's sputum has become thicker and more difficult to suction through the catheter. Which of the following should the therapist recommend at this time?

   A. Replace the HME with a heated humidifier.
   B. Suction the patient more frequently.
   C. Increase the suction pressure to −140 mm Hg.
   D. Use a larger suction catheter.

95. While making O_2 rounds, the respiratory therapist notices very little mist being produced by a jet nebulizer attached to an aerosol mask. Which of the following may be causing this?

   1. **The capillary tube filter is clogged.**
   2. **The jet is obstructed.**
   3. **The liter flow is too low.**

   A. 1 only
   B. 1 and 2 only
   C. 2 and 3 only
   D. 1, 2, and 3

96. The respiratory therapist is using a size 12 Fr suction catheter to suction a female patient who is intubated with a 6.5-mm ET tube. The therapist is having difficulty aspirating the thick secretions. Which of the following is the most appropriate action to take?

   A. Change to a coudé suction catheter.
   B. Increase the suction pressure to −160 mm Hg.
   C. Instill 5 mL of normal saline down the ET tube.
   D. Change to a size 14 Fr suction catheter.

97. The respiratory therapist has instilled air into a ventilator patient's ET-tube cuff so that a slight leak is heard with a stethoscope at peak inspiration. The peak inspiratory pressure is 30 cm H_2O at the time. Four hours later, after suctioning the patient and draining H_2O from the ventilator tubing, the therapist notes that the peak inspiratory pressure is 40 cm H_2O. Which of the following is true regarding this patient's ET-tube cuff care?

   1. **The leak around the cuff is larger.**
   2. **Air should be removed from the cuff.**
   3. **Minimal leak technique should be used at 40 cm H_2O.**

   A. 1 only
   B. 2 only
   C. 1 and 3 only
   D. 2 and 3 only

98. While a patient's lungs are being ventilated with a manual resuscitator, ABG results indicate a PaO_2 of 50 torr. Which of the following would increase the O_2 being delivered by the bag?

   1. **Adding a reservoir to the bag.**
   2. **Increasing the O_2 flow to the bag.**
   3. **Increasing the ventilation rate.**

   A. 1 only
   B. 1 and 2 only
   C. 2 and 3 only
   D. 1, 2, and 3

99. The peak inspiratory pressure has dropped from 34 cm H_2O to 5 cm H_2O on a volume ventilator operating in the assist/control mode. The respiratory therapist notices the exhaled volume spirometer is filling during inspiration. Which of the following is the most likely cause of this?

   A. The exhalation valve is malfunctioning.
   B. There is a leak around the ET-tube cuff.
   C. The pressure manometer is malfunctioning.
   D. No problem exists because this is a normal occurrence.

100. A patient is receiving mechanical ventilation with a volume ventilator set on a VT of 700 mL, but the exhaled volume display reads 400 mL. After finding no leaks in the tubing and connections, the respiratory therapist wants to determine the volume the ventilator is actually delivering. To most accurately measure this volume, the therapist should place a respirometer

   A. At the exhalation valve.
   B. At the ventilator outlet.
   C. At the humidifier outlet.
   D. At the patient wye connector.

101. A 32-year-old woman enters the emergency department complaining of shortness of breath. A CBC reveals a hemoglobin level of 8 vol%. The respiratory therapist determines that her SpO_2 is 99%. Which of the following statements are true regarding this patient's condition?

   1. **The patient is hypoxic.**
   2. **The patient is most likely cyanotic.**
   3. **Oxygen is not indicated at this time.**

   A. 1 only
   B. 3 only
   C. 1 and 2 only
   D. 2 and 3 only

102. A patient with ARDS is receiving mechanical ventilation with PEEP. The PEEP level is increased from 5 cm H_2O to 10 cm H_2O. Which of the following should be monitored by the respiratory therapist to evaluate the patient's response?

   1. **Blood pressure**
   2. **Heart rate**
   3. **Body temperature**
   4. **Fluid intake and output**

   A. 1 and 2 only
   B. 1, 2, and 3 only
   C. 1, 2, and 4 only
   D. 2, 3, and 4 only

103. A patient using a 35% Venturi mask has the following arterial blood gas values

pH	7.48
$PaCO_2$	30 torr
PaO_2	53 torr
HCO_3^-	25 mEq/L
BE	+2

The respiratory therapist increases the oxygen to 40%. Which of the following blood gas values should *increase* after this change?

1. pH
2. $PaCO_2$
3. PaO_2
4. HCO_3^-

A. 3 only
B. 2 and 3 only
C. 1, 2, and 3 only
D. 2, 3, and 4 only

104. The following arterial blood gas results are recorded for a patient with COPD who is breathing spontaneously. The FiO_2 the patient is receiving is not noted:

pH	7.25
$PaCO_2$	80 torr
PaO_2	74 torr
HCO_3^-	38 mEq/L
BE	+14
pH	7.48

The respiratory therapist should conclude from this information which of the following?

A. The patient has acute respiratory acidemia and is breathing room air.
B. The patient is not chronically retaining CO_2.
C. The patient is breathing supplemental oxygen.
D. The blood gas sample is most likely venous blood.

105. A patient receiving mechanical ventilation with a volume ventilator has a PaO_2 of 58 torr with a PEEP of 5 cm H_2O and an FiO_2 of 0.50. After the PEEP is increased to 10 cm H_2O, the cardiac output decreases from 4.1 L/min to 3.2 L/min. The most appropriate recommendation is to

A. Discontinue PEEP and increase the FiO_2 to 0.70.
B. Increase PEEP to 12 cm H_2O.
C. Decrease PEEP to 5 cm H_2O and increase the FiO_2 to 0.60.
D. Maintain the current settings and measure cardiac output in 1 h.

106. A patient is receiving IPPB therapy at a peak inspiratory pressure of 25 cm H_2O. The patient begins having bronchospasms during the treatment. Which of the following is true regarding this situation?

1. **The peak inspiratory pressure will increase.**
2. **The delivered tidal volume will decrease.**
3. **The inspiratory time will increase.**

A. 1 only
B. 2 only
C. 1 and 3 only
D. 2 and 3

107. A 65-kg (143-lb) female patient arrives in the emergency department intubated and receiving manual ventilation with 100% oxygen. The respiratory therapist should select which of the following ventilator settings to best ventilate the lungs of this patient?

A. Mode, assist/control; VT, 700 mL; rate, 12/min; FiO_2, 1.0
B. Mode, control; VT, 550 mL; rate, 12/min; FiO_2, 0.60
C. Mode, SIMV; VT, 700 mL; rate, 6/min; FiO_2, 1.0
D. Mode, SIMV; VT, 650 mL; rate, 12/min; FiO_2, 0.80

108. The following data are collected from a 70-kg (154-lb) male patient receiving mechanical ventilation

Mode	SIMV
Rate	12/min
VT	600 mL
FiO_2	0.40
Flow rate	60 L/min
PEEP	5 cm H_2O
Mechanical dead space	200 mL
pH	7.24
$PaCO_2$	58 torr
PaO_2	62 torr
HCO_3^-	23 mEq/L
BE	−2

The respiratory therapist should recommend which of the following?

A. Increase the tidal volume to 700 mL.
B. Remove the dead space.
C. Increase the FiO_2.
D. Increase the inspiratory flow rate.

109. The following data are collected for an 80-kg (176-lb) patient with ARDS receiving volume-controlled ventilation:

Mode	A/C
Rate	18/min
VT	800 mL
PEEP	15 cm H_2O
FiO_2	0.90
PIP	53 cm H_2O
pH	7.35
$PaCO_2$	47 torr
PaO_2	53 torr
HCO_3^-	26 mEq/L
BE	+2

    Which of the following is the most appropriate recommendation?

    A. Increase PEEP to 20 cm H_2O.
    B. Switch to pressure-control ventilation.
    C. Increase the FiO_2 to 1.0.
    D. Increase the tidal volume to 900 mL.

110. The following data are obtained from a 75-kg (165-lb) patient with postoperative atelectasis:

Mode	SIMV
Ventilator rate	10/min
VT	700 mL
Total rate	28/min
FiO_2	0.35
Peak flow	25 L/min
PEEP	5 cm H_2O
Pressure support	10 cm H_2O
pH	7.24
$PaCO_2$	57 torr
PaO_2	66 torr
HCO_3^-	23 mEq/L
BE	0

    The patient is tachypneic and agitated and the high-pressure alarm is triggering with each breath. On the basis of this information, the respiratory therapist should recommend which of the following?

    A. Increase the peak flow.
    B. Increase the FiO_2.
    C. Increase the pressure support.
    D. Increase the tidal volume.

111. Which of the following is most likely to increase the possibility of tracheal wall damage caused by excessive E-T tube cuff pressures?

    A. Using minimal occluding volume technique.
    B. Maintaining cuff pressure at 25 cm H_2O.
    C. Using minimal leak technique.
    D. Maintaining cuff pressure at 32 mm Hg.

112. Venous return is least impaired by which of the following ventilator settings?

    A. SIMV mode; rate, 12/min
    B. Control mode; rate, 10/min
    C. Assist/control mode; rate, 10/min
    D. SIMV mode; rate, 8/min

113. The following data are collected for a 75-kg (165-lb) patient receiving ventilation in the pressure-control mode:

Peak inspiratory pressure	22 cm H_2O
PEEP	5 cm H_2O
Rate	12/min
FiO_2	0.50
Exhaled tidal volume	300 mL
ABGs:	
pH	7.27
PaO_2	54 torr
PaO_2	68 torr
HCO_3^-	24 mEq/L
BE	0

    The respiratory therapist should recommend which of the following?

    A. Increase the PIP to 26 cm H_2O.
    B. Increase the FiO_2 to 0.70.
    C. Increase PEEP to 10 cm H_2O.
    D. Increase the rate to 15/min.

114. The secretions of a tracheotomized patient are thick and difficult to mobilize. Which of the following should the respiratory therapist recommend?

    A. Add a heater to the nebulizer.
    B. Suction the patient every hour.
    C. Restrict fluid intake.
    D. Suction with a pressure of −160 mm Hg.

115. The following data are collected for a 70-kg (154-lb) female receiving mechanical ventilation with a volume ventilator:

Mode	SIMV
Ventilator rate	15/min
Total rate	26/min
VT	700 mL
FiO_2	0.65
Pressure support	10 cm H_2O
PEEP	5 cm H_2O
ABGs:	
pH	7.48
$PaCO_2$	30 torr
PaO_2	62 torr
HCO_3^-	23 mEq/L
BE	−2

Which of the following ventilator changes are appropriate at this time?

A. Increase the PEEP to 10 cm H_2O.
B. Decrease the tidal volume to 650 mL.
C. Decrease the SIMV rate to 10/min.
D. Decrease the pressure support to 5 cm H_2O.

END OF ADVANCED PRACTITIONER WRITTEN REGISTRY EXAM. FOR ANSWER KEY/RATIONALES, GO TO THIS SECTION ON EVOLVE EXAM REVIEW.

PRETEST ANSWERS AND RATIONALES

CHAPTER ONE

1. C;

$$\frac{1900 \times 0.28}{4} = \frac{532}{4} = \frac{133\,\text{min}}{60} = 2.2\,\text{h}$$

2. D; The reservoir bag on a partial or non-rebreathing mask should remain one-third to one-half full at all times. If the bag contains less gas, then it is an indication of inadequate flow to the mask and the flow from the flowmeter must be increased. Typically, flows of 10 to 15 L/min are necessary to maintain adequate flow. The non-rebreathing mask provides an oxygen percent of approximately 60% to 80%.

3. B; Hemoglobin has a greater affinity for carbon monoxide (CO) than it does for oxygen, but its affinity decreases as the oxygen level in the blood increases. Therefore, the higher the PaO_2, the less affinity Hb has for CO, and oxygen is then able to combine with Hb. Hyperbaric oxygen, or 100% oxygen delivered under 2 to 3 atmospheres of pressure, can elevate PaO_2 levels to approximately 1800 mm Hg, or three times what can be achieved at 100% oxygen at atmospheric pressure, and is the most useful in this situation. If hyperbaric oxygen is not available, a non-rebreathing mask or 100% CPAP should be administered.

4. A; Hyperventilation with a PaO_2 of only 58 mm Hg while receiving 60% oxygen indicates intrapulmonary shunting with refractory hypoxemia. Intrapulmonary shunting is caused by atelectasis, pulmonary edema, or consolidated alveoli, none of which will improve by a simple increase in the oxygen level. If the alveoli are collapsed or full of fluid or consolidated material, oxygen will not be able to enter these alveoli and diffuse into the blood, and no matter how high the oxygen level is increased, the PaO_2 will not increase significantly. To deliver more O_2 into the alveoli, apply pressure to increase the surface area for gas exchange to take place. This is accomplished with CPAP. **In almost all cases on the exam, if the patient in the question is hyperventilating in response to hypoxemia with 60% oxygen or higher, do not increase the FiO_2. Apply CPAP**.

5. D; Oxygen content is the amount of oxygen in the blood, both bound to hemoglobin and dissolved in the plasma. It is calculated from the following formula

$$CaO_2 = (1.34 \times Hb \times O_2\ \text{sat}) + (PaO_2 \times 0.003)$$
$$= (1.34 \times 14 \times 0.95) + (88 \times 0.003)$$
$$= 17.8 + 0.26 = 18\ \text{g/dL}$$

Note: Because the amount of oxygen dissolved in plasma is always such a small number (0.26 gm/dL in this problem), I suggest not even figuring it on the exam so that you can save time. You will still get an answer close enough to the correct answer.

6. B; To calculate the total flow delivered by a high-flow oxygen delivery device, the sum of the air/O_2 ratio parts for the O_2 percentage of the device is multiplied by the flow from the flowmeter supplying the device. The air/O_2 ratio for 30% is 8:1. In other words, for every 1 L of O_2 flow from the flowmeter, 8 L of air is being entrained into the device. Add the ratio parts together, $8 + 1 = 9$, and then multiply by the liter flow of 5 L/min: $9 \times 5 = 45$ L/min.

CHAPTER TWO

1. B; Pulmonary secretions will become thicker and harder to mobilize from the airway when the inspired air reaches the lower airway holding an insufficient volume of water. By the time the air reaches the carina, it should be close to fully saturated at body temperature. This represents 44 mg of water/liter of gas, which exerts a water vapor pressure of 47 mm Hg. Therefore, a water content of less than 44 mg/L at body temperature represents a humidity deficit, which will result in secretions becoming drier and thicker.

2. A; Air fully humidified at body temperature holds 44 mg of water/liter of air. Air holding less than this value represents a humidity deficit. The deficit is calculated by subtracting the volume of water in the inspired air from 44 mg/L. In this question, the inspired air contains 38 mg/L: $44 - 38 = 6$ mg/L.

3. C; The whistling noise is the pressure pop-off valve opening as a result of excessive pressure in the humidifier caused by kinking in the cannula tubing. Because pressure built up in the humidifier has opened the pop-off valve, no leaks are present in the setup. If the tubing is kinked and no noise is heard from the humidifier, a leak exists somewhere in the setup. Check all tubing connections and make sure the top of the humidifier is tight. Typically, pop-off valves on humidifiers open at a pressure of 2 psi.

4. D; Heat moisture exchangers (HMEs) provide approximately 70% to 90% body humidity, as opposed to 100% when heated humidifiers are used. Patients who develop thick secretions should not have their inspired air humidified with an HME. More water delivery is necessary to help moisten the secretions. This is best accomplished with the use of a heated humidifier.

5. D; Bland aerosol therapy, or delivery of sterile water through a nebulizer, is often irritating to the airway, which results in coughing. This may be used to induce coughing to obtain a sputum sample. Adding water to the airway will also help liquefy the secretions, which makes them easier to mobilize from the airway. After extubation, inflammation of the glottic area may occur as a result of irritation from the ET tube. Inflammation leads to vasodilation, causing swelling of the glottic area and producing upper airway resistance, inspiratory stridor, and increased work of breathing. Cool bland aerosol delivery results in vasoconstriction or shrinking of these blood vessels, causing a decreased airway resistance and work of breathing.

6. D; Aerosol is produced by a nebulizer when water is drawn up the capillary tube and into the path of a high-velocity flow of gas. Anything that prevents the water from being drawn up the tube or flowing through the jet will diminish the mist output. *Too low* of a liter flow will also result in decreased mist production.

CHAPTER THREE

1. C; Yellow sputum indicates an increased number of white blood cells in the sputum. This indicates that infection is present. Yellow sputum is often referred to as being *purulent*. When yellow sputum is collected, the respiratory therapist should recommend a sputum culture and sensitivity test, chest x-ray film, and complete blood count (CBC) to determine the WBC level.

2. A; Patients who have difficulty breathing while lying down (supine) are said to have orthopnea. This is commonly observed in patients with COPD, in patients with chronic cardiac conditions, and in obese patients.

3. C; Paradoxical respirations occur when a portion of the chest wall moves inward (instead of outward) when the patient inhales and outward (instead of inward) with exhalation. This is generally observed in patients with chest trauma, flail chest, or paralysis of the diaphragm.

4. C; Determining how well the extremities are being perfused may be assessed by compression of the nailbed on the patient's index finger until it turns white.

The pressure should then be released and the time noted for how long it takes the nailbed to return to its original color. This is referred to as capillary refill time and should be no longer than 3 s. A capillary refill time of longer than 3 s indicates inadequate perfusion to the extremities, which could be the result of decreased cardiac output, hypotension, or cold extremities.

5. C; Decreased vibrations, or *tactile fremitus,* are felt over fluid, such as a pleural effusion and pulmonary edema, and over a pneumothorax.

6. D; The carina is located on a chest film at the level of the fourth rib. In this question, the tip of the tube is resting on the carina. The tube needs to be withdrawn until the tip is resting 2 to 5 cm above the carina.

7. A; PET is an imaging technique that is able to distinguish between benign and malignant tumors, especially those in the thorax.

8. A; Both a CT scan and an MRI are capable of diagnosing a pulmonary embolism.

CHAPTER FOUR

1. C; If the ET tube is in the trachea, the CO_2 detector should read approximately 5% to 6%. A level of only 1.5% indicates that the tube cannot be in the trachea but is in the esophagus.

2. D; In an unconscious patient, the most common cause of upper airway obstruction is the tongue falling against the posterior wall of the pharynx. The oropharyngeal airway will pull the tongue forward, relieving the obstruction. The oropharyngeal airway should be used in *unconscious patients only*.

3. A; Magill forceps are a curved instrument used to grasp the ET tube and advance it through the vocal cords during nasotracheal intubation.

4. B; A fenestrated tracheostomy tube has a hole in the outer cannula that the patient may breathe through when the inner cannula is removed, the cuff is deflated, and the proximal end of the tube is plugged. This allows for the patient to begin inhaling through the nose or mouth and through the fenestration and exhaling through the fenestration and upward through the vocal cords just as in normal breathing.

5. C; Although a cuff pressure of 12 mm Hg may be adequate in some instances to seal the airway effectively, in this question, 12 mm Hg is inadequate and a leak is present around the cuff. Increasing the pressure in the cuff slowly and stopping just at the point where a small leak is heard ensures that the least amount of pressure is being placed on the wall of the trachea with only a minimal leak. This is referred to as the *minimal leak technique*. Generally, it is safe to use cuff pressures of up to 20 mm Hg (27 cm H_2O) without causing pressure damage to the tracheal wall.

6. C; Although having a patient turn his or her head to the right may increase the chances of advancing a suction catheter into the left mainstem bronchus, the most effective method is to use an angle-tip catheter known as a *coudé catheter*. The distal end is angled to the left to increase the potential for entering the left mainstem bronchus so that the left lung may be suctioned.

CHAPTER FIVE

1. D; The placing of a bronchoscope into a patient's airway has several complications including pulmonary hemorrhage, pneumothorax, hypoxemia, laryngospasm (nonintubated patient), bronchospasm, cardiac arrhythmia, and hypotension.

2. C; As the physician attempts to advance the bronchoscope tube through the vocal cords in nonintubated patients, the irritation of the tube on the cords can result in laryngospasm, making it difficult to enter the trachea. *Do not be fooled on the exam. This is not a concern if the patient is intubated because the bronchoscope tube passes through the ET tube without coming in contact with the vocal cords.*

3. C; After a bronchoscopy, complications that may have occurred as a result of the procedure that would result in higher ventilator pressures than before the procedure are bronchospasm or pulmonary hemorrhage caused by an increased airway resistance and a pneumothorax resulting in decreased lung compliance.

4. B; Because air tends to gravitate upward in the thorax, placing the chest tube in the second intercostal space is indicated. To drain fluid from the pleural space, which tends to gravitate downward, insert the chest tube lower, generally in the seventh or eighth intercostal space.

5. D; It is normal for the water level in the water-seal chamber to fluctuate as the patient inhales and exhales. Bubbling that occurs only in the suction control chamber under −15 cm H_2O pressure—and not in the water-seal chamber—indicates that the pneumothorax is resolving. Excessive or persistent bubbling occurring in the water-seal chamber may be an indication of a leak in the system or that air is still being removed from the pleural space.

6. B; As mentioned in the previous explanation, it is normal for the water level in the water-seal chamber to fluctuate as the patient inhales and exhales. The absence of fluctuation may indicate an obstruction in the chest tube, for example, from a blood clot. To remove the obstruction, "milk" or "strip" the tube. This technique involves compressing the tube briefly, which allows pressure to build up, and then releasing it so that the gush of pressure will remove the obstruction.

CHAPTER SIX

1. D; Opening the airway is the first step to follow if a patient is assessed to be apneic. If the airway is not opened properly with the use of the head tilt/chin lift method, artificial breaths may be obstructed and ventilation may fail. An oropharyngeal airway may also be used in unconscious apneic patients to maintain a patent upper airway during rescue breathing.

2. D; Rescue breathing for an infant is performed at a rate of 20/min or one breath every 3 s.

3. C; Epinephrine is a cardiac stimulant that is indicated for asystole. It may be instilled directly down the patient's ET tube when an IV line is not available.

4. C; Epinephrine and lidocaine are both indicated when ventricular fibrillation is present. Both of these drugs may be instilled down the ET tube when an IV or central line is not available.

5. A; According to advanced cardiac life support (ACLS) guidelines, if ventricular fibrillation is not reversed with an initial defibrillation level of 200 J from a biphasic defibrillator, then 300 J is indicated. Up to 360 J may be used in an attempt to reverse ventricular fibrillation. When a monophasic defibrillator is used, 360 J is indicated.

6. A; To reverse atrial fibrillation, use a lower level of energy. Generally, 25 to 100 J is used to restore normal cardiac function. Emergency airway equipment such as a laryngoscope, blades, ET tubes, and suction equipment, along with oxygen and a manual resuscitator, should be set up at the bedside during this procedure.

CHAPTER SEVEN

1. C; On a pressure-cycled ventilator like the Bird Mark 7, tidal volume is increased by increasing the peak inspiratory pressure. The more pressure delivered to the lungs, the higher the tidal volume. When inspiratory flow rate is decreased, the delivered tidal volume increases slightly. The lower the flow rate, the less turbulent the flow through the tubing; therefore less volume is compressed into the sides of the tubing and airway.

2. B; Generally, a pneumothorax is not a common hazard associated with IPPB, but it can occur when excessively high pressures are used during the treatment. It is most commonly observed with patients who have bullous emphysema. The bullae are weak air spaces that may rupture if excessive pressure is delivered.

3. A; One of the common complications of IPPB is dizziness or lightheadedness. This symptom is the result of hyperventilation, which reduces the blood flow to the head. To prevent this problem from occurring, instruct patients to slow their breathing rate down by pausing longer between breaths.

4. D; Although an uncommon hazard of IPPB, hemoptysis can occur as a result of excessive inspiratory pressure. Pulmonary hemorrhage may occur from pneumonia or a lung tumor. If such occurs, the treatment must be stopped immediately to avoid the possibility of air entering a blood vessel and resulting in an air embolism.

5. A; Excessive ventilation resulting in dizziness is the only hazard of IPPB in this question. IPPB results in a *decreased* cardiac output and an *increased* ICP as the positive pressure in the chest reduces blood flow back to the heart.

6. C; As mentioned in the previous explanation, positive pressure prevents blood from returning to the heart. Therefore, blood circulating from the upper body cannot get back to the heart, which normally causes ICP to increase. This is not a concern for most patients, except for those who have head trauma, in whom elevated ICP levels may pose a dangerous risk. The lower the inspiratory pressure delivered and the less time with positive pressure in the airway, the less potential for increasing the ICP. Because increasing the flow shortens the inspiratory time, high flow rates along with lower inspiratory pressures are indicated.

7. C; It is important to use language that the patient can understand when therapy is described. The use of medical terms such as *atelectasis* or *inspiratory capacity* most likely will not be understood by the patient.

8. D; Although incentive spirometry may be beneficial in the treatment of atelectasis, it's greatest benefit is preventing atelectasis.

9. A; For incentive spirometry to be beneficial in preventing atelectasis, the patient must have a VC of greater than 10 mL/kg of ideal body weight. Of these choices, twice the patient's tidal volume is most appropriate.

CHAPTER EIGHT

1. C; Postural drainage and percussion are indicated to help mobilize thick pulmonary secretions that the patient cannot remove with deep breathing and coughing techniques. The secretions observed with pulmonary edema are thin, watery, and frothy secretions that do not require special techniques for removal. Postural drainage and percussion may even worsen the condition by placing the patient in various positions that may further compromise the cardiac status and further increase airway resistance.

2. B; Autogenic drainage is a modified coughing technique that may be as beneficial in mobilizing secretions as postural drainage and percussion. The breathing technique used in this technique helps move secretions into the upper airway so that they can be more easily removed with coughing.

3. A; To drain anterior segments, place the patient in a supine position (lying on the back) with the bed flat and pillows under the knees. This position promotes drainage from the anterior portion of the chest into the larger upper airways for easier mobilization with coughing.

4. B; In this question, the patient is lying on his right side, the same side as his pneumonia, and he becomes hypoxemic and short of breath. This results from gravity draining blood to the bad lung because of the position, which causes increased ventilation/perfusion mismatching. In other words, more blood is circulating through the bad lung than through the good lung. The patient needs to be placed with his left lung, or good lung, down to promote more circulation to the good lung, which would result in improvement of his oxygenation status.

CHAPTER NINE

1. D; The P wave of the cardiac cycle is a positive wave that represents atrial depolarization, or atrial contraction. The normal duration of the P wave is 0.06 to 0.10 s.

2. D; Artifacts show a misrepresentation of the cardiac waveform on the cardiac monitor and may be caused by electrical interference, poor electrode contact with the skin, or excessive movement of the patient.

3. B; PVCs are the result of ventricular irritability caused by hypoxemia, acid–base disturbances, electrolyte abnormalities, CHF, myocardial inflammation, coronary artery disease, and an excessive dosage of digitalis. PVCs are characterized by abnormally shaped QRS complexes, which are wider than normal. Lidocaine, procainamide, or propranolol is administered to treat PVCs.

4. C; Pulse pressure is the difference between the systolic and diastolic pressures. Normal is 40 mm Hg. In this question, the patient's blood pressure was 110/50, and the difference is 60 mm Hg (110−50).

5. C; One of the complications of arterial lines is a thrombosis distal to the puncture site. If thrombosis and embolization occur, a weak pulse would be palpated distal to the puncture site. A continuous flush of saline and heparin through the system helps prevent clot formation.

6. D; CVP is the measurement of right atrial pressure. The normal value is less than 6 mm Hg. Decreased values are seen with leaks in the CVP measuring line and low blood volume (hypovolemia).

CHAPTER TEN

1. B; Alveolar ventilation is best determined by observation of the patient's $PaCO_2$ value. The normal arterial value is 35 to 45 mm Hg. A value less than 35 mm Hg indicates hyperventilation; a value of greater than 45 mm Hg is indicative of hypoventilation. Changing tidal volume, respiratory rate, and dead space alters $PaCO_2$ levels.

2. D; Mixed venous PO_2 (PvO_2) is the amount of oxygen found in the pulmonary artery. A normal value is 35 to 45 mm Hg. A decreased PvO_2 indicates inadequate oxygenation of the tissues most commonly caused by a decreased cardiac output. As cardiac output drops, blood flow to the tissues slows while tissue oxygen uptake remains at the same rate. Therefore, some tissues take more oxygen from the blood than normal, which deprives other tissues of the normal amount of oxygen. When the blood returns from the body to the pulmonary artery, it contains less oxygen than it should and is reflected by a drop in the PvO_2.

3. C; $P(A–a)O_2$, or the A–a gradient, is the difference between alveolar PO_2 (PAO_2) and arterial PO_2 (PaO_2).

$$PAO_2 = (PB - 47\ mm\ Hg) \times (FiO_2 + 10)$$

Note: 47 mm Hg represents water vapor pressure.

$$PAO_2 = (747 - 47) \times 0.40 - (36 + 10)$$
$$= (700 \times 0.40) - 46 = 280 - 46$$
$$= 234\ mm\ Hg$$

$$234\ mm\ Hg - 122\ mm\ Hg = 112\ mm\ Hg$$

(With the use of the traditional equation, the answer is 113 mm Hg.)

4. A; A shift of the oxyhemoglobin curve to the right indicates that hemoglobin has less affinity for oxygen and releases it more readily to the tissues, thus increasing tissue oxygenation. Conditions that shift the curve to the right include hypercapnia, acidemia, hyperthermia, and increased levels of 2,3-DPG.

5. D; Decreased $PaCO_2$ levels indicate less acid in the blood; therefore, an increase in the pH occurs. This blood gas result indicates respiratory alkalemia. It is an acute condition because the HCO_3^- level is normal and has not begun to decrease, which would lower the pH back to normal. This is considered an acute or uncompensated respiratory alkalosis.

6. D; An Allen test should always be performed to determine collateral circulation to the hand. If there is inadequate perfusion to the hand from the ulnar artery, the radial artery of that hand should not be punctured. The appropriate action to take is to check for adequate ulnar blood flow in the other wrist.

CHAPTER ELEVEN

1. D;

$$\text{Static CL} = \frac{\text{Tidal volume}}{\text{Plateau pressure} - \text{PEEP}}$$
$$= \frac{850\ mL}{27 - 4} = \frac{850\ mL}{23\ cm\ H_2O}$$
$$= 37\ mL/cm\ H_2O$$

2. D; The I:E time alarm is triggered when the ventilator settings are delivering ventilator breaths with an inverse I:E time or when the inspiratory time is longer than the expiratory time. The potential hazards of an inverse I:E time include decreased cardiac output, barotrauma, and intrinsic PEEP. To return the I:E time to a normal condition of 1:2 or 1:3, increase the inspiratory flow. If the flow is increased, the tidal volume is delivered faster, which results in a decreased inspiratory time.

3. B; Complications of mechanical ventilation include barotrauma, *decreased* renal output, decreased venous blood return, and *decreased* cardiac output. Positive pressure ventilation results in decreased venous return and cardiac output by compressing the blood vessels returning blood to the heart (superior and inferior vena cavae). Renal output may decrease because of hypotension resulting from decreased cardiac output and an increased production of antidiuretic hormone (ADH). As venous blood returns to the heart, pressure receptors in the right atrium sense the drop in blood return and send a signal to the hypothalamus. The pituitary gland is then stimulated to release more ADH, which causes the kidneys to hold on to more fluid to increase the fluid level in the blood. It is one of the body's ways of compensating for hypovolemia.

4. C; Static lung compliance is the measurement of how easily the lung is stretched. The higher the compliance, the more easily it stretches. The lower the lung compliance, the less easily it stretches or the stiffer and harder it is to ventilate. Conditions that decrease compliance include atelectasis, pulmonary edema, pulmonary fibrosis, consolidation, pneumonia, pleural effusion, ARDS, and pneumothorax. The stiffer or less compliant the lung is, the more pressure is needed to ventilate the lung, which is observed by increasing peak and plateau pressures. If peak pressure increases with little or no change in the plateau pressure, airway resistance has increased. Increased airway resistance results from bronchospasm, airway secretions, water or kinks in the ventilator tubing, and patient coughing.

5. B;

$$\text{Desired rate} = \frac{\text{rate (current)} \times PaCO_2\ \text{(current)}}{PaCO_2\ \text{(desired)}}$$
$$= \frac{15 \times 30}{40} = \frac{450}{40} = 11/min$$

6. A; The blood gas results in the question reveal a normal ventilatory status (PaCO$_2$, 42 mm Hg) with hypoxemia (PaO$_2$, 58 mm Hg). Because the patient's lungs are being well ventilated, changes in rate and tidal volume are not necessary. For the PaO$_2$ to increase, the FiO$_2$ must be increased.

CHAPTER TWELVE

1. A; The upper airways of patients with emphysema collapse during exhalation, which traps air in the lungs. If patients exhale through pursed or puckered lips, back pressure is generated in the airways, keeping them open longer so that more air is exhaled and less air stays trapped in the lungs.
2. B; Eosinophil levels are increased in allergic conditions such as asthma.
3. C; The inflammatory process seen with pneumonia results in consolidated material being produced in the gas exchange areas of the lung, which are evident on a chest film.
4. C; During an asthma attack, the patient first becomes hypoxemic. As a result of the low PaO$_2$ level, the patient begins to hyperventilate, which lowers the PaCO$_2$ level and increases the pH level. This is an example of acute respiratory alkalosis with hypoxemia. If the attack is not reversed in 1 to 2 h, the patient begins to tire and will go into respiratory acidemia—her PaCO$_2$ levels will begin to increase and pH will decrease.
5. A; AIDS patients often contract pneumonia caused by the *Pneumocystis carinii* bacteria. These bacteria are often treated with the aerosolized drug pentamidine.
6. D; Streptokinase is an anticoagulant drug used to prevent and treat blood clots.

CHAPTER THIRTEEN

1. A; The Apgar score assesses the neonate in five areas: heart rate, respiratory effort, color, reflex irritability, and muscle tone. Each area is scored 0, 1, or 2 points, and the higher the score, the better. A score of **7 to 10** is normal, and the infant is observed, the upper airway is suctioned with a bulb syringe, and the baby is placed in a warmer. A score of **4 to 6,** as seen in this question, indicates moderate asphyxia, which requires stimulation and oxygen administration. A score of **0 to 3** indicates severe asphyxia, which requires immediate resuscitation with ventilator assistance.
2. B; High pulmonary artery pressures (pulmonary hypertension) are normal in utero. After birth, the infant breathes in air containing oxygen, a pulmonary vasodilator, which dilates the pulmonary vessels and results in a drop in pulmonary artery pressures. As the pressure drops, the foramen ovale and ductus arteriosus gradually close. If pulmonary pressures

remain elevated, such as in persistent fetal circulation (PFC), the high pressure keeps the foramen ovale and ductus arteriosus open, which results in blood shunting through these openings from the right side of the heart to the left, bypassing the lungs and resulting in hypoxemia.
3. B; CPAP *increases* FRC by keeping alveoli from collapsing and maintaining more air in the lungs after exhalation occurs. CPAP is used to improve oxygenation. If atelectasis and intrapulmonary shunting are reduced and lung compliance is increased, PaO$_2$ increases. Pulmonary vascular resistance begins to decrease as the PaO$_2$ level increases by dilation of the pulmonary vasculature.
4. D; Complications of a UAC include infection, thromboembolism, air embolism, and hemorrhage. UACs should be left in place no longer than 7 to 10 days so that these complications are avoided.
5. C; An infant that is cold stressed generates heat by breaking down brown fat. As brown fat is metabolized, oxygen consumption increases, which often results in hypoxemia. This leads to lactic acidosis (metabolic acidosis). Cold stress may also result in hypoglycemia (decreased glucose) and apnea.
6. B; A diagnostic tool for cystic fibrosis is an elevated sweat chloride level.

CHAPTER FOURTEEN

1. B; Acetylcysteine is a mucolytic drug that chemically reduces the viscosity of secretions, which makes them easier to expel from the airway. Its use is indicated for lung conditions that are characterized by thick, tenacious sputum, such as bronchiectasis and cystic fibrosis. Another commonly used mucolytic is pancreatic dornase or Pulmozyme.
2. C; Racemic epinephrine stimulates alpha-receptors, which results in constriction of blood vessels, reducing the swelling observed with glottic edema.
3. A; Succinylcholine is fast-acting, short-lasting paralytic agent often used to paralyze combative patients who are difficult to intubate. The patient should be administered a sedative before being given any paralytic drug.
4. C; Decadron is a steroid that exhibits antiinflammatory properties. It is useful in the treatment of asthma and glottic edema.

CHAPTER FIFTEEN

1. B; Portable liquid oxygen containers make it much easier for patients receiving continuous oxygen to travel and be active. They are lightweight, and much

more oxygen can be stored in liquid than in gaseous form.

2. A; It is much more important to make sure that home care patients are familiar with the equipment, medications, medication side effects, and proper treatment administration than the pathology of their disease. An improved quality of life is dependent on their knowledge of treatment modalities.

3. D; Because the Bennett AP-5 is the only choice of the four in this question that is an IPPB machine powered by electricity, it is the most convenient for use in the home. The other choices operate on compressed gas, which is not as safe or convenient as using an electric-powered IPPB machine.

4. B; Diaphragmatic breathing exercises are beneficial for patients with emphysema. Air-trapping caused by the disease increases FRC and lung volume, which pushes the diaphragm down and makes it flat rather than maintaining its normal dome-shape. This renders the diaphragm almost useless, and the accessory muscles become the primary muscles of ventilation. Teaching the patient to concentrate on using the diaphragm through exercises will increase tidal volume and reduce respiratory rate. Diaphragmatic exercises are coupled with pursed-lip breathing so that FRC also *decreases*.

CHAPTER SIXTEEN

1. C; A 15% improvement in a before-and-after bronchodilator study indicates that significant improvement was achieved with the bronchodilator.

2. B; Functional residual capacity (FRC) is the amount of air left in the lungs after a normal exhalation. This capacity increases in any condition in which air-trapping occurs, such as in emphysema and cystic fibrosis.

3. D; Maximal inspiratory pressure (MIP) is the maximum amount of negative pressure a patient can generate during inspiration. It determines how deep a breath the patient can take, which is essential for an adequate cough. Normal MIP is −50 to −100 cm H_2O. An MIP of less than −20 cm H_2O indicates that the patient has not produced enough negative pressure to cough adequately and ventilator assistance is necessary.

4. C; Xenon is a radioactive isotope that the patient inhales. Photoscintigrams are used to determine how well the xenon was distributed in the lung.

Photoscintigraphy evaluates the relationship of the distribution of ventilation to pulmonary perfusion.

5. B; The flow studies in this question are all below normal, indicating obstructive disease. Because the values improve more than 15% after a bronchodilator is administered, there is significant improvement. Obstructive diseases are characterized by decreased flows and increased capacities, whereas restrictive diseases are characterized by normal flows (FEV/FVC) and decreased capacities.

CHAPTER SEVENTEEN

1. B; Autoclaving sterilizes equipment in only 15 minutes at 121° C and 2 atmospheres of pressure. Because of their hard plastic construction, bacterial filters can tolerate the high temperature produced by autoclaving.

2. D; Tuberculosis, legionellosis, and histoplasmosis are all spread by the airborne route. Standard precautions must be followed, and the patient must be placed in a private room, often equipped with a negative pressure ventilation system. All persons entering the room should wear HEPA masks for protection.

3. C; Immersing equipment in glutaraldehyde (Cidex) for 15 min disinfects equipment. Immersion for 3 to 10 h results in sterilization. Equipment exposed to ethylene oxide gas for 4 h at 50° to 56° C will be sterilized. Acetic acid (vinegar), which is commonly used in the home for cleaning equipment, disinfects but does not sterilize. Pasteurization exposes equipment to water at 60° to 70° C and disinfects in 20 to 30 min. It does not have the capability to sterilize.

4. D; Gowns, gloves, and goggles should be worn when changing ventilator tubing to protect against the splashing of water from the circuit.

5. A; Tuberculosis is spread by the airborne route. Standard precautions must be followed, and the patient must be placed in a private room, often equipped with a negative pressure ventilation system. All persons entering the room should wear HEPA masks for protection.

6. D; Biologic indicators consist of strips of paper impregnated with bacteria that are placed in a glass ampule with a culture medium. The ampule is then placed in the sterilizer with the equipment to determine whether the procedure sterilized the equipment.

ANSWERS TO POSTCHAPTER STUDY QUESTIONS

CHAPTER ONE

1. 60%, 1:1; 40%, 3:1; 35%, 5:1; 30%, 8:1; and 24%, 25:1
2. Venturi mask, aerosol mask, T-piece (Briggs adapter), face tent, tracheostomy collar
3. Conserves O_2 by storing it in the reservoir
4. 17 vol%,

$$1.34 \times 13 \times 0.96 = 16.7$$
$$0.003 \times 82 = \frac{+0.25}{16.95} \text{ or } 17 \text{ vol\%}$$

5. 24 L/min,

$$60\% \text{ (1:1 air/}O_2 \text{ ratio)}$$
$$1 + 1 = 2, 2 \times 12 \text{ L/min} = 24 \text{ L/min}$$

6. Consistent ventilatory pattern, VT 300 to 700 mL, respiratory rate of less than 25/min
7. 10.8 L/min,

$$1.8 \times 6 = 10.8 \text{ L/min}$$

8. 1 h, 46 min,

$$\frac{1900 \times 0.28}{5} = \frac{532}{5} = 106 \text{ min} = 1 \text{ h } 46 \text{ min}$$

9. Nasal cannula, simple O_2 mask, partial rebreathing mask
10. Poor perfusion, severe anemia, hypotension, elevated HbCO level, direct light, phototherapy and fluorescent light sources, nail polish, dark skin pigmentation
11. CO poisoning, cyanide poisoning, decompression sickness, gas gangrene, gas embolism
12. Increases FiO_2
13. 48 L/min,

$$\text{Insp. flow rate} = \frac{VT}{\text{Insp. time}} = \frac{0.4 \text{ L}}{0.5 \text{ s}}$$
$$= 0.8 \text{ L/s} \times 60$$
$$= 48 \text{ L/min}$$

CHAPTER TWO

1. Bronchospasm; overhydration; overheating of inspired gases; tubing condensation affecting FiO_2 or draining into patient's airway; delivering contaminated water to the patient.
2. 25%
3. 14 mg/L
4. Heated cascade or wick humidifier
5. Overhydration, bronchospasm, sudden mobilization of secretions, electrical hazard, condensation in tubing, swelling of secretions resulting in airway obstruction, drug reconcentration
6. Decreased water output
7. Improve secretion mobilization, increase delivery of aerosolized medications, prevent dehydration, induce cough, relieve upper airway inflammation, and hydrate airways
8. Slow, moderately deep breaths, with a 2- to 3-s breath hold at the end of inspiration
9. 70% to 90%

CHAPTER THREE

1. Infection (increased WBC count)
2. *Pseudomonas* species
3. Increased airway resistance, COPD, upper airway obstruction, decreased lung compliance, pulmonary fibrosis, pneumothorax, pleural effusion, abnormal chest wall, anxiety
4. Difficulty breathing while lying down (supine); COPD, chronic cardiac disease, obese patients
5. Deep, rapid breathing pattern (hyperventilation); patients with diabetic ketoacidosis (DKA)
6. Atelectasis, pneumothorax, chest deformities, flail chest
7. Chest moves in during inspiration and out during expiration; flail chest or other chest trauma
8. Fluid around the ankles that results from right-sided or left-sided heart failure
9. Massive atelectasis
10. Tension pneumothorax
11. Diaphragm, external intercostal muscles
12. Air-trapping, enlarged accessory muscles of the chest
13. Pneumothorax, emphysema
14. Atelectasis, consolidation, pleural effusion, pleural thickening, pulmonary edema

15. Aortic valve disease, mitral valve disease, pulmonic valve stenosis, tricuspid valve insufficiency
16. Na^+, 135 to 145 mEq/L; K^+, 3.5 to 5.0 mEq/L; Cl^-, 95 to 105 mEq/L
17. Both result in muscle weakness
18. Renal failure
19. Alveolar hyperventilation
20. RBCs, 4 to 6 million/mm^3; Hb, males 13 to 18 g/dL, females 12 to 16 g/dL; Hct, 35% to 45%; WBC 5000 to 10,000/mm^3
21. Inadequate oxygen-carrying capacity
22. Bone marrow diseases, DIC
23. Hemorrhaging

CHAPTER FOUR

1. 20 mm Hg (27 cm H_2O)
2. Glottic edema
3. Passy-Muir speaking valve
4. The oropharyngeal airway is used to prevent upper airway obstruction, mainly from the tongue, in unconscious patients only. It may be used as a bite block for unconscious, intubated patients.
5. A fenestrated tracheostomy tube is used to wean a patient from a conventional tracheostomy tube and allow the patient to speak.
6. Poorly tolerated by conscious or semiconscious patients, biting the tube, increased production of oral secretions, easier inadvertent extubation, harder to communicate, gagging, tube not as stable, difficulty passing suction catheter because of curvature of tube
7. Diminished breath sounds in the left lung, asymmetrical chest movement
8. To suction the oropharynx
9. −120 mm Hg
10. At peak inspiration

CHAPTER FIVE

1. Removal of foreign bodies and mucus plugs to treat atelectasis; pulmonary hemorrhage; difficult tracheal intubation; biopsy of airway tumors; sputum collection for culture and sensitivity
2. Hypoxemia, laryngospasm, bronchospasm, arrhythmias, hemorrhage, respiratory depression, hypotension, pneumothorax
3. Diazepam (Valium) or midazolam (Versed)
4. To dry out the airway
5. Soak in glutaraldehyde (Cidex) solution for 3 to 10 h to disinfect or sterilize
6. To drain fluid or air from the pleural space so the lung may reexpand
7. Obstruction of the tube

8. Tension pneumothorax
9. Clamp the tube and identify the source of the leak.
10. −15 cm H_2O

CHAPTER SIX

1. Atropine, epinephrine, lidocaine
2. Hypotension
3. Ventricular fibrillation, ventricular tachycardia
4. Hypertension
5. Intubate and suction the airway
6. Ventilatory rate: 40/min; peak inspiratory pressure: initially 30 to 40 cm H_2O and subsequent pressure of 15 to 20 cm H_2O
7. Add O_2 reservoir, use high O_2 flow rate (10 to 15 L/min), use slower ventilation rate (10 to 20/min), and avoid excessive volumes if reservoir attachment is not used
8. Monophasic: 360 J; biphasic: 200 J
9. 360 J
10. Lidocaine, epinephrine
11. Atrial flutter, atrial fibrillation, ventricular tachycardia, paroxysmal supraventricular tachycardia, ventricular fibrillation
12. 25 to 100 J
13. Decreased PaO_2, increased size of pneumothorax, increased ET tube cuff pressure

CHAPTER SEVEN

1. Increased mean airway pressure, increased VT, decreased work of breathing, alteration of I:E times, mechanical bronchodilation, reduced cerebral blood flow
2. Increased work of breathing, hypoventilation, inadequate cough effort, increased airway resistance, atelectasis, pulmonary edema, weaning from ventilator
3. Hyperventilation, hyperoxygenation, decreased cardiac output, increased ICP, pneumothorax, hemoptysis, gastric distention, nosocomial infection
4. Pulmonary hemorrhage, untreated pneumothorax
5. 20 beats/min
6. Decreased VT
7. Increased VT
8. Decreased inspiratory time
9. Tighten tubing connections; check for leaks around mouthpiece, mask, or ET tube; check expiratory valve function
10. Increased inspiratory flow, decreased peak inspiratory pressure
11. 10 mL/kg of body weight
12. Sustained maximal inspiration (SMI)
13. Cooperative patient, motivated patient, respiratory rate less than 25/min

CHAPTER EIGHT

1. 10 to 20 cm H_2O
2. 10 to 25 cm H_2O
3. Patients with cystic fibrosis
4. Postural drainage and percussion
5. Hypoxemia, rib fractures, increased airway resistance, increased ICP, hemorrhage, decreased cardiac output, aspiration
6. Prone, with head down
7. Sinusitis; middle ear infection; epistaxis; facial, oral, or skull surgery or trauma

CHAPTER NINE

1. Clot in catheter, tip of catheter up against vessel wall, clot in transducer, air bubbles in the line
2. Hypervolemia, pulmonary hypertension, right ventricular failure, pulmonary valve stenosis, tricuspid valve stenosis, pulmonary embolism, arterial vasodilation, left-sided heart failure, improper transducer placement, positive pressure ventilator breath, severe flail chest, pneumothorax
3. Hypovolemia, vasodilation, leaks or air in line, improper transducer placement
4. Lidocaine, propranolol, procainamide
5. Defibrillation, chest compressions, lidocaine
6. Pulmonary hypertension, mitral valve stenosis, left ventricular failure
7. Decreased PVR, hypovolemia
8. Left atrial pressure
9. Left ventricular failure, mitral valve stenosis, aortic stenosis, systemic hypertension
10. Hypovolemia, pulmonary embolus (PAWP could also be normal)
11. CVP, less than 8 cm H_2O or less than 6 mm Hg; PAP,

$$\frac{20 - 30 \text{ mm Hg}}{5 - 15 \text{ mm Hg}}$$

or a mean of 10 to 20 mm Hg; PAWP, 4 to 12 mm Hg
12. 4 L/min;

$$\frac{240 \text{ mL/min}}{6 \times 10} = \frac{240}{60} = 4 \text{ L/min}$$

13. 2% to 5%
14. 4.4 mL/dL;

$$CaO_2 = (1.34 \times 14 \times 0.95) + (82 \times 0.003) = 18$$

$$CvO_2 = (1.34 \times 14 \times 0.72) + (37 \times 0.003) = 13.6$$

$$18 - 13.6 = 4.4 \text{ mL/dL}$$

15. Pneumonia, pneumothorax, pulmonary edema, atelectasis
16. 11%;

$$PaO_2 = [(747 - 47) \times 0.50] - 40 \times 1.25 = 300$$

$$PaO_2 - PaO_2 = 300 - 122 = 178$$

$$\frac{QS}{QT} = \frac{178 \times 0.003}{4.5 + (178 \times 0.003)} = 11\%$$

17. Vasoconstrictors (dopamine, epinephrine), hypovolemia, decreased $PaCO_2$, septic shock (late stages)
18. Vasodilators (nitroprusside sodium, morphine, nitroglycerin), increased $PaCO_2$, septic shock (early stages)
19. Vasoconstrictors, increased $PaCO_2$, hypoxemia, acidemia, pulmonary embolism, pneumothorax, positive pressure ventilation, PEEP, CPAP
20. Vasodilators, hyperoxemia, decreased $PaCO_2$, alkalemia
21. $4.5 (5) \times 10 = 225 \text{ mL/min}$
22. Hyperthermia, exercise, seizures, shivering
23. Hypothermia, cyanide poisoning, musculoskeletal relaxation

CHAPTER TEN

1. Interpretation is as follows
   A. Uncompensated metabolic acidemia, normal oxygenation
   B. Fully compensated (chronic) respiratory acidemia, moderate hypoxemia
   C. Uncompensated respiratory alkalemia, normal oxygenation
   D. Combined respiratory and metabolic acidemia, mild hypoxemia
   E. Fully compensated respiratory alkalemia, normal oxygenation
   F. Partially compensated respiratory acidemia, normal oxygenation
2. An Allen test is done before radial artery puncture to determine collateral blood flow to the hand. It is essential to determine if ulnar blood flow is present, in case the radial artery spasms or clots.
3. Hypercapnia, acidosis, hyperthermia, increased 2,3-DPG
4. When the curve shifts to the right, the Hb affinity for O_2 decreases, which makes O_2 binding more difficult; however, the O_2 that does bind with Hb will be released more easily to the tissues.

5. 144 mm Hg;

$$PAO_2 = [(747 - 47) \times 0.40] - (45 \times 1.25)$$

$$280 - 56 = 224$$

$$PAO_2 - PaO_2 = 224 - 80 = 144$$

6. $PaCO_2$

7. pH, 7.25; $PaCO_2$, 23 mm Hg; PaO_2, 80 mm Hg; HCO_3^-, 12 mEq/L; partially compensated metabolic acidemia. The initial problem is metabolic acidemia. The patient responds to this acidemia by hyperventilation to remove CO_2, which begins bringing the pH back up toward normal levels. Your answer should show that the levels of pH, $PaCO_2$, and HCO_3^- all decreased.

CHAPTER ELEVEN

1. ARDS
2. Decreases VT
3. 5 to 10 cm H_2O
4. If 60% O_2 still results in hypoxemia (and $PaCO_2$ is normal or low)
5. $VT \times RR$
6. $(VT - VD) \times RR$
7. 4 mL/cm H_2O;

$$\frac{volume}{pressure} = \frac{200\ mL}{50\ cm\ H_2O} = 4\ mL/cm\ H_2O$$

8. 620 mL;

$$\begin{aligned} lost\ volume &= PIP \times tubing\ compliance \\ &= 20 \times 4 = 80\ mL \\ &= 700\ mL - 80\ mL = 620\ mL \end{aligned}$$

9. 8/min to 12/min
10. 10 to 12 mL/kg of ideal body weight
11. Atelectasis, hypoxemia with the use of 60% O_2 or more, decreased FRC, to prevent the use of more than 60% O_2 to maintain normal PaO_2 level, decreased lung compliance, pulmonary edema
12. Barotrauma, decreased venous return, decreased cardiac output, decreased urinary output
13. The level of PEEP that improves lung compliance without decreasing cardiac output
14. Decreasing PvO_2 levels and a drop in blood pressure
15. Leaks in the circuit, patient disconnection
16. Decreasing lung compliance, airway secretions, bronchospasm, water in the ventilator tubing, kink in the ventilator tubing, coughing
17. 5 to 15 cm H_2O above average peak inspiratory pressure
18. Bronchospasm, water in the ventilator tubing, mucosal edema, secretions

19. 35 to 45 mm Hg, or 4.5% to 5.5%
20. Hyperventilation, apnea, total airway obstruction, hypotension, pulmonary embolism, decreased cardiac output
21. Hypoventilation, hyperthermia
22. VC < 15 mL/kg, $P(A-a)O_2$ > 450 mm Hg with the use of 100% O_2, VD/VT > 60%, unable to obtain an MIP of at least −20 cm H_2O, PEP < 40 cm H_2O, respiratory rate > 35/min
23. Barotrauma, pulmonary infection, atelectasis, tracheal damage, decreased venous return, decreased urinary output, lack of nutrition, pulmonary O_2 toxicity
24. 37.5 mL/cm H_2O;

$$\frac{750\ mL}{20\ cm\ H_2O} = 37.5\ mL/cm\ H_2O$$

25. Pneumonia, pulmonary edema, consolidation, atelectasis, air-trapping, pleural effusion, pneumothorax, ARDS
26. R_{AW} is increasing.
27. VC > 15 mL/kg, VT three times body weight (kg), able to obtain a MIP of at least −20 cm H_2O, VD/VT <60%, $P(A-a)O_2$ < 350 mm Hg with the use of 100% O_2, respiratory rate < 25/min, and life-threatening conditions, anemia, fever, or electrolyte imbalances not present
28. 100 to 600 cycles/min
29. Reduced risk of barotrauma, reduced risk of cardiac side effects, less fluctuation in ICP, improvement in mucociliary clearance
30. Increase the FiO_2 to 0.40;

$$80 \times 0.3 \div 60 = 0.40$$

31. Increase the ventilator rate to 11/min;

$$8 \times 55 \div 40 = 11$$

32. Increase the VT or ventilator rate (to decrease $PaCO_2$).
33. Decrease the FiO_2 to 0.60.
34. Leaks in the tubing or around the ET tube or chest tube; air-trapping

CHAPTER TWELVE

1. Emphysema, chronic bronchitis, asthmatic bronchitis
2. Flattened diaphragm, increased lung markings (hyperinflation), reduced vascular markings, bullae or bleb formation
3. 50 to 65 mm Hg
4. Pedal edema, distended jugular (neck) veins, enlarged liver
5. By causing pulmonary vasodilation of pulmonary vessels, thereby decreasing pulmonary hypertension

6. Eosinophils
7. Pentamidine
8. Left ventricular failure, mitral valve stenosis, aortic stenosis, systemic hypertension
9. Dyspnea; pink, frothy secretions; crackles; tachypnea; cyanosis; diaphoresis; distended neck veins; arrhythmias
10. Supplemental O_2, cardiac medications, ventilatory support, airway maintenance, morphine, IPPB with ethyl alcohol, diuretics
11. Sepsis, aspiration, near-drowning, O_2 toxicity, shock, thoracic trauma, extensive burns, toxic gas inhalation, fluid overload, fat embolism, narcotic overdose
12. Hypoxemia (often not responsive to O_2), cyanosis, severe dyspnea, decreased lung compliance, retractions, widened $P(A-a)O_2$ gradient, tachypnea
13. Mechanical ventilation with PEEP, diuretics, airway maintenance, monitoring of cardiac pressures
14. Air in the pleural space
15. Needle aspiration in the second or third intercostal space
16. CPAP or Bi-PAP
17. Eye movement, EEG, ECG, apnea, chest or abdominal movement, SpO_2

CHAPTER THIRTEEN

1. Heart rate, respiratory effort, color, reflex irritability, muscle tone
2. Apgar score 0 to 3: immediate resuscitation with ventilatory assistance; 4 to 6: stimulation and O_2 administration; 7 to 10: routine observation, suction upper airway with bulb syringe, dry infant, and place under warmer.
3. Nasal flaring
4. pH, 7.35 to 7.45; $PaCO_2$, 35 to 45 mm Hg; PaO_2, 50 to 70 mm Hg; HCO_3^-, 20 to 26 mEq/L; BE, −5 to +5
5. To improve oxygenation, to increase static lung compliance, to increase FRC, to decrease the work of breathing, to decrease intrapulmonary shunting, and to decrease pulmonary vascular resistance
6. Barotrauma, decreased venous return, air-trapping, pressure necrosis, loss of CPAP from crying or displacement
7. Neonatal retinopathy, BPD
8. In the descending aorta at x-ray level: T6 to T10 or L3 to L4
9. Easily obtained ABG levels, avoidance of frequent arterial punctures, continuous monitoring of blood pressure, infusion of drugs and fluids
10. Infection, thromboembolism, air embolism, hemorrhage
11. Nasal flaring, grunting, retractions, tachypnea, cyanosis, mixed respiratory and metabolic acidosis with hypoxemia

12. High O_2 concentrations, high ventilatory pressures
13. Increased airway resistance, normal or increased static lung compliance, V/Q mismatching, hypoxemia while breathing room air, tachypnea, barrel chest, retractions, hypercapnia
14. "Ground glass" appearance, opacification, atelectasis, hyperlucency, bullae
15. O_2 therapy, positive pressure ventilation, adequate humidification of inspired gases, CPT, adequate nutrition, maintenance of fluid balance, bronchodilator therapy, airway suctioning
16. Stress or hypoxia in utero of postmature infants leads to expulsion of meconium into the amniotic fluid, where it may be aspirated with the infant's first breath
17. Long fingernails, peeling skin, hypoxemia, hypercarbia, tachypnea, retractions, nasal flaring, grunting, barrel chest, cyanosis, crackles and rhonchi on auscultation
18. Perinatal asphyxia, meconium aspiration, pneumonia, sepsis, congenital heart defects, diaphragmatic hernia, hypoplastic lungs, hypoglycemia
19. Tachypnea, hypoxemia, cyanosis, more than a 15-mm Hg difference in preductal and postductal PaO_2 on 100% O_2, increase in PaO_2 over 100 mm Hg when $PaCO_2$ is maintained between 20 and 25 mm Hg
20. Mechanical hyperventilation, PaO_2 of more than 100 mm Hg, tolazoline, nitroprusside sodium, $NaHCO_3$, dopamine
21. Bacterial infection (*H. influenzae,* streptococci, staphylococci, pneumococci)
22. High fever, drooling, sore throat, dyspnea, tachycardia, inspiratory stridor, retractions, accessory muscle use, hoarseness, swollen epiglottis, hypoxemia, and respiratory alkalosis, followed by respiratory acidosis if not reversed
23. "Thumb sign"
24. Intubation, if possible; tracheotomy, if intubation is not possible; O_2 therapy; antibiotics; mechanical ventilation, if necessary
25. Tachypnea, tachycardia, productive cough with thick secretions, increased AP chest diameter, digital clubbing, increased chloride level in sweat, accessory muscle use, hypoxemia with respiratory alkalosis in early stages, chronic ventilatory failure in late stages, cyanosis, cor pulmonale in late stages, decreased result on flow studies and increased FRC on pulmonary function tests
26. Aerosolized acetylcysteine, CPT, O_2 therapy, expectorants, antibiotics, continuous aerosol therapy

CHAPTER FOURTEEN

1. Thick secretions
2. Upper airway edema (swelling)
3. Epinephrine, racemic epinephrine, isoproterenol, metaproterenol, terbutaline, albuterol
4. Atropine, ipratropium (Atrovent)

5. Succinylcholine
6. Prevents attacks by stabilizing mast cells
7. Gentamicin, cystic fibrosis (*Pseudomonas* species); amoxicillin, bronchiectasis; amphotericin B, fungal infections; pentamidine, *Pneumocystis carinii;* ribavirin, RSV and bronchiolitis
8. Dexamethasone, beclomethasone, flunisolide
9. Edema, moon face, adrenal suppression, oral candidiasis (thrush mouth)
10. Zafirlukast (Accolate), montelukast (Singulair), zileuton (Zyflo)
11. To prevent asthma attacks

CHAPTER FIFTEEN

1. To help the patient become independent, cope with the disease, understand the disease and its limitations, and set realistic goals and find ways to attain them
2. Pulmonary function tests, sputum collection and analysis, ABG collection and analysis, exercise tolerance testing, chest x-ray films
3. Creates a subtle back pressure into the larger airways, which reduces the volume of trapped air and helps to reduce the feeling of dyspnea
4. Membrane concentrator, 40%; molecular sieve concentrator, 90% to 95%
5. FiO$_2$ analysis, alarm checks, flow measurement, filter and battery checks

6.
$$\frac{3 \times 860}{2.5} = \frac{2580}{2.5} = 1032\,L;$$
$$\frac{1032\,L}{2\,L/min} = 516\,min\ or\ 8.6\,h$$

CHAPTER SIXTEEN

1. Emphysema (or other obstructive lung diseases)
2. Restrictive lung conditions (e.g., pulmonary fibrosis, scoliosis, pneumonia)
3. Respirometer
4. FEV$_1$/FVC
5. FEV$_1$, FEF$_{25\%-75\%}$, FEF$_{200-1200}$
6. Obstructive
7. PIF, PEF, FVC, FEV$_1$, FEF$_{25\%-75\%}$
8. O$_2$ toxicity, emphysema, pulmonary edema, asbestosis, sarcoidosis, pulmonary fibrosis
9. The response to the bronchodilating agent (an increase in flow study results of at least 15% indicates a significant response)
10. The maximum amount of negative pressure the patient can generate during inspiration; determines the level of respiratory muscle strength

CHAPTER SEVENTEEN

1. Tuberculosis, histoplasmosis, legionellosis, measles
2. HEPA filter
3. Autoclave, ethylene oxide gas, glutaraldehyde solution
4. Streptococcal pneumonia, epiglottitis, adenovirus, meningitis, pertussis, *H. influenzae*
5. Hospital-acquired infection
6. *Pseudomonas, Klebsiella, Serratia,* and *Legionella* species
7. Chemical and biologic indicators, culture and swab sampling

INDEX

A

Abdominal thrusts, performing, 75–76
ABG. *See* Arterial blood gas
Abnormal heart sounds (murmurs), 42
Absolute humidity, 24
  relative humidity, relationship, 24b
Absorption atelectasis, 162
Acapella oscillatory PEP device, 102
Accelerating ramp wave, 147f
Acetic acid (vinegar), 201
Acetylcysteine (Mucomyst), 179–180
  indication, 179
Acid-base balance (pH), 124–126
  compensation, 125–126
  measurement, Sanz electrode (usage), 128
  relationships, 125
Acidemia, 125. *See also* Respiratory acidemia
  occurrence
Acrocyanosis, 168b
Acute respiratory distress syndrome (ARDS), 19
  chest x-ray films, characteristics, 160
  clinical signs/symptoms, 160
  definition, 160–161
  mechanical ventilation, PEEP (usage of), 160–161
  network, guidelines, 131
  pathophysiology, 160
  treatment, 160–161
Acute ventilatory failure, 139. *See also* Impending acute
    ventilatory failure
ADH. *See* Antidiuretic hormone
Adrenalin Chloride. *See* Epinephrine hydrochloride
Adult CPR modifications, 77
Adult patients. *See* One-rescuer CPR; Two-rescuer CPR
Advance directives, 82
Adventitious breath sounds, 41
Aerosol
  pretest questions, 23
  postchapter study questions, 31
  review, 23–31
Aerosolized antibiotics, 183–184
Aerosolized corticosteroids, 184
Aerosol mask
  illustration, 15f
  placement, 14b
  usage, 96
    example, 121
Aerosol particles, characteristics, 27
Aerosol therapy, 27–31
  clinical uses, 27
  hazards, 27
Afebrile characteristic, 44
Afterload, 118
Airborne infections, precautions, 202
Air bubbles, presence, 112
Air entrapment mask, 13–17
  illustration, 13f
  setting, 14b
Air/O_2 entrainment ratios, calculation, 14t

Air/O_2 ratios, calculation, 14b
  magic box method, usage, 14t
Air trapping, presence, 88
Airway clearance techniques, 96
Airway disorders (treatment success), Dexamethasone (usage),
  179
Airway humidification, 24
Airway management
  postchapter questions, 67
  pretest questions, 49
  review, 49–67
Airway obstruction, 50. *See also* Upper airway obstruction
  treatment
Airway resistance (RAW), calculation, 142
Airway suctioning, 64–66
Albuterol (Proventil) (Ventolin), 180
Alcohol poisoning, 9
Alcohols (sterilization/disinfection), 201
Alkalemia. *See* Respiratory alkalemia
  indication, 125
  occurrence, 125
Allen test, 111
Alupent. *See* Metaproterenol
Alveolar air equation, 18
Alveolar dead space, 140
Alveolar hypoventilation, 7
Alveolar PO_2 (PAO_2), 122–123
Alveolar ventilation, 124
  changes, 145
  decrease, 133
  improvement, 133b
Aminophylline. *See* Theophylline
Amoxicillin, 183
Amphotericin B, 183
Analgesics, 184. *See also* Narcotic analgesics; Nonnarcotic
    analgesics
Anatomic dead space, 134b, 140–141
Anectine. *See* Succinylcholine
Anemic hypoxia, 8
Angina pectoris, 34–35
Anteroposterior (AP) chest radiograph positions, 42
Antibiotics. *See* Aerosolized antibiotics
Antidiuretic hormone (ADH), production (increase),
  140
Antimicrobial action, conditions, 200
Apgar
  results, 168
  score, determination, 167
  scoring system, 168
    assessed signs, 168
    example, 168t
Apical lordotic chest radiograph position, 42
Apnea, 35
  alarm, 138
  mechanical ventilation, indication, 139
  monitoring. *See* Home apnea monitoring
ARDS. *See* Acute respiratory distress syndrome
Arformoterol (Brovana), 181
Arrhythmias, 71
  termination, cardioversion (usage), 82
Arterial blood, (sites) obtaining, 122. *See also* Neonates

Page numbers followed by *f, b* and *t* indicate figure, boxes and
   es, respectively.

54

Arterial blood gas (ABG)
  analysis, 121–128
  example problems, 126–127
  levels, 47
    example, 126–127
  normal value chart summary, 126t
  sampling, 122
  values, 146t
Arterial blood gas (ABG) interpretation, 126
  chart, 127t
  postchapter study questions, 128
  pretest question, 121
  review, 121–128
  steps, 126
Arterial catheter (arterial line), 111–112
  complications, 112
Arterialized capillary blood sampling, 171
Arterial lines, troubleshooting, 112
Arterial oxygenation, 122–124
Arterial oxygen content
  determination, 9b
    pretest question, 1
  measurement, 116
Arteriovenous oxygen content, difference, 116
Artificial airways, 50–51
  maintenance, 64–66
Aspiration, 100
Assist-control mode. *See* Volume ventilator
Asthma
  attack, treatment, 155
  causes, 153
  chest x-ray films, characteristics, 154
  classifications, 153–154
  clinical signs/symptoms, 154
  definition, 153–155
  pathophysiology, 154
  preventive treatment, 154–155
  pulmonary function studies, characteristics, 154
  status asthmaticus, 155
  treatment, 154–155
Atelectasis, 7, 43
  causes, 162
  chest x-ray films, characteristics, 162
  clinical signs/symptoms, 162
  definition, 162–163
  mechanical ventilation complication, 140
  pathophysiology, 162
  treatment, 162–163
Atrial depolarization, 106–107
Atrial fibrillation, 109
  coarse waves, 109f
Atrial flutter, 109
  response, 109f
Atrial impulses, blockage, 109
Atropine, 70. *See also* Naloxone atropine vasopressin epinephrine lidocaine
Atropine sulfate, 181
  administration route, 80
  CPR administration, 80
  dosage, 80
  indications, 80
  pharmacologic actions, 80
Atrovent. *See* Ipratropium bromide
Augmented leads, 104
Autoclave (pressurized steam), 200

Autogenic drainage, 100
  phases, 100

B
Babington nebulizer. *See* Hydrosphere
Bacilli, 200
  examples, 200
Bacteria, classes, 200
Bacterial pneumonia, 156
Barometric pressure, usage, 18b
Barotrauma, 139
Barrel chest, 39
  AP diameter, increase, 39f
Bedside spirometers (portable spirometers), 198
Before-and-after bronchodilator studies, 196
Bennett AP-5, 92
  components, 92f
  unit, usage, 187–188
Bennett PR-2 ventilator, 91–92
  components, 91f
  controls, 92
  diluter regulator, 91
  dilution control, 92
  inspiratory pressure control, 92
  nebulization control, 92
  peak flow control, 92
  sensitivity control, 92
  terminal flow control, 92
Bennett valve, 92
Bicarbonate (HCO_3^-), 46
Bigeminy, 109b
Bilevel positive airway pressure (Bi-PAP), use of, 131, 163
Biologic indicators, 201
  usage, 199
Biot respiration, 35
  wave formation, 35f
Bird Mark 7, 89–91
  air mix control, 90–91
  controls, 90–91
  expiratory timing device, 91
  flow control, 90
  flow wave patterns, 90f
  gas flow, 89–90
  hand timer rod, 91
  inspiratory pressure control, 91
  sensitivity control, 91
  ventilator, 89f
Bland aerosol therapy, indications, 23
Blebs, definition, 152
Blender/nebulizer, usage, 18
Blood, carbon dioxide entry, 124
Blood gas
  analysis, monitoring, 121
  analyzers, 128
    capabilities, 128
    quality control procedures, 128
  electrodes, 128
  levels, obtaining (pretest question), 1
  measurements, 121
Blood loss, excess, 8
Blood pressure, 44
  factors, 44
Blood urea nitrogen (BUN), 46
Body humidity, 24

Body plethysmography, usage, 193
Body surface area (BSA), 118
Body temperature, 44
Bohr effect, 124
Bourdon gauge, 6f
  advantage, 6
  flowmeter, calibration, 6
  outlet, humidifier/nebulizer attachment, 6
  regulator, 4f
BPD. *See* Bronchopulmonary dysplasia
Brachial artery, palpation, 76
Bradycardia, 44
Bradypnea, 35
Breathing. *See* Diaphragmatic breathing; Pursed-lip breathing;
  Segmental breathing
  cycle, 69
  difficulty, 32
  exercises, 188
  patterns, 35
  work, 36
    decrease, 86
Breathlessness, determination, 76
Breath sounds, 41
  auscultation, 41
Brethine. *See* Terbutaline sulfate
Bricanyl. *See* Terbutaline sulfate
Briggs adaptor, 16
  illustration, 16f
Bronchi, chronic dilation, 157–158
Bronchial breath sounds, 41
Bronchial tree, mast cells stimulation, 154
Bronchiectasis
  causes, 155
  chest x-ray films, characteristics, 156
  clinical signs/symptoms, 156
  definition, 155–156
  pathophysiology, 155–156
  pulmonary function studies, characteristics, 156
  treatment, 156
Bronchiolitis, 176–177
  causes, 176
  chest x-ray findings, 177
  clinical manifestations, 177
  definition, 176–177
  pathophysiology, 176
  severity, 177
  treatment, 177
Bronchoalveolar lavage (BAL), 157
Bronchodilators, 191. *See also* Parasympatholytic bronchodilators;
  Sympathomimetic bronchodilators
  studies; Before-and-after bronchodilator studies
  therapy, spirometry test
Bronchopulmonary dysplasia (BPD), 170, 172–173
  causes, 172
  chest x-ray findings, 173
  clinical manifestations, 173
  definition, 172–173
  impact, 170b
  pathophysiology, 172–173
  stages, 172–173
  treatment, 173
Bronchopulmonary hygiene techniques, 100–102
  postchapter study questions, 102
  pretest questions, 96
  review, 96–102

Bronchoscopes. *See* Fiberoptic bronchoscopes; Rigid
  bronchoscope
  types, 70
Bronchoscopy, 69–74
  assistance, trachea entry difficulty, 69
  complications, 69, 71
  indications, 70–71
  respiratory therapist responsibility, 71
  ventilator pressure, increase, 69
Bronchospasm, 27, 71
  acetylcysteine side effect, 179–180
Bronchovesicular breath sounds, 41
Brovana. *See* Arformoterol
Brownian motion, 27
BSA. *See* Body surface area
Bubble humidifiers (nonheated humidifiers), 25
  components, 25f
Bullae, definition, 152
Bullous disease, relative IPPB contraindication, 88
Bullous emphysema, 152
BUN. *See* Blood urea nitrogen
Bundle of His, division, 103–104

C
Calcium (Ca), 46
Calcium chloride, 81
  indications, 81
Capillary blood sampling. *See* Arterialized capillary blood
  sampling
Capillary hydrostatic pressure, 158
Capillary refill, 37
Capnography. *See* End-tidal CO_2 monitoring
Carbon dioxide (CO_2)
  detection, disposable colorimetric device (usage), 58f
  transport, 124
Carbon monoxide (CO) poisoning, 8
  treatment, pretest question, 1
Cardiac arrhythmias, 45
  encounter, 108
  QRS complex, abnormal shape, 103
Cardiac cycle, example, 105f
Cardiac index (CI)
  decrease, factors, 118
  increase, factors, 118
  measurement, 118
Cardiac insufficiency, relative IPPB contraindication, 88
Cardiac ischemia, 106
Cardiac monitoring
  postchapter study questions, 120
  pretest questions, 103
  review, 103–120
Cardiac output
  calculation, 116b
  decrease, 9, 87, 100
  intrapulmonary shunting, 117
  measurement, 115–116
  usage, 142b
Cardiac stress test, 119
Cardiogenic pulmonary edema, 158–163
Cardiopulmonary patient assessment
  patient history, 33–48
  postchapter study questions, 48
  pretest questions, 32
  review, 33–48
  symptoms, assessment, 33–35

Cardiopulmonary resuscitation (CPR), 75–83
  administration, routes, 79–80
  adult/child modifications, 77
  considerations, 77
  drugs
    administration, 80–81
    usage, 75
  ECG strip indication, 75
  hazards, 77
  infant modifications, 77
  infant pulse, return, 75
  performing, 75
  pharmacologic intervention, 79–81
Cardiopulmonary resuscitation (CPR) techniques
  postchapter study questions, 83
  pretest questions, 75
  review, 75–83
Cardiopulmonary stress test, 119–120
Cardiopulmonary stress testing, 119–120
Cardioversion, 81–82
Carotid artery, palpation, 76
Cascade humidifiers (heated humidifiers), 26
  components, 26f
Catheters
  size, selection, 65
  tip
    occlusion, 112
    rest, 112
  types, 66
Central apnea, 164f–165f
Central sleep apnea, 163
  symptoms, 163
Central venous pressure (CVP), 113
  decrease, 103
  decrease, conditions, 115
  monitoring, 114–115
    pulmonary artery catheter, usage, 114–115
  PEEP, impact (determination), 114b
  water manometer, usage, 114b
Centrilobular emphysema (centriacinar emphysema), 152
Cerebral blood flow
  alteration, 87
  reduction, hyperventilation (usage problems), 143b
Chemical agents (sterilization/disinfection), 200–201
Chemical indicators, 201
Chest
  consolidation, 42
  deformities, 37–39
  infiltrates, 42
  inspection, 35–36
  leads. See Precordial leads
  pain, 34–35
  palpation, 40
    assessment, 39f
  radiograph positions, 42–43
  radiolucency, 42
  radiopaque, 42
  symmetry, 36
  vibrations, 40
  wall, percussion, 40
  X-ray film interpretation, 42–43
Chest physical therapy (CPT), 96–102
  complications, 100
  contraindications, 97
  goals, 96

Chest physical therapy (CPT) (Continued)
  indications, 96–97
  techniques, 96
Chest tube
  drainage considerations, 74
  drainage system, 72–73
    water level fluctuation, 69
  insertion/monitoring, 71–74
  one-bottle system, 72
  three-bottle system, 73
  two-bottle system, 72
Cheyne-Stokes respiration, 35
  wave formation, 35f
Child CPR modifications, 77
Chloride (Cl⁻), 45–46
  levels, elevation, 167, 177
Chronic bronchitis, 153
  cause, 153
  chest x-ray films, characteristics, 153
  clinical signs/symptoms, 153
  pathophysiology, 153
  pulmonary function studies, characteristics, 153
  treatment, 153
Chronic hypoxemia, 36–37
Chronic obstructive pulmonary disease (COPD), air trapping (presence), 88
Chronic respiratory acidemia, 125b
Chronic respiratory alkalemia, 125b
CI. See Cardiac index
Circulatory hypoxia. See Stagnant hypoxia
CL. See Lung compliance
Clark electrode, usage, 128
Closed head injury, relative IPPB contraindication, 88
Closed suction catheter, 65f
Coagulation studies, 46–47
Cocci, 200
Collar. See Tracheostomy mask
Collateral circulation (determination), modified Allen test (usage), 122
Collection bottles, 66
Combative patient, intubation difficulty, 179
Combination drugs, 184
Combitube, 54f. See also Esophageal-tracheal Combitube insertion
Compensated blood gas measurement, interpretation, 126b
Compensated flowmeter, 5f
  needle valve, location, 5–6
Compensated metabolic acidemia, 126b
Compensated metabolic alkalemia, 126b
Compensated respiratory acidemia, 125b
Compensated respiratory alkalemia, 125b
Compensation, 125–126. See also Acid-base balance
Complete upper airway obstruction, signs, 50
Compressed GAs Association (CGA), color code system development, 2t
Compression depth, 77
Compression/ventilation ratios
  one rescuer, 77
  two rescuers, 77
Computed tomography (CT), 43
  usage, 43
Computerized charting, 47
Computerized monitoring, 47–48
Computers, clinical application, 47–48
Condensation, occurrence, 26

Conscious adult, obstructed airway, 75–77
Consciousness
  cooperation ability, 45
  emotional state, 45
  level, 44–45
  time/place orientation, 45
Conscious sedation, 70
Contact precautions, 202
Contaminated equipment, handling, 202
Continuous positive airway pressure (CPAP), use of, 132, 163
  receiving, 140–141
  ventilator separation, 132
Contraction. See Ventricular depolarization
Co-oximetry (hemoximetry), 21
COPD. See Chronic obstructive pulmonary disease
Cor pulmonale. See Right-sided heart failure
Corticosteroids. See Aerosolized corticosteroids
Coudé suction catheter, 66
Cough ability (determination), pulmonary function tests (usage), 191
Cough instruction, 188
Cough technique, 100
CPAP. See Continuous positive airway pressure
CPR. See Cardiopulmonary resuscitation
CPT. See Chest physical therapy
Crackles, 41
Critically ill patient, transportation, 82–83
Cromolyn sodium (Intal), 182
Croup. See Laryngotracheobronchitis
Cuff care, 64–66
Cuff deflation, 64
Cuff pressure, maintenance, 64
Culture sampling, 201
Curved blade. See McIntosh blade
CVP. See Central venous pressure
Cyanide poisoning, 9
Cyanosis, 37
Cylinder color code system, CGA development, 2t
Cylinder factors, 4
Cylinder markings, 2f
Cylinder testing, 3
Cylinder valves
  regulator attachment, 2
  safety relief devices, 2
Cystic fibrosis, 177
  causes, 177
  chest x-ray findings, 177
  clinical manifestations, 177
  definition, 177
  pathophysiology, 177
  treatment, 177

D

Dead space (VD), 140–141
  addition, rarity, 141b
  removal, 141b
  types, 140–141
Decadron. See Dexamethasone
Decelerating ramp wave, 147f
Defibrillation, 81–82
Delivered VT, effects, 92–93
Dexamethasone (Decadron), usage, 179
Diagnostic sleep studies, 163–165
Diameter Index Safety System, usage, 5

Diaphragm
  characteristics, 43
  ventilation muscle, 39
Diaphragmatic breathing, 188
  exercises, 187
Diaphragm compressor, 7f
Diaphragm oscillating device, 144
Diastole, 103–104
Diastolic pressure, 112
Diazepam (Valium), usage, 70
Diffusion capacity. See Normal diffusion capacity
Diffusion capacity of the lungs (DL), 195–196
Diffusion defects, 7
Digital clubbing, 36–37
  indications, 36
Digit configuration, 36f
Diluents, 179–185
Disaster management, participation, 83
Diseases, transmission, 199
Disinfection, 199–200
  techniques, 200–201
Disulfide bonds, breakage, 179–180
Diuretics, 185
DL. See Diffusion capacity of the lungs
Dobutamine hydrochloride, 81
  pharmacologic actions, 81
Do-not-resuscitate (DNR) protocols, 82
Dopamine hydrochloride, 81
  pharmacologic actions, 81
Dornase alfa (Pulmozyme) (RhDNase), 180
Dosage calculations. See Drugs
Double-stage reducing valve, 3
DPIs. See Dry powder inhalers
Droplet spreading, precautions, 202
Drugs, 185–186. See also Combination drugs
  calculations
    dosage calculations, 186
    percentage strength, 185–186
      calculation, 186
      ratio strength conversion, 186
Dry powder inhalers (DPIs), 185
  types, 185
Dubowitz scoring system, 168
Ductus arteriosus, patency, 167
Dullness, 40
Dynamic lung compliance, 141
  calculation, 141b
Dyspnea, 34. See also exertional dyspnea; Paroxysmal nocturnal dyspnea
  causes, 34
  oxygen therapy indication, 7
  types, 34

E

ECMO. See Extracorporeal membrane oxygenation
Edema. See Glottic edema; Subglottic edema
Electric cardiac pacemakers, 111
  illustration, 111f
Electric nebulizers, 29–30
Electrocardiogram (ECG)
  artifacts, discovery, 103
  graph paper, 105
  interpretation, steps, 107
  leads, 103–104
  monitoring. See Long-term ECG monitoring

Electrocardiogram (ECG) (Continued)
   normal pattern, 105f
   P wave, characteristic, 103
   strip, indications, 75
   three-lead systems, 104
   tracing, 106f
     interpretation, 120f
     PR interval, prolongation, 106f
     ST segment depression, 106f
   waves, 105–106
Electrocardiography, 103–120
Embolism, 9
Embolus, 159–160
Emotional state, 45
Emphysema, 151–153
   causes, 152
   centrilobular type (centriacinar type), 152
   chest x-ray films, characteristics, 152
   clinical signs/symptoms, 152
   definition, 151–153
   panlobular type (panacinar type), 151–152
   pathophysiology, 152
   pulmonary function studies, characteristics, 152
   treatment, 152–153
Empyema, 157b
Endotracheal (ET) intubation, 32
   performing, steps, 56–58
Endotracheal (ET) tubes, 55–59
   complications, 58
   components, 58f
   drugs, usage, 80
   extubation, 66–67
   hazards, 55
   indications, 55
   laryngeal/tracheal complications, 67
   markings, 58
   placement, 43
   sizes, 57t
End-tidal CO_2 ($PETCO_2$) monitoring (capnography), 138
   illustration, 139f
   readings
     decrease, 138
     increase, 138
Entrainment
   mask. See Air entrapment mask
   port, impact, 13–14
EPAP. See Expiratory positive airway pressure
Epiglottis, infection, 175–176
   causes, 175
   clinical manifestations, 175
   definition, 175–176
   pathophysiology, 175
   treatment, 175–176
   x-ray findings, 175
Epinephrine. See Naloxone atropine vasopressin epinephrine
     lidocaine
   administration route, 80
   cardiac stimulant, 76–77
   CPR administration, 80
   indications, 80
   pharmacologic actions, 80
Epinephrine hydrochloride (Adrenalin Chloride) (Sus-Phrine), 180
Equipment decontamination
   consideration, 201–202
   postchapter study questions, 203

Equipment decontamination (Continued)
   pretest questions, 199
   review, 199–202
   terminology, 199–202
Equipment handling. See Contaminated equipment
Equipment quality control, 201–202
Equipment sterilization, 199
   autoclaving, usage, 200
   ethylene oxide gas sterilization, 200–201
ERV. See Expiratory reserve volume
Esophageal pressure measurements, 164
Esophageal-tracheal Combitube (ETC), 55
   advantages, 55
   contraindications, 55
   disadvantages, 55
   indications, 55
ET. See Endotracheal
Ethanol (ethyl alcohol), 182
Ethylene oxide gas sterilization, 200–201
Euspnea, 35
Exercise-induced asthma (EIA), 155
   cause, 155
   incidence reduction, nonpharmacologic measures,
     155
Exercise stress testing, 119
Exertional dyspnea, 34
Exhaled VT, measurement, 134
Expiratory positive airway pressure (EPAP), 131
Expiratory reserve volume (ERV), 192
Expiratory retard (expiratory resistance), 136
Expiratory time, alteration, 87
Expiratory timing device. See Bird Mark 7
External intercostals, ventilation muscle, 39
Extracorporeal membrane oxygenation (ECMO), 175
Extremities
   inspection, 36–37
   perfusion, 32
Extubation
   complications, 66–67
   procedure, 66

F
Face tent, 16
   illustration, 16f
Febrile characteristic, 44
FEF. See Forced expiratory flow
Fenestrated tracheostomy tube, 61
   components, 61f
Fetal circulation, normalcy, 174
FEV. See Forced expiratory volume
Fiberoptic bronchoscope, 70f
Fick equation, 115–116
FiO_2. See Fraction of inspired oxygen
First-degree heart block, 110
   representation, 110f
Fixed hyperbaric chambers, 20f
Fixed multiplace chamber, 20
Flatness, 40
Flow-directed pulmonary artery catheter, 113
Flow interrupter oscillating device, 144
Flowmeter, 5. See also Compensated flowmeter; Uncompensated
     flowmeter outlets, Diameter Index Safety System usage
   pressure compensation, determination
Flow rate control, 134
Flow-sensing devices, 197–198

Flow studies, 194–196
Flow volume loop/curve, 195
  comparison, 195f
Flow waveforms, 147
Flutter valve, 102
  illustration, 102f
Foradil. *See* Formoterol
Foramen ovale, patency, 167
Forced expiratory flow (FEF), 194
Forced expiratory volume (FEV), 194
  decrease, 194b, 196–197
  FEV/FVC ratio, 194
Forced vital capacity (FVC), 193
  ratio. *See* Forced expiratory volume
Foreign body aspiration, 176
  causes, 176
  chest x-ray findings, 176
  clinical manifestations, 176
  definition, 176
  pathophysiology, 176
  treatment, 176
Formoterol (Foradil), 181
Four-channel Swan-Ganz catheter. *See* Quadruple Swan-Ganz
  catheter
Fraction of inspired oxygen (FiO$_2$), changes, 145
FRC. *See* Functional residual capacity
Functional residual capacity (FRC), increase of, 152, 192–194
  body plethysmography, usage, 193
  calculations, 192
  increase, 191
  measurement
    helium dilution test, usage, 192
    nitrogen washout test, usage, 192–193
Funnel chest, 38
Furosemide (Lasix), 185
FVC. *See* Forced vital capacity

G

Galvanic cell oxygen analyzers, 20
Gas inspiration, 24b
Gas-powered resuscitators, 79
  expiration/inspiration, 79f
Gastric distention, 88
Gentamicin, 183
Glottic edema, 66
  ET tube complications, 67
  post-extubation respiratory distress, 179
Gloves/gown, usage, 202
Glucose, 46
Glutaraldehydes, 201
Gram's stain method, 199–200
Gravitational sedimentation, 27

H

Haldane effect, 124
Hand washing, 202
HBO. *See* Hyperbaric oxygen
HbO$_2$. *See* Oxyhemoglobin
HCO$_3^-$, level, shift, 125
HCO$_3^-$, relationships, 125
Hct. *See* Hematocrit
Head trauma, ventilation (usage), 143
Heart
  block. *See* First-degree heart block; Second-degree heart block;
    Third-degree heart block

Heart *(Continued)*
  blood supply, 106
  electrical conduction, 103–111
  primary arteries, 107f
  rate, 47
    calculation, 107
    decrease, 9
  rhythm
    regularity, determination, 107
    representation, 106f
  secondary arteries, 107f
  shadow, 43
  sounds, 41–42. *See also* Abnormal heart sounds; Normal
    heart sounds
    auscultation
    lubb-dubb sound
  venous blood return (decrease), mechanical ventilation
    (complication), 140
Heated humidifiers, 26b. *See also* Cascade humidifiers; Wick
    humidifiers
  bacteria, growth
Heat moisture exchanger (HME), 26–27
  components, 26f
  usage, 23
Helium dilution test, usage, 192
Helium/oxygen (70:30 mixture), 19
Helium/oxygen (80:20 mixture), 19b
  delivery, 19b
Helium/oxygen mixtures, delivery, 19
Helium/oxygen therapy, 19
Hematocrit (Hct), 46
Hematology tests, 46
Hemodynamic monitoring, 111–119
Hemoglobin (Hb), 46
  level, decrease, 8
Hemoptysis, 34
  blood, coughing, 88
  causes, 34
  relative IPPB contraindication, 88
Hemorrhage, 71
Hemoximetry. *See* Co-oximetry
Henderson-Hasselbalch equation, 124–125
HEPA. *See* High-efficiency particulate air
HFCWO. *See* High-frequency chest wall oscillation
HFJV. *See* High-frequency jet ventilation
HFO. *See* High-frequency oscillation
HFPPV. *See* High-frequency positive pressure ventilation
HFV. *See* High-frequency ventilation
High-efficiency particulate air (HEPA) filter, usage, 199
High-flow cannula, 17
High-flow devices, consideration, 17–18
High-flow oxygen delivery devices, 13
High-flow oxygen devices, setting, 17–18
High-flow therapy (HFT), cannula (usage), 17
High-frequency chest wall oscillation (HFCWO), 101
High-frequency jet ventilation (HFJV), 144
High-frequency oscillation (HFO), 144–145
  types, 144
High-frequency positive pressure ventilation (HFPPV), usage, 144
High-frequency ventilation (HFV), 144–145
  advantages, 145
High-pressure alarm. *See* Ventilator
High-pressure cuff, 64
High-risk infant, 167–172
  factors, 167–168

High-risk infant *(Continued)*
  maternal factors, 167
  term, description, 167–168
High-volume low-pressure cuff, usage, 64
Hi-Low Evac tube, 59f
Histotoxic hypoxia, 9
HME. *See* Heat moisture exchanger
Holding chambers
  types, 29f
  usage, 29
Holter monitoring, 111
Home apnea monitoring, 190
Home cleaning equipment, 189–190
Home oxygen administration, 188–189
Home rehabilitation, 187–190
  goals, 187
Humidification. *See* Airway humidification
Humidifiers. *See* Bubble humidifiers; Pass-over humidifiers; Wick
    humidifiers
  consideration, 23
  efficiency, 25
  factors, 25
  outlet, nasal cannula (connection), 23
  types, 25–26
Humidity. *See* Absolute humidity; Body humidity; Relative humidity
  clinical uses, 24
  deficit, 24–25
  definition, 23–27
  postchapter study questions, 31
  therapy, 23–31
Humidity/aerosol
  pretest questions, 23
  review, 23–31
Hydrosphere (Babington nebulizer), 28
  components, 28f
Hygroscopic properties, 27
Hyperbaric chambers, 20
Hyperbaric oxygen (HBO)
  physiologic effects, 20
  therapy, 20
    indications, 20
Hypercalcemia, 46
  clinical symptoms, 46
Hyperchloremia, 46
  clinical symptoms, 46
Hyperinflation therapy
  postchapter study questions, 95
  pretest questions, 85–86
  review, 86–94
Hyperkalemia, 45
  clinical symptoms, 45
Hypernatremia, 45
  clinical symptoms, 45
Hyperpnea, 35
Hyperresonance, 40
Hypertension, 44
Hyperthermia, 44
Hypertonic saline solution (1.8% NaCl), 179
Hyperventilation, 124
Hyperventilation, usage (problems), 143b
Hypocalcemia, 46
  clinical symptoms, 46
Hypocapnia, 124
Hypochloremia, 45–46
  clinical symptoms, 46

Hypokalemia, 45
  clinical symptoms, 45
Hyponatremia, 45
  clinical symptoms, 45
Hypopnea, 35
Hypotension, 44, 71
Hypothermia, 44
Hypotonic saline solution (0.4% NaCl), 179
Hypoventilation, 124, 162
Hypoxemia, 71, 100
  levels, 124
  oxygen therapy indication, 7
  signs/symptoms, 7
Hypoxia. *See* Anemic hypoxia; Histotoxic hypoxia; Hypoxemic
    hypoxia; Stagnant hypoxia
  types, 7–9

I

IBW. *See* Ideal body weight
IC. *See* Inspiratory capacity
ICP. *See* Intracranial pressure
Ideal body weight (IBW), 130
  calculation, 132–133
  determination, 133b
I:E inspiratory/expiratory ratio, 134–135
  alarm, sounding, 129
  calculation, 134b
Imaging studies, 43–44
Imaging studies, usefulness, 32
Impeller nebulizer (spinning disk nebulizer), 30
  components, 29f
Impending acute ventilatory failure, 139
Incentive spirometers, 94f
Incentive spirometry
  devices, 94
  goals, 93
  hazards, 93
  order, 85
  performing, steps, 94
  requirements, 93
  sustained maximal inspiratory therapy, 93–94
Increased mean airway pressure, 86
Incubator, usage, 169
Inertial impaction, 27
Infant CPR modifications, 77
Infant respiratory distress syndrome (IRDS), 172
  causes, 172
  chest x-ray findings, 172
  clinical manifestations, 172
  definition, 172
  pathophysiology, 172
  treatment, 172
Infants. *See* High-risk infant
  clinical assessments, 168–169
  ductal shunt, 170
Infarction, 106
Infection control
  postchapter study questions, 203
  pretest questions, 199
  review, 199–202
  standard precautions (universal precautions),
    202
  terminology, 199–202
Infiltrates, 42
Inflation hold control, 135–136

Influenza vaccine, 185
Inhaled steroids, side effects, 184
Initial inspiratory goal, 86
Inspiration, initiation, 86
Inspiratory capacity (IC), 193
Inspiratory flow
    control, 134
    minimum percent increase, 191
Inspiratory positive airway pressure (IPAP), 131
Inspiratory pressure control. See Bennett PR-2 ventilator; Bird Mark 7
Inspiratory reserve volume (IRV), 192
Inspiratory stridor, 67
Inspiratory time
    alteration, 87
    calculation, 135b
    effects, 93
Inspired gas, overheating, 27
Intal. See Cromolyn sodium
Intermittent positive pressure breathing (IPPB), 28
    administration, 85
    corrective actions, 93
    definition, 86
    delivery, 85
    effectiveness, 86
    factors, 86
    machines
        convenience, 187
        operation, 89–92
        usage, factors. See Pressure-limited IPPB machine
    machine variables, setting, 89
    patients, cooperation (absence), 88
    physiologic effects, 86–87
    problems, 93
    proper administration, 89
    respiratory therapist administration, 85
    therapy, 94
        contraindications, 88
        hazards, 85, 87–88
        indications, 87
        introduction, 86–94
    treatment, 85
        patient complaints, 85
    units, characteristics, 89–92
Intracardiac administration, 80
Intracranial pressure (ICP), increase, 87, 100
Intrapulmonary percussive ventilation, 101
Intrapulmonary shunting, 116–118
Intrathoracic metastatic nodal disease, imaging study selection, 32
Inverse I:E ratio, 135
    ventilation, combination. See Pressure control ventilation
IPAP. See Inspiratory positive airway pressure
IPPB. See Intermittent positive pressure breathing
Ipratropium bromide (Atrovent), 181
IRDS. See Infant respiratory distress syndrome
Iron deficiency, impact, 8
IRV. See Inspiratory reserve volume
Isoproterenol hydrochloride, 81
    indications, 81
    pharmacologic actions, 81

J
Jet nebulizers, 27–28
    components, 27f
Jet size, impact, 13–14

K
Kistner tracheostomy tube, 62
    cannula/flange/valve, usage, 62f
Kussmaul respirations, 35
    wave formation, 35f
Kyphoscoliosis, 38
Kyphosis, 37

L
Laboratory test results, assessment, 45–47
Labored breathing, oxygen therapy indication, 7
Laryngeal mask airway (LMA), 52–54
    advantages, 52
    components, 52f
    contraindications, 52
    disadvantages, 53
    indications, 52
    insertion, 53f
        technique, 55
Laryngoscope, 56f
    insertion, 56f
Laryngospasm, 66, 71
Laryngotracheal web, 67
Laryngotracheobronchitis (LTB) (croup), 27, 176
    causes, 176
    clinical manifestations, 176
    definition, 176
    pathophysiology, 176
    treatment, 176
    x-ray findings, 176
Larynx, laryngoscopic view, 57f
Lasix. See Furosemide
Lateral chest radiograph position, 42
Lateral decubitus chest radiograph position, 42–43
Lead aVF, 104
Lead aVL, 104
Lead aVR, 104
Lead placements, 104
Lecithin-sphingomyelin (L:S) ratio, 172
Left-to-right shunt (production), PDA (impact), 175b
Left ventricular end-diastolic pressure (LVEDP), 115
Lethal fibrillation. See Ventricular fibrillation
Lethal tachycardia. See Ventricular tachycardia
Leukotriene modifiers, 182
Levabuterol (Xopenex), 180–181
Lidocaine (Xylocaine), 70. See also Naloxone atropine vasopressin epinephrine lidocaine
    administration route, 80
    CPR administration, 80
    indications, 80
Limb leads, 104. See also Standard limb leads
Liquid gas systems, 3
Liquid oxygen
    system, 188
        flow duration, calculation, 4b
    tank, duration (calculation), 5b
    weight, 4
LMA. See Laryngeal mask airway
Long-term ECG monitoring, 104
Loop diuretic, 185
Lordosis, 37
Low-flow oxygen systems, 9–17
Low PEEP/CPAP alarm, 138
Low-pressure alarm. See Ventilator

Low tidal volume alarm, 138
Lower respiratory tract infections, 156–158
L:S ratio. *See* Lecithin-sphingomyelin ratio
LTB. *See* Laryngotracheobronchitis
Lung abscess
    causes, 157
    chest x-ray films, characteristics, 157
    clinical signs/symptoms, 157
    definition, 157
    laboratory findings, characteristics, 157
    pathophysiology, 157
    treatment, 157
Lung compliance (CL), 141–142
    calculation, 141–142
        importance, 142b
    consideration, 142
    data, usage, 142b
    decrease, 158
    definition, 141
    dynamic lung compliance, 141
        accuracy, 141
    increase, 152
    peak pressures, 142b
    plateau pressures, 142b
    static lung compliance, 141–142
Lung condition, consolidation characteristic, 151
Lung consolidation, 156
Lung disorders, 158–163
    streptokinase, usage, 151
Lungs
    capacities, 191–198, 191f. *See also* Total lung capacity
        measurement
    diffusion capacity (DL), 195–196
    diseases
        contrast, 196
        severity, 196
    flow-sensing devices, 197–198
    flow studies, 194–196
    lower lobe
        anterior basal segment, drainage position, 98f
        lateral basal segment, drainage position, 97f
        posterior basal segment, drainage position, 97f
        superior segment, drainage position, 98f
    normal diffusion capacity, 196
    peak flow, 194–195
    peak flowmeter, usage, 195b
    predicted values, determination, 196
    recoil properties, 39
    right middle lobe, lateral/medial segments (drainage position),
        98f
    studies, 194–196
    superior/inferior lingular segments, drainage position, 98f
    upper lobe
        anterior segment, drainage position, 99f
        apical segment, drainage position, 99f
        posterior segment, drainage position, 99f
    volumes, 191–198
        decrease, 196
        measurement, 191f
LVEDP. *See* Left ventricular end-diastolic pressure

M

Magic box method, usage, 14t
Magill forceps, 58

Magnetic resonance imaging (MRI), 43–44
    disadvantages, 43–44
    usage, 43
Major arrhythmia, 108
Malnutrition, impact, 140
Manual resuscitators, 77–79
    components, 78f
    usage, hazards, 78–79
    uses, 77
Maximal inspiratory maneuvers, sustaining,
    86
Maximal inspiratory pressure (MIP), 197
    determination, methods, 197
    measurement, 139, 197
    relationship, 139b
Maximum voluntary ventilation (MVV), 119–120,
    195
McGill forceps, usage, 49
McIntosh blade (curved blade), 56–57
MDI. *See* Metered-dose inhaler
Mean airway pressure (Paw)
    impact, 138
    increase, 86
    monitoring, 138
Mean pulmonary artery pressure (MPAP), 118
Mechanical bronchodilation, 87
Mechanical dead space, 140–141
Mechanical ventilation
    complications, 129, 139–140
    indications, 139
    initiation, criteria, 139
    time on-time off method, 143
    weaning, 143
        criteria, 143
        techniques, 143
Mechanical ventilators, 129–150
Meconium aspiration, 173
    causes, 173
    chest x-ray findings, 173
    clinical manifestations, 173
    definition, 173
    pathophysiology, 173
    treatment, 173
Medical emergency team (MET), 81
Medical gases
    control, 3–7
        review, 1–21
    storage, review, 1–21
Mental status, assessment, 44–45
MET. *See* Medical emergency team
Metabolic acidemia, 125. *See also* Compensated metabolic
    acidemia
Metabolic alkalemia, 125. *See also* Compensated metabolic
    alkalemia
Metabolic components, respiratory components (contrast),
    125
Metaproterenol (Alupent) (Metaprel), 180
Metered-dose inhaler (MDI), 29
    activation, 29
    components, 28f
    popularity, 29
Methacholine challenge test, 196–197
Methemoglobin, impact, 8
microNefrin. *See* Racemic epinephrine

Midazolam (Versed), 70, 184–185
Mild intermittent asthma, 153
Mild persistent asthma, 153–154
Miller blade (straight blade), 56–57
Minimal leak technique, 64
Minimal occluding volume technique, 64
Minor arrhythmia, 108
Minute volume (MV)
  changes, 145
  measurement, 194b
  study, 194
MIP. *See* Maximal inspiratory pressure
Mist
  production, reduction, 23
  visibility, 16
Mixed gas therapy, 19
Mixed respiratory/metabolic acidemia, 126
Mixed respiratory/metabolic component, 126
Mixed sleep apnea, 163
Mixed venous blood gas sampling, 113
Moderate persistent asthma, 154
Modified Allen test, usage, 122
Moisture, amount (example), 24b
Mouth-to-valve mask ventilation, 79
MPAP. *See* Mean pulmonary artery pressure
MRI. *See* Magnetic resonance imaging
Mucociliary activity, reduction, 7
Mucolytics, 179–180
Mucomyst. *See* Acetylcysteine
Multidose DPI devices, 185
Murmurs. *See* Abnormal heart sounds
MV. *See* Minute volume
MVV. *See* Maximum voluntary ventilation
Myocardial work (increase), oxygen therapy
  (indications), 7

N

Naloxone atropine vasopressin epinephrine lidocaine (NAVEL),
  80
Naloxone hydrochloride (Narcan), administration,
  77
Narcotic analgesics, 184
Nasal cannula, 10f
  ABG results, 121
  usage, 169
Nasal catheter, usage, 169
Nasal CPAP, 170
  complications, 170
  indications, 170
   absence, 167
Nasal reservoir cannula, 10
  illustration, 10f
Nasopharyngeal airway, 52
  hazards, 52
  tip/flange, usage, 51f
Nasotracheal intubation, 58
Nasotracheal tubes, 58–59
  advantages, 59
  complications, 59
Nebulization control, 92
Nebulizers. *See* Impeller nebulizer; Small-volume nebulizer;
  Spinning disk nebulizer; Ultrasonic nebulizer
  considerations, 30–31
  dilution mode, 18b
  gas, receiving, 23

Nebulizers *(Continued)*
  nosocomial infection source, 26b
  types, 27–30
Negative pleural pressure, loss, 162
Neonatal cardiopulmonary disorders, 172–175
Neonatal respiratory care, 167–177
  postchapter study questions, 177–178
  pretest questions, 167
  review, 167–177
Neonatal resuscitation, 76–77
Neonatal retinopathy, 7
Neonates
  Apgar scoring system, 168
  arterial blood, sites (obtaining), 170–171
  assessment, 168–169
  clinical assessments, 168–169
  Dubowitz scoring system, 168
  oxygen delivery devices, 169–170
  oxygen therapy, hazards, 170
  Silverman scoring system, 168
Neuromuscular blocking agents, 182–183
Newborn. *See* Persistent pulmonary hypertension of the
  newborn
Nitric oxide (NO), 19
  rebound effects, prevention, 19
  toxicity levels, 19
Nitrogen washout test, usage, 192–193
Nocturnal asthma, 155
Nonheated humidifiers. *See* Bubble humidifiers; Pass-over
  humidifiers
Nonnarcotic analgesics, 184
Non-rebreathing mask, 12–13
  illustration, 12f
Norcuron. *See* Vecuronium
Normal diffusion capacity, 196
Normal fetal circulation, 174
Normal heart sounds, 41–42
Normal PvO_2, 115
Normal saline solution (0.9% NaCl), 179
Nosocomial infection, 88, 199–200
  nebulizer source, 26b
Nutrition (absence), mechanical ventilation (complication),
  140

O

Oblique chest radiograph position, 42
Obstructed airway. *See* Conscious adult; Unconscious adult
Obstructive apnea, 164f–165f
Obstructive lung diseases, 196
  restrictive lung diseases, contrast, 196
Obstructive sleep apnea, 163
  symptoms, 163
Occupational asthma, 155
One-bottle system, 72
  water seal, 72f
One-rescuer CPR (adult patient), 76
One-way valve system, 79f
Optimal PEEP, 136–137
  determination, 136b
  representation, 142b
Oropharyngeal airway, 50–64
  consideration, 51
  flange/channel, usage, 50f
  hazards, 51
  insertion, 51f

Orthopnea, 34, 159
Oscillating devices, types, 144
Oximetry, 172
Oxygen
    administration, 20. *See also* Home oxygen administration
    analyzers; Galvanic cell oxygen analyzers; Polarographic
        oxygen analyzers
    blender, 18
        components, 18f
    cannula, usage, 17
    carry, blood capacity, 8
    concentrator, 189
        photograph, 189f
        portable units, availability, 189
    cylinders, 188
        disadvantages, 188
        pressure, pretest question, 1
    delivery
        devices. *See* Neonates
        low-flow device, usage, 13
    delivery devices, 9–17
    flowmeter, gas mixtures, 19
    hemoglobin (Hb), affinity (shift), 124
    hood, 169
        components, 169f
    inadequacy, 7
    levels, achievement, 78
    mask, usage, 132
    percentage control, 135
    physician order, example, 15b
    systems, indication, 187
    tent, 17
        components, 17f
    therapy
        complications, 7
        hazards. *See* Neonates
        indications, 7–18
    toxicity, 7
Oxygenated Hb, decrease, 37
Oxygenation
    excess, 87
    mechanical ventilation indication, 139
    target, 131
Oxygen consumption (V̇O₂)
    calculation, 119b
    decrease, factors, 119
    increase, factors, 119
Oxygen (O₂) therapy, requirement, 152
Oxygen/medical gas therapy
    cylinder markings, 2f
    postchapter study questions, 21
    pretest questions, 1
Oxygen saturation (SaO₂), 124
    monitoring (pulse oximetry), 20–21
        readings, inaccuracy (causes), 21
Oxyhemoglobin (HbO₂) dissociation curve, 123–124
    affinities, 123f
    shift, 121

P

P wave, 105
    observation, 107
P-50, 124
PA. *See* Pulmonary artery
PAC. *See* Premature atrial contraction

PaCO₂. *See* Partial pressure of carbon dioxide in arterial blood
Pancuronium bromide (Pavulon), 183
Panlobular emphysema (panacinar emphysema), 151–152
PAO₂. *See* Alveolar PO₂
PaO₂. *See* Partial pressure of oxygen in arterial blood
PAP. *See* Pulmonary artery pressure
Paradoxical pulse (pulsus paradoxus), 44
Paradoxical respirations, 36
    respiratory therapist observation, 32
Parasympatholytic bronchodilators, 181
Paroxysmal nocturnal dyspnea, 34, 159
Partially compensated metabolic acidemia, 126b
Partially compensated metabolic alkalemia, 126b
Partially compensated respiratory acidemia, 125b
Partially compensated respiratory alkalemia, 125b
Partial pressure of carbon dioxide in arterial blood (PaCO₂),
        160
    decrease, 87, 133b
        high-frequency ventilation/oscillation, usage, 145b
        ventilator rate, increase, 143b
    increase, 133
    level, alteration, 134, 134b
    low levels, maintenance, 174b
    maintenance, 174b
    monitoring. *See* Transcutaneous PaCO₂/PaO₂ monitoring
Partial pressure of carbon dioxide (PCO₂) measurement,
        Severinghaus electrode (usage), 128
Partial pressure of oxygen in arterial blood (PaO₂), 122
    levels, 124
    maintenance, 174b
    monitoring. *See* Transcutaneous PaCO₂/PaO₂ monitoring
Partial pressure of oxygen (PO₂) measurement, Clark electrode
        (usage), 128
Partial rebreathing mask, 12
    illustration, 12f
    setup, pretest question, 1
Partial thrombopastin time (PTT), 47
Partial upper airway obstruction, signs, 50
Pass-over humidifiers (nonheated humidifiers), 25
    inlet/outlet, 25f
Passy-Muir speaking valve, 64
Passy-Muir tracheostomy, 63f
Passy-Muir valve, 64
Passy-Muir valve in-line, mechanical ventilation, 63f
Pasteurization, 200
Patients
    airway, opening, 49
    care plan. *See* Respiratory home care
    chart, review, 47
    cross-contamination, prevention, 140b
    history, 33–48
    interview, 33
        techniques, 33
    intubation, 49
    land/air transportation, 82–83
    transportation, respiratory care equipment (usage), 83
    ventilators
        circuit, precautions, 199
        control mode, 129
Pavulon. *See* Pancuronium bromide
Paw. *See* Mean airway pressure
PAWP. *See* Pulmonary artery wedge pressure
PCO₂. *See* Partial pressure of carbon dioxide
PCV. *See* Pressure control ventilation
PCWP. *See* Pulmonary capillary wedge pressure

PDA, impact. *See* Left-to-right shunt
PEA. *See* Pulseless electrical activity
Peak flow, 194–195
Pectus carinatum, 38
  illustration, 38f
Pectus excavatum, 38
  illustration, 38f
Pedal edema, 36–37
Pediatric patient, airway disorders, 175–177
Pediatric respiratory care
  postchapter study questions, 165
  pretest questions, 151
  review, 151–165
PEEP. *See* Positive end expiratory pressure
Pendant reservoir cannula, 10
  illustration, 10f
Pentamidine, 183
Pentamidine, usage of, 156–157, 183
Percussion, 100. *See also* Chest
  dullness, 40
  flatness, 40
  hyperresonance, 40
  indication, absence, 96
  resonance, 40
  sounds, 40
  tympany, 40
Peripheral artery puncture, 171
Peripheral artery sites, 111
Peripheral edema, 44
  cor pulmonale, impact, 152
Permissive hypercapnia, 131, 160–161
Persistent fetal circulation (PFC), 174
  PVR, impact, 174b
Persistent pulmonary hypertension of the newborn (PPHN),
    174–175
  causes, 174
  chest x-ray findings, 174
  clinical manifestations, 174
  conditions, 174
  definition, 174–175
  drug therapy, 174–175
  evidence, 19
  normal fetal circulation, 174
  pathophysiology, 174
  treatment, 174–175
PET. *See* Position emission tomography
PETCO$_2$. *See* End-tidal CO$_2$
PFC. *See* Persistent fetal circulation
pH. *See* Acid-base balance
Phosphodiesterase inhibitors, 181–182
Physical agents (sterilization/disinfection), 200–201
Physical assessments, 35–45
Physiologic dead space, 140
Physiologic shunting, increase (conditions), 117
Pilot tube, usage, 27–28
PIP, 130b
  levels, 137f
    maintenance, 138b
Piston compressor, 6f
  air, entry, 6–7
Piston oscillating device, 144
Plasma oncotic pressure, 158
Plateau pressure
  increase, 142b
  occurrence, 141–142

Platelet count, 46
Pleural effusion, 161–162
  causes, 161
  chest x-ray films, characteristics, 162
  clinical signs/symptoms, 161
  definition, 161
  pathophysiology, 161
  treatment, 162
Pleural friction rub, 41
Pleural space, air evacuation, 69
Pleur-Evac System, 73f
Pneumococcal vaccine (Pneumovax), 185
Pneumocystis carinii pneumonia (PCP), 156–157
Pneumonia, 43
  causative organisms, 151
  cause, 156
  chest x-ray films, characteristics, 156
  clinical signs/symptoms, 156
  definition, 156–157
  pathophysiology, 156
  treatment, 157
  types, 156–157
Pneumotachometers, 198
Pneumothorax, 43, 71, 87–88. *See also* Untreated
    pneumothorax
  absolute contraindication, 88
  assessment, transillumination (usage), 170b
  causes, 161
  chest x-ray films, characteristics, 161
  clinical signs/symptoms, 161
  definition, 160–161
  diagnostic procedures, 161
  immediate action, 161
  pathophysiology, 161
  treatment, 161
  treatment, absence, 88
PO$_2$. *See* Partial pressure of oxygen
Point of care (POC) analyzers, 128
Polarographic oxygen analyzers, 20
Polysomnogram, continuous recordings, 163–165
Polysomnography, 163–165
Portable spirometers. *See* Bedside spirometers
Position emission tomography (PET), 44
Positive airway pressures, transfer, 140
Positive end expiratory pressure (PEEP), 136–137, 160–161
  curves, comparisons, 136f
  hazards, 136
  impact, determination, 114b
  indications, 136
  levels, 130
    optimum, 137f
  optimum, 136–137
    determination, 136b
Positive expiratory pressure (PEP)
  contraindications, 101
  device. *See* Acapella oscillatory PEP device;
      Single-use PEP device
  mask therapy, performing (steps), 101
  therapeutic effects, 101
  therapy, 101–102
Positive pressure ventilation, 130–131
Positive pressure ventilators, types, 130–131
Postanterior (PA) chest radiograph position, 42–43
Posterior chest, symmetry (assessment), 39f
Postterm infant, meconium aspiration risk, 173

Postural drainage
  indication, absence, 96
  order, 96
  positions, 99–100
Potassium (K⁺), 45
PPHN. *See* Persistent pulmonary hypertension of the
  newborn
Precordial leads (chest leads), 104
  placement, 104f
Precordial thump, 81–82
Premature atrial contraction (PAC), 108
  arrhythmias, relationship, 108
  representation, 108f
Premature ventricular contraction (PVC), 109
  representation, 109f
Prematurity, retinopathy, 7
Preset machine VT, volume loss, 133–134
Preset pressure ventilators, 130
Preset regulator, mechanics, 3–4
Preset volume ventilators, 130
Pressure chamber, constant pressure (trap), 4
Pressure control ventilation (PCV), 130–131
  inverse I:E ratio ventilation, combination, 130b
Pressure-cycled ventilators, 130–131
Pressure-limited IPPB machine, usage (factors), 92–93
Pressure support ventilation (PSV), 132
  receiving, 140–141
Pressure waveforms, 147–149
  example, 148f
  tracings, 114f
Primary arteries, 107f
PR interval, 106
  observation, 107
  prolongation, 106f
Procainamide
  administration route, 80
  CPR administration, 80
  dosage, 80
  indications, 80
  pharmacologic actions, 80
Processing indicators, 201
Propranolol hydrochloride
  CPR administration, 80–81
  indications, 80–81
  pharmacologic actions, 81
Prothrombin time (PT), 47
Proventil. *See* Albuterol
PSV. *See* Pressure support ventilation
PTT. *See* Partial thrombopastin time
Pulmonary angiography, 159–160
Pulmonary artery (PA), pressure waveform tracing, 114f
Pulmonary artery (PA) catheter. *See* Flow-directed pulmonary
    artery catheter
  insertion, 113
  insertion, complications, 115
Pulmonary artery pressure (PAP), increase of, 113, 158
  measurement, 115
  monitoring, 114–115
Pulmonary artery wedge pressure (PAWP), 118
  pressure waveform tracing, 114f
Pulmonary blood flow, decrease of, 162
Pulmonary capillary wedge pressure (PCWP), 113, 115
Pulmonary capillary wedge pressure (PCWP) level of, 158
  decrease, conditions, 115
  increase, conditions, 115

Pulmonary capillary wedge pressure (PCWP) level of *(Continued)*
  monitoring, 114–115
  value, 115
Pulmonary disease, symptoms, 33–35
Pulmonary edema
  IPPB, positive effects, 88–89
  secretions, observation, 182
  treatment, IPPB (usage), 88–89
Pulmonary edema (cardiogenic), 158–163
  causes, 158
  chest x-ray films, characteristics, 159
  clinical signs/symptoms, 159
  definition, 158–159
  pathophysiology, 158
  treatment, 159
Pulmonary embolism (PE)
  anticoagulation (antithrombus) therapy, 160
  causes, 159
  chest x-ray films, characteristics, 159
  clinical signs/symptoms, 159
  definition, 159–160
  diagnostic procedures, 159–160
  pathophysiology, 159
  prevention, 160
  treatment, 160
Pulmonary function studies, 196–197
Pulmonary function testing
  postchapter study questions, 198
  pretest questions, 191
  review, 191–198
Pulmonary function tests
  interpretation, 196
  usage. *See* Cough ability
Pulmonary hemorrhage, absolute contraindication, 88
Pulmonary hypertension, 34–35
Pulmonary infarction, 113
Pulmonary infection, 139–140
Pulmonary oxygen toxicity, mechanical ventilation complication,
    140
Pulmonary patient home care, respiratory therapist
    responsibilities, 190
Pulmonary rehabilitation, conditions, 187
Pulmonary tissue damage, prevention, 170b
Pulmonary vascular resistance (PVR)
  decrease, factors, 118
  increase
    factors, 118
    impact, 174b
  measurement, 118
Pulmozyme. *See* Dornase alfa
Pulse
  detection, 103
  pressure, 112
    presence, 103
  rate, 103
Pulse-dose oxygen delivery systems, 11b
  usage, 187–188
Pulseless electrical activity (PEA), 110–111
Pulse oximeter, usage, 20–21
Pulse oximetry. *See* Oxygen saturation
Pulsus alternans, 44
Pulsus paradoxus. *See* Paradoxical pulse
Purkinje fibers, 103–104
Pursed-lip breathing, 153, 188
  benefit, 151

PVC. *See* Premature ventricular contraction
PVR. *See* Pulmonary vascular resistance

Q

Q wave, 105
QRS complex, 105–106
   distance, variation, 108
   length, determination, 107
   widening, 106
Quadruple Swan-Ganz catheter (four-channel Swan-Ganz catheter), 113f
Quality control procedures, 128

R

R wave, 103
   distance, variation, 108
   number, counting, 107
RA. *See* Right atrium
Racemic epinephrine (microNefrin) (Vaponefrin), 180
Radial artery puncture, 122
Radiolucency, 42
Radiopaque, 42
Ramp wave
   acceleration, 147
   deceleration, 147
Rapid response team, 81
RAW. *See* Airway resistance
Red blood cells (RBCs), 46
Reducing valve
   gas entry, 3f
   technical problems, 4
   types, 3
Regulators, technical problems, 4
Rehabilitation, 187–190. *See also* Home rehabilitation conditions; Pulmonary rehabilitation
   patient, care
Relative humidity, 24
   absolute humidity, relationship, 24b
Rescue breathing, 77
Reservoir cannulas, usage, 187–188
Residual volume (RV), 192
   RV/TLC ratio, 194
Resonance, 40
Respiratory acidemia, 125. *See also* Chronic respiratory acidemia; Compensated respiratory acidemia
Respiratory alkalemia, 125. *See also* Chronic respiratory alkalemia; Compensated respiratory alkalemia
Respiratory care equipment, usage, 83
Respiratory care orders, 47
Respiratory care plans/protocols, development, 48
Respiratory care procedures
   postchapter study questions, 74
   pretest questions, 69
   review, 69–74
Respiratory components, metabolic components (contrast), 125
Respiratory depression, 71
   oxygen therapy complication, 7
Respiratory distress, example, 151
Respiratory drugs, miscellany, 182
Respiratory home care
   postchapter study questions, 190
   pretest questions, 187
   review, 187–190

Respiratory home care patient
   care plan, 187–188
   periodic evaluations, 188
   respiratory therapist discussion area, 187
Respiratory medications
   classification, 179–186
   postchapter study questions, 186
   pretest questions, 179
   review, 179–186
Respiratory rate
   control, 134
   study, 194
Respiratory system disorders
   postchapter study questions, 165
   pretest questions, 151
   review, 151–165
Respirometer. *See* Wright respirometer
Restrictive disease, 38
Restrictive lung diseases, 196
   obstructive lung diseases, contrast, 196
Resuscitators. *See* Manual resuscitators
   design, 78
   self-inflating bags, usage, 78
Retinopathy of prematurity (ROP), 170
RhDNase. *See* Dornase alfa
Ribavirin (Virazole), 184
Rib fractures, 100
Right atrium (RA), pressure waveform tracing, 114f
Right bundle-branch block, QRS widening, 106
Right mainstem bronchus, entry, 43
Right mainstem bronchus intubation, 162
Right-sided heart failure (cor pulmonale), 152
   impact. *See also* Peripheral edema
Right ventricle (RV), pressure waveform tracing, 114f
Rigid bronchoscope, 70f
Rocuronium (Zemuron), 183
Room humidifier, 30
ROP. *See* Retinopathy of prematurity
RV. *See* Residual volume; Right ventricle

S

S wave, 105
SA. *See* Sinoatrial
Safety relief devices, 2
Saline solution. *See* Hypertonic saline solution; Hypotonic saline solution; Normal saline solution
Salmeterol (Serevent), 181
Sanz electrode, 128
SaO$_2$. *See* Oxygen saturation
Scoliosis, 37–38
Secondary arteries, 107f
Second-degree heart block, 110
   representation, 110f
Secretions, thickening, 23
Sedatives, 184–185
Segmental breathing, 188
Self-cycling, 86
Sensitivity control, 135–137
Serevent. *See* Salmeterol
Serum electrolytes, 45–46
Severe persistent asthma, 154
Severinghaus electrode, usage, 128
Shunt percentage, calculation, 117b
Shunt values, calculation (interpretation), 118
Sigh controls, 135

Silverman scoring system, 168
Simple oxygen mask, 11
   illustration, 11f
SIMV. *See* Synchronized intermittent mandatory ventilation
Sine flow wave, 147f
Sine wave, 147
Single-dose DPI devices, 185
Single-stage reducing valve, 3
Single-use PEP device, 101f
Sinoatrial (SA) node, 103–104
Sinus arrhythmia, 108
   representation, 108f
Sinus bradycardia, 108–111
   representation, 108f
Sinus tachycardia, 108
   representation, 108f
Sleep apnea, 163–165
   types, 163
Sleep-related upper airway obstruction, spectrum, 164f–165f
Sleep studies. *See* Diagnostic sleep studies
Small-volume nebulizer, 28
   components, 28f
Sodium bicarbonate
   indication, 77
   2% $NaHCO_3$, 180
Sodium (Na^+), serum electrolyte, 45
Sodium nitroprusside (Nipride), 81
   pharmacologic actions, 81
Sore throat, ET tube complication, 67
Spacers
   effectiveness, 29
   types, 29f
Speaking tracheostomy tubes, 63
Special tracheostomy tubes, 61–64
Spinal conformations, 37f
Spinning disk nebulizer. *See* Impeller neublizer
Spirillum, 200
Spirometers. *See* Bedside spirometers; Wright respirometer
Spirometry test, 191
Spontaneous breath, 136f
Spontaneous pneumothorax, 161
Spores, 199–200
Square flow wave, 147f
Square wave (constant flow), 147
Stagnant hypoxia (circulatory hypoxia), 9
Standard limb leads, 104
Static lung compliance, 141–142
   actual volume, usage, 141b
   approximation, 129
   calculation, 141b
   decrease, 129
      result, 142
Static pressure, occurrence, 141–142
Status asthmaticus, 155
Sterile distilled water, 179
Sterilization, 199–200
   techniques, 200–201
Stopcock, clot, 112
Straight blade. *See* Miller blade
Strain gauge pressure transducer, 111
Streptococcus pneumoniae, 156
Streptokinase, usage, 151
Stridor, 41. *See also* Inspiratory stridor
Stroke volume (SV), 118
   measurement, 118

ST segment, 106
   depression, 106f
Subcutaneous emphysema, 139
   relative IPPB contraindication, 88
Subglottic edema, 67
Succinylcholine (Anectine), 182–183
Suction catheter, passage, 49
Suctioning technique, 64–65
Surfactant, deficiency/loss, 162
Sus-Phrine. *See* Epinephrine hydrochloride
SVR. *See* Systemic vascular resistance
Swab sampling, 201
Swan-Ganz catheter, 113
Sympathomimetic bronchodilators, 180–181
Synchronized intermittent mandatory ventilation (SIMV),
   132
   receiving, 140–141
   usage, 143
Systemic vascular resistance (SVR)
   decrease, factors, 118
   increase, factors, 118
Systemic vascular resistance (SVR), measurement, 118
Systolic PAP, 115
Systolic pressure, 112

T

T wave, 106
Tachycardia, 44
Tachypnea, 35
Talking tracheostomy tube, 63f
TDPs. *See* Therapist-driven protocols
Temporary internal pacemaker, 111
Tension pneumothorax, 43, 161
   needle aspiration, usage, 161
   result, 74
Terbutaline sulfate (Brethine) (Bricanyl), 180
Theophylline (aminophylline), 181–182
Therapist-driven protocols (TDPs), 48
Thermodilution technique, 115–116
Third-degree heart block, 110
   representation, 110f
Three-bottle system, 73
   water seal, 73f
Tidal volume (VT), 192, 194
Tidal volume (VT)
   control, 132–134
      sensitivity control, 135–137
   decrease, 133
   delivery, 86
   effects. *See* Delivered VT
   increase, 86
   measurement. *See* Exhaled VT
Time on-time off method. *See* Mechanical ventilation
TLC. *See* Total lung capacity
Tobramycin (TOBI), 183
Total arterial oxygen content, calculation, 116b
Total lung capacity (TLC), 193
   decrease, 193b
   ratio. *See* Residual volume
Total lung compliance, 141
Total venous oxygen, calculation, 116b
Trachea, shift, 40
Tracheal breath sounds, 41
Tracheal damage, mechanical ventilation complication, 140
Tracheal malacia, 67

Tracheal mucosal ulceration, 67
Tracheal position, palpation, 40f
Tracheal stenosis, 67
Tracheal stoma care, 60–61
Tracheal suctioning
  hazards, 66
  indications, 66
Tracheostomies
  complications, 60
  indications, 60
Tracheostomy button, 62
  cannula, usage, 62f
Tracheostomy mask (collar), 17
  illustration, 17f
Tracheostomy tubes, 60–64. *See also* Fenestrated tracheostomy
    tube; Special tracheostomy tubes
  complications, 60
  components, 60f
  late complication, 60
  weaning, 49
Transcutaneous $PaCO_2/PaO_2$ monitoring, 171–172
  disadvantages, 171
Transducer clot, 112
Transducer position, 112
Transilluminator
  placement, 171
  usage, 170b
Transmission-based precautions, 202
Transtracheal catheter, 9f
Transvenous pacemaker, 111
Traumatic pneumothorax, 161
Triple-stage reducing valve, 3
T-tube flow-by, 16
  illustration, 16f
Tuberculosis (TB)
  cause, 157–158
  chest x-ray films, characteristics, 158
  clinical signs/symptoms, 158
  definition, 157–158
  pathophysiology, 157–158
  pulmonary function studies, characteristics, 158
  treatment, 158
Tuberculosis, relative IPPB contraindication, 88
Tubocurarine chloride, 183
12-lead ECG, three-lead system, 104
Two-bottle system, 72
  water seal, 72f
Two-rescuer CPR (adult patient), 76
Tympany, 40

U

UAP. *See* Umbilical artery catheter
Ultrasonic nebulizer, 30
  components, 30f
Ultrasonic therapy, hazards, 30
Umbilical artery, 170–171
Umbilical artery catheter (UAC)
  advantages, 171
  complications, 167, 171
  placement, 170–171
Uncompensated flowmeter, 5f
  needle valve, location, 5
  outlet, humidifier/nebulizer attachment, 5
Unconscious adult, obstructed airway, 76
Unconscious patients, 75

Untreated pneumothorax, absolute contraindication, 88
Upper airway edema (cool aerosol), 27
Upper airway obstruction, 49–67
  causes, 49–50
  signs. *See* Complete upper airway obstruction; Partial upper
    airway obstruction
Upper chest, assessment, 39f
Urinalysis, 47
Urinary output (decrease), mechanical ventilation complication,
  140

V

Vaccines, 185. *See also* Influenza vaccine; Pneumococcal
  vaccine
Vacuum systems, 66
Vaponefrin. *See* Racemic epinephrine
Vasopressin, 81. *See also* Naloxone atropine vasopressin
  epinephrine lidocaine
  indications, 81
VC. *See* Vital capacity
VD. *See* Dead space
VD/VT ratio, 139
Vecuronium (Norcuron), 183
Vegetative organisms, 199–200
Venous blood return (decrease), mechanical ventilation
  (complication), 140
Venous engorgement, 44
Venous oxygen content, measurement, 116
Venous return
  decrease, 170
  PEEP, impact, 114b
Ventilation
  adequacy, determination, 124
  control mode, settings, 146t
  excess, 87
  studies, 194
Ventilation/perfusion (V/Q) scan of, 159–160
  distribution, evaluation, 191
  mismatch, 7
  scanning, 43, 196
Ventilator
  adjustments, 149t
  alarm, 137–138
    sounding, 49
  circuit, maintenance, 149
  controls, 131–135
  flow, 147–149
    waveforms, 147
  high-pressure alarm, 137–138
  humidifier, replacement, 23
  low-pressure alarm, 137
  modes, 131–132
  monitoring, 137–138
  patient information, 129
  pressure waveforms, 147–149
  problems, practice, 146–147
  scenario, example, 130b, 133b
  square wave (constant flow), 147
  variable changes, estimation, 145
  volume, 147–149
  VT setting, recommendation, 133b
  weaning, difficulty, 45–46
Ventilator-associated pneumonia (VAP), 59, 149–150
  reduction, methods, 149–150
Ventilator-dependent patients, MDI (usage), 29

Ventilator management
    postchapter study questions, 150
    pretest questions, 129
    review, 129–150
Ventilator speaking valves, 63f
Ventilatory effort (PES), increase, 164f–165f
Ventilatory pattern, 27
Ventilatory rates, HFPPV (usage), 144
Ventolin. *See* Albuterol
Ventricular depolarization (contraction), representation, 105–106
Ventricular fibrillation (lethal fibrillation), 110
    representation, 110f
Ventricular irritability, 109
Ventricular tachycardia (lethal tachycardia), 109
    representation, 110f
Venturi mask
    setting, 14b
    usage, 1
        example, 123b
Venturi tube, usage, 27–28
Vesicular breath sounds, 41
Vibrations, 100
    decrease, 40
        determination, 32
Vinegar. *See* Acetic acid
Viral pneumonia, 156
Virazole. *See* Ribavirin
Vital capacity (VC), 193
    decrease, 193b
    measurement, 139
Vital signs, 47
Vocal cords
    paralysis, 67
    ulceration, 67

Volume-cycled ventilator, control mode, 129
Volume expanders, 75
Volume ventilator, 130–132
    assist-control mode, 131
    control mode, 129, 131
        data collection, 145b–146b
    usage, 143b
        example, 145b
Volume waveform, 148
    difference, 148f
    example, 148f
VT. *See* Tidal volume

W
Water, capacity, 24
Wave pattern abnormalities, 109
WBCs. *See* White blood cells
Wheezes, 41
White blood cells (WBCs), 46
Wick humidifiers (heated humidifiers), 26
    components, 25f
Wright respirometer, 198
    components, 197f

X
Xopenex. *See* Levabuterol
X-ray exposure, determination, 43

Y
Yankauer suction, 66
    illustration, 66f

Z
Zemuron. *See* Rocuronium

ABBREVIATIONS

ABG	arterial blood gas
ACLS	advanced cardiac life support
ADH	antidiuretic hormone
AGA	appropriate for gestational age
AIDS	acquired immunodeficiency syndrome
AP	anteroposterior
ARDS	acute respiratory distress syndrome
atm	standard atmosphere
AV	atrioventricular
BAL	bronchoalveolar lavage
BD	base deficit
BE	base excess
Bi-PAP	bilevel positive airway pressure
BPD	bronchopulmonary dysplasia
BSA	body surface area
BTPS	body temperature and pressure saturation (correction factor)
BUN	blood urea nitrogen
Ca	calcium
CaO$_2$	total arterial oxygen content
C(a-v)O$_2$	arterial–venous oxygen content difference
CBC	complete blood count
CCU	coronary care unit
CGA	Compressed Gas Association
CHF	congestive heart failure
CI	cardiac index
CL	lung compliance
Cl$^-$	chloride ion
CMV	continuous mechanical ventilation
CNS	central nervous system
CO	carbon monoxide
CO$_2$	carbon dioxide
COPD	chronic obstructive pulmonary disease
CPAP	continuous positive airway pressure
CPR	cardiopulmonary resuscitation
CPT	chest physical therapy
CRT	certified respiratory therapist
CT	computed tomography
CVO$_2$	total oxygen content of mixed venous blood
CVP	central venous pressure
DIC	disseminated intravascular coagulation
DISS	Diameter Index Safety System
DKA	diabetic ketoacidosis
DL	diffusion capacity of the lung
DLCO	carbon monoxide diffusion capacity
DNR	do-not-resuscitate
DPG	diphosphoglycerate
DPI	dry powder inhaler
ECF-A	eosinophilic chemotactic factor of anaphylaxis
ECG	electrocardiography, -phic, -gram
ECMO	extracorporeal membrane oxygenation
EEG	electroencephalogram
EIA	exercise-induced asthma
EMD	electromechanical dissociation
~~S	emergency medical service

EOA	esophageal obturator airway
EPAP	expiratory positive airway pressure
ERV	expiratory reserve volume
ET	endotracheal
ETC	esophageal–tracheal combitube
FEF$_{200-1200}$	forced expiratory flow after first 200 mL
FEF$_{25\%-75\%}$	forced expiratory flow, midexpiratory phase
FET	forced expiratory technique
FEV$_{0.5}$	forced expiratory volume in 0.5 s
FEV$_1$	forced expiratory volume in 1 s
FEV$_3$	forced expiratory volume in 3 s
FEV$_6$	forced expiratory volume in 6 s
FiO$_2$	fractional inspired O$_2$ concentration
Fr	French
FRC	functional residual capacity
FVC	forced vital capacity
GI	gastrointestinal
Hb	hemoglobin
HbCO	carboxyhemoglobin
HBO	hyperbaric oxygen
HbO$_2$	oxyhemoglobin
HCO$_3^-$	bicarbonate
Hct	hematocrit
HEPA	high-efficiency particulate air (filter)
HFCWO	high-frequency chest wall oscillation
HFJV	high-frequency jet ventilation
HFO	high-frequency oscillation
HFPPV	high-frequency positive pressure ventilation
HFT	high-flow therapy
HFV	high-frequency ventilation
HHN	handheld nebulizer
HIV	human immunodeficiency virus
HMD	hyaline membrane disease
HME	heat moisture exchanger
IBW	ideal body weight
IC	inspiratory capacity
ICP	intracranial pressure
ICU	intensive care unit
ID	internal diameter
I:E	inspiratory:expiratory (ratio)
IMV	intermittent mandatory ventilation
INH	isoniazid
IO	intraosseous infusion
IPAP	inspiratory positive airway pressure
IPPB	intermittent positive pressure breathing
IPV	intrapulmonary percussive ventilation
IRDS	infant respiratory distress syndrome
IRV	inspiratory reserve volume
IT	implantation tested
IV	intravenous
J	joules
JVD	jugular venous distention
K$^+$	potassium ion
LGA	large for gestational age
LMA	laryngeal mask airway

LTB	laryngotracheobronchitis
LVEDP	left ventricular end-diastolic pressure
LVF	left ventricular failure
MAP	mean airway pressure
Mc	megacycle
MDI	metered-dose inhaler
MEP	maximal expiratory pressure
MET	medical emergency team
MI	myocardial infarction
MIP	maximal inspiratory pressure
MPAP	mean pulmonary artery pressure
MRI	magnetic resonance imaging
MSAP	mean systemic arterial pressure
MVV	maximum voluntary ventilation
Na$^+$	sodium ion
NBRC	National Board for Respiratory Care
NG	nasogastric
NIF	negative inspiratory force
NO	nitric oxide
NSAID	nonsteroidal antiinflammatory drug
O$_2$	oxygen
OD	outside diameter
PA	posteroanterior
P(A-a)O$_2$	alveolar-arterial oxygen pressure difference
PAC	premature atrial contraction
PaCO$_2$	partial pressure of carbon dioxide, arterial
PALS	pediatric advanced life support
PAO$_2$	partial pressure of oxygen, alveolar
PaO$_2$	partial pressure of oxygen, arterial
PAP	pulmonary artery pressure
P̄aw	mean airway pressure
PAWP	pulmonary artery wedge pressure
PB	barometric pressure
PCO$_2$	partial pressure of carbon dioxide
PCV	pressure control ventilation
PCWP	pulmonary capillary wedge pressure
PDA	patent ductus arteriosus
PE	pulmonary embolism
PEA	pulseless electrical activity
PEEP	positive end-expiratory pressure
PEF	peak expiratory flow
PEP	positive expiratory pressure
PET	positron emission tomography
PETCO$_2$	end-tidal carbon dioxide tension
PFC	persistent fetal circulation
PFT	pulmonary function test
PIF	peak inspiratory flow
PIP	peak inspiratory pressure
pK	dissociation constant (6.1)
PO$_2$	partial pressure of oxygen
POC	point of care
PPHN	persistent pulmonary hypertension of the newborn

ppm	parts per million
PROM	premature rupture of membranes
psi	pounds per square inch
psig	pounds per square inch, gauge
PSV	pressure support ventilation
PT	prothrombin time
PtcPO$_2$	transcutaneous PO2
PTT	partial thromboplastin time
PVC	premature ventricular contraction
PvO$_2$	partial pressure of oxygen, mixed venous blood
PVR	pulmonary vascular resistance
QS	shunted blood
QT	cardiac output (L/min)
RBC	red blood cell
RCP	respiratory care practitioner
RDS	respiratory distress syndrome
RLF	retrolental fibroplasia
ROP	retinopathy of prematurity
RR	respiratory rate
RRT	registered respiratory therapist
RSV	respiratory syncytial virus
RV	residual volume
SA	sinoatrial
SaO$_2$	hemoglobin saturation with oxygen, arterial blood
SARS	severe acute respiratory syndrome
SGA	small for gestational age
SIDS	sudden infant death syndrome
SIM	sustained maximal inspiration
SIMV	synchronized intermittent mandatory ventilation
SPAG	small particle aerosol generator
SpO$_2$	pulse oximetry
SRS-A	slow-reacting substance of anaphylaxis
SV	stroke volume
SvO$_2$	hemoglobin saturation with oxygen, mixed venous blood
SVR	systemic vascular resistance
TB	tuberculosis
TDP	therapist-driven protocol
TLC	total lung capacity
UAC	umbilical artery catheter
μm	micrometer
USN	ultrasonic nebulizer
V̇A	alveolar minute volume
VAP	ventilator-associated pneumonia
VC	vital capacity
VD	dead space volume
V̇E	minute volume
V̇O$_2$	oxygen consumption per unit of time
V/Q	ventilation/perfusion (ratio)
VT	tidal volume
VTG	thoracic gas volume
WBC	white blood cell

COMMONLY USED EQUATIONS

1. Calculating minutes remaining in an oxygen cylinder

$$\text{Minutes remaining} = \frac{\text{Cylinder pressure} \times \text{cylinder factor}}{\text{Liter flow}}$$

Cylinder factors:
"H" cylinder: 3.14 L/psig
"E" cylinder: 0.28 L/psig

For exam purposes, you may use the factor 3 for the "H" cylinder and 0.3 for the "E" cylinder.

2. Calculating the duration of flow for a liquid O_2 system

Note: 1 L of liquid oxygen weighs 2.5 lb (1.1 kg)

$$\text{Gas remaining in liquid container} = \frac{\text{Liquid wt (lb)} \times 860}{2.5\ \text{lb/L}}$$

Shortcut equation for gas remaining in a liquid container: $344 \times$ liquid wt (lb)

$$\text{Minutes remaining in liquid container} = \frac{\text{Gas remaining (L)}}{\text{Flow (L/min)}}$$

3. Calculating total arterial oxygen content (CaO_2), total venous oxygen content (CVO_2), and arterial venous oxygen content difference $C(a\text{-}v)O_2$

The sum total of oxygen bound to hemoglobin and dissolved in the plasma

$$O_2 \text{ bound to Hb} = 1.34 \times Hb \times SaO_2$$

$$O_2 \text{ dissolved in plasma} = PaO_2 \times 0.0003$$

Note: Use the fractional concentration for the SaO_2, for example, 0.95 instead of 95%.

Add the answers to each to determine the CaO_2

Use the same equation for calculating venous content but substitute SvO_2 for SaO_2 and PvO_2 for PaO_2.

Subtract the CVO_2 from the CaO_2 to determine the content difference.

For exam purposes, because the amount of dissolved O_2 is so small, do not take the time to calculate it. Calculate the amount bound to Hb and select the answer on the exam that is slightly higher than your answer.

4. Calculating total flow delivered by a high-flow oxygen delivery device

Add the air/O_2 entrainment ratio parts together and multiply by the flowmeter setting

EXAMPLE:

40% air entrainment mask running at 8 L/min.
40% air/O_2 ratio = 3:1; 3 + 1 = 4; 4 × 8 = 32 L/min

5. Determining the actual flow rate of He/O_2 mixtures through an O_2 flowmeter

80/20 heliox mixture: multiply flowmeter reading by 1.8
70/30 heliox mixture: multiply flowmeter reading by 1.6

To determine what to set the O_2 flowmeter on to deliver the ordered heliox flow, divide the factor 1.8 or 1.6 into the ordered flow.

6. Calculating relative humidity (RH)

$$RH = \frac{\text{Absolute humidity}}{\text{Capacity}} \times 100$$

Absolute humidity is the amount of water in a given volume of gas.

Capacity is the total amount of water capable of being held in the gas at a given temperature.

7. Calculating body humidity (BH)

$$BH = \frac{\text{Absolute humidity}}{44\ \text{mg/L}} \times 100$$

8. Calculating humidity deficit (HD)

$$HD = 44\ \text{mg/L} - \text{absolute humidity}$$

Expressed as a percentage:

$$\frac{\text{Humidity deficit (mg/L)}}{44\ \text{mg/L}}$$

9. Calculating alveolar PO_2 (PAO_2) using the alveolar air equation.

Shortcut equation for the exam when the barometric pressure is 747 torr:

$$PAO_2 = (7 \times O_2\%) - (PaCO_2 + 10)$$

10. Calculating $P(A\text{-}a)O_2$
(Referred to as the A-a gradient)

$$PAO_2 - PaO_2$$

11. Calculating intrapulmonary shunt

$$\frac{QS}{QT} = \frac{(PAO_2 - PaO_2) \times 0.003}{(CaO_2 - CVO_2) + (PAO_2 - PaO_2)(0.003)}$$

Shortcut equation for the exam:

$$\frac{PAO_2 - PaO_2}{20} + 3\% - 4\%$$

12. Calculating systemic vascular resistance (SVR)

$$\frac{MSAP - CVP\ (mm\ Hg)}{QT}$$

QT = cardiac output
MSAP = mean systemic arterial pressure

The answer is in the units mm Hg/L/min. Multiply by 80 to convert to dyne $\times$ s $\times$ cm^{-5}.